ANATOMY MUSEUM

ANATOMY MUSEUM

Death and the Body Displayed

Elizabeth Hallam

REAKTION BOOKS

To Ian, with love
And in memory of Beatrice Selina Hallam, 1908–1988

Published by Reaktion Books Ltd
Unit 32, Waterside
44–48 Wharf Road
London N1 7UX, UK
www.reaktionbooks.co.uk

First published 2016
Copyright © Elizabeth Hallam 2016

Printed and bound in China by 1010 Printing International Ltd

A catalogue record for this book is available from the British Library

ISBN 978 1 86189 375 8

CONTENTS

Introduction:
Articulating Anatomy 7

One Hand and Eye:
Dynamics of Tactile Display 46

Two Animations:
Relics, Rarities and Anatomical Preparations 97

Three Nerve Centre:
Museum Formation I 133

Four Skeletal Growth:
Museum Formation II 157

Five Visualizing the Interior 199

Six Living Anatomy 238

Seven Paper, Wax and Plastic 278

Eight Relocations and Memorials 316

Abbreviations 353
References 354
Select Bibliography 423
Acknowledgements 425
Photo Acknowledgements 427
Index 429

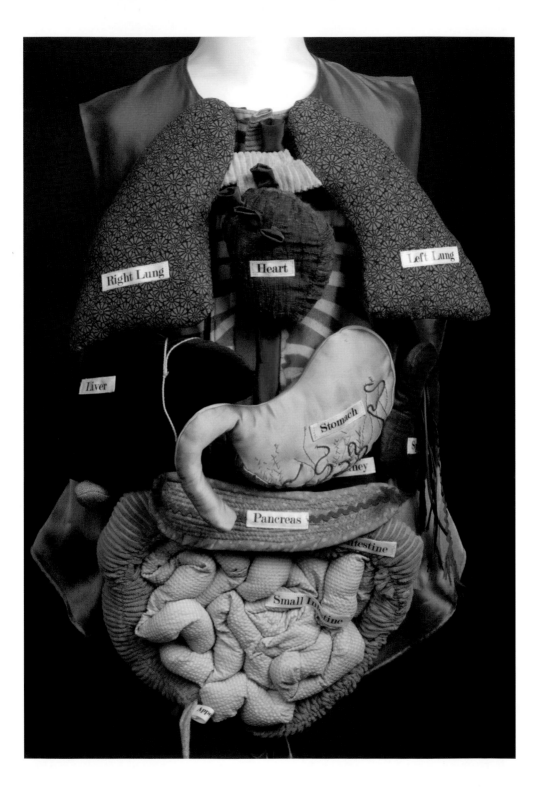

INTRODUCTION:
ARTICULATING ANATOMY

Almost immediately, he dreamt of a beating heart.

He dreamt it as active, warm, secret, the size of a closed fist, of garnet colour in the penumbra of a human body as yet without face or sex; with minute love he dreamt it, for fourteen lucid nights. Each night he perceived it with greater clarity. He did not touch it, but limited himself to witnessing it, observing it, perhaps correcting it with his eyes. He perceived it, lived it, from many distances and many angles.

Jorge Luis Borges, 'The Circular Ruins', in *Labyrinths*[1]

This book is about human bodies: how they have been imagined, made visible and tangible in museums of anatomy and other related sites of display. It explores the collection and exhibition of bodies after death in historical and contemporary settings, asking how and why human remains have been acquired and preserved, and examining what these practices entail for the people involved in them. In Western societies deceased bodies have been significant in shaping perceptions of the human form and this study focuses on interactions that are sustained between the living and the dead in the pursuit of knowledge, especially knowledge of anatomy. Preserved human remains exhibited for visual contemplation and tactile examination have taken a diversity of forms, from saints' relics and personal mementoes to works of art and anatomical specimens, or preparations, as they have also been termed.[2] Deceased bodies and body parts, along with related visual images and three-dimensional models, are explored throughout this study, which analyses twenty-first-century anatomical displays as well as tracing aspects of their histories. These histories encompass medieval reliquaries and early modern cabinets of curiosities, anatomical theatres, the private collections of medical practitioners and enduring body

1
Jo Sheffield, textile anatomy: 'Organ Waistcoat', in the Hunterian Museum, Royal College of Surgeons of England, London, 2005.

fragments, such as locks of hair, kept as emotive reminders of the deceased. Human bodies after death have been the focus of intensive anatomical investigation as well as ritualized action and memorialization – all involving modes of display that hold the dead in proximity to the living.

Death is not always the end of social life for bodies.[3] Preserved in parts, and their treatment now regulated by law, many continue to have presence and purpose in the museums or collections of university medical schools, colleges and hospitals. The functions of and audiences for these bodies are varied: in Britain, many museums of anatomy and of pathology – the former concerned with bodies defined as 'normal', the latter with those deemed 'diseased' – are reserved for use by professionals and students in the fields of medicine, science and health, while others are open to the general public.[4] By placing these museums in historical perspective, it is possible to see how human and other animal bodies have entered varied and changing post-mortem lives. How and why bodies have been acquired, preserved, dissected and otherwise crafted within processes of display, especially in medical education, are central concerns here.[5] For bodies embark upon many trajectories as they are anatomized, observed, photographed and drawn, kept in storage or disposed of, in the dynamics of anatomical exposition.

Anatomy is a shifting, not fixed, field of knowledge that is constituted and communicated in practice within particular social and cultural contexts.[6] Differing methods of anatomical exploration are historically emergent, encouraging particular ways of seeing, handling and conceptualizing the human body.[7] How has the collection and display of bodies figured in this field of knowledge production and dissemination? How have anatomy museums been formed and transformed, and what kinds of cultural practices and social relationships are entailed? These museums operate within social networks of people that have included not only anatomists and their assistants, but artists, technicians, doctors, students, travellers, wealthy collectors, naturalists, taxidermists, model makers, anthropologists, architects, photographers and many other experts and non-specialists. Wide-ranging social connections, through which body parts have been transacted, are just as crucial in the development of anatomy museums as the intensive work on site to display and maintain those bodies.

Containing the remains of once-living persons and animals, collections in anatomy museums are both grown and made; they cut across the categories of the organic and the artefactual.[8] The labour invested in anatomical display has been considerable – from embalming to dissection, and from painting to film-making – as has the labour of viewing, interpreting and learning from such display. This book probes perceptions

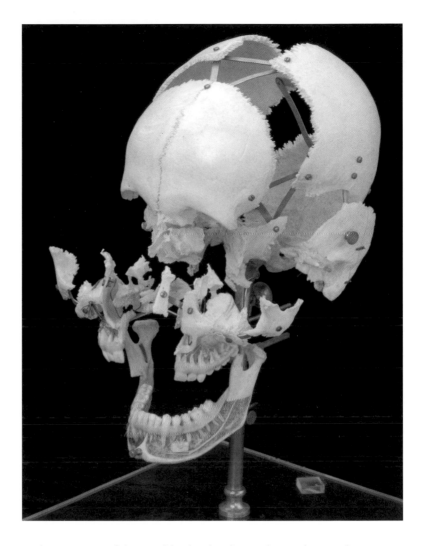

2
Exploded human
skull, *c.* 1920,
by N. Rouppert
(successor to Maison
Tramond), Paris.

and treatments of deceased bodies by those who work in and visit museums of anatomy, attending to the embodied practices of the living alongside the bodies of the dead.[9] The lives of those deceased and those alive become entwined in anatomical displays, just as those displays engage both their makers and their users/visitors. These engagements can be complex and potent, especially as the material objects comprising these anatomical displays are often difficult entities whose very substance has the capacity to provoke anxieties and whose form, matter and meanings are often unstable, ambiguous and changing.

Exploring bodies, of the anatomized and of those involved in anatomizing, this book attends to material and visual aspects of displays as well as the relations that enable, and are forged by, processes of body collecting and display. An initial example, a preserved 'exploded' human skull, is telling with regard to these issues (illus. 2). This striking object was exhibited in the Anatomy Museum (or the Anatomical Museum, as it was known from its foundation in the mid-nineteenth century until the early twentieth century) of the Anatomy Department at Marischal College, University of Aberdeen, in northeast Scotland – the main museum analysed in the chapters to follow.[10] Visitors permitted to enter the Anatomy Museum – which was dedicated to medical education, not open to the general public – would walk through its main double doors with ornate brass handles and were immediately faced by the exploded skull. Prior to the radical changes that the museum underwent in 2009, the exploded skull was one of four arranged in a row on top of a central display case and kept in transparent Perspex boxes to protect them from dust and to exert curatorial control over the handling of these delicate exhibits (see illus. 34).

The adult skull's white bones are pristine with skin and muscle removed; there is no blood, no visible decay. Eyes and brain have long been separated from the skull, which was originally prepared for a particular purpose – to show the bony components of the head without any messy matter to obscure them. Only neat lines of coloured, waxed fibres in the upper and lower jaw, standing for blood vessels and nerves, thread through this ossified structure. Bones in the skull have been carefully prized apart along suture lines, or 'serrated seams', and the fragments held together by a brass framework.[11] This system of brass supports, strips, wires, screws and hooks, separates the skull into its constituent parts while keeping it intact. Thus the skull's parts are articulated – connected together – by its brass system, which is designed to be opened and closed so that the size and shape of bones as well as their spatial relationships are made clearly visible from different angles. Produced through both growth and deliberate, intricate crafting, the skull – like many 'biological artefacts' in medical collections – is at once natural and artificial, categories that are themselves historically and culturally variable.[12]

The anonymous skull, removed from the person within whose body it once lived, is stripped of the skin and facial features so closely associated with particular individuals and culturally valued as indicators of gender, age and ethnicity.[13] Without these the skull has become depersonalized and generalized; it is made to appear not as one person's skull but rather as a human skull. This body part has been radically redefined so that the deceased person's remains have become museum specimens – a redefinition undergone by innumerable portions of bodies in museums of anatomy. Often, (although not always) without name, museum specimens have come to be associated not with those within whom they developed throughout life, but with those who acquired, preserved, dissected, collected and exhibited them after death.[14] These shifts in associations have frequently been informed by relations of power and inequality, as discussed in this book. For many of those whose bodies have been acquired for anatomical purposes – prior to the mid-twentieth-century rise in whole- body donors bequeathing themselves to medical schools – were from particular social groups: the poor and disadvantaged, criminals and colonized peoples.[15] Given the extent to which, within medical domains, human remains have been acquired, worked on and invested in, complex and unresolved questions arise regarding issues of ownership and the appropriate treatment of bodies after death.[16]

The exploded skull is marked with inscriptions, indicators of the meanings and associations it has accrued through its post-mortem life. The label *N. Rouppert à Paris* refers to the commercial firm which preserved and sold it – an hisorically well-reputed supplier of osteological specimens and maker of anatomical models.[17] The year of its purchase, 1920, was written in black ink by Robert William Reid (1851–1939), professor of anatomy at Marischal College and curator of the Anatomy Museum at the time. The inscriptions register some of the social relations in which the skull has been entangled as it passed from a deceased person though a specialist business in Paris and on to Aberdeen for use in teaching anatomy. Such a route taken by a body part is just one among a multitude of movements, all varying according to historical period and place, involved in the formation of anatomy, pathology and other medical museums.

The skull has also entered the lives of students who have interacted with it during their medical training. According to Robert Douglas Lockhart (1894–1987), one of Reid's successors as professor of anatomy, each human skull was like a jigsaw that required 'an eye for shape and position' in order to understand it from an anatomical point of view.[18] Developing this 'eye' was a process of visual education that taught students how to see human bodies in anatomical terms, a process which drew learners into particular kinds of embodied encounters with a range of anatomical displays.[19] In this context, the exploded skull would have been studied through observation conducted within a disciplined, physically and imaginatively active learning process.

Embodied practices – such as observation – which generate and augment knowledge and skills in anatomy, develop within particular sites and spaces. They are indivisibly physical, mental, sensory, emotional and social; as Rachel Prentice notes in her study of contemporary anatomical and surgical learning in the USA, 'a practitioner's entire body participates in medical education.'[20] Such participation is contextually dependent, as are the attitudes and values that emerge from, or are reinforced by, teaching and learning as modes of situated social interaction.[21] Just as displays of anatomy (and hence the knowledges they help to disseminate) change, so do embodied engagements with them. For anatomical displays have often been devised to elicit interaction with them not only through sight, but through touch, while smell and sound have also come into play for both display producers and users. Sensory involvement with such displays is, again, variable, but there is often a strong emphasis on tactility – as in some contemporary anatomy museums reserved for medical education, for example – and this marks these exhibitionary sites as somewhat different to public museums that have tended to be predominantly, although not exclusively, 'visual, don't-touch places' especially for visitors (rather than conservators and curators).[22]

Returning to the exploded skull, when it is observed in terms of its anatomy, this objectifying stance can still slip into a more empathetic mode, generating an interplay in the perception of the specimen as both dead physical matter and as once part of a living person. Although most evidently dead and no longer sentient, viewers might see an animated expression in its composition – could it be laughing, or dropping its jaw in shock? To see aspects of life in a dead skull is not unusual within anatomical practices that display deceased bodies in order to impart knowledge of the living. Anatomical images and exhibits have presented – and encouraged the imagining of – bodies after death as though alive, so that the anatomized yet living corpse is a figure that reoccurs in many modified forms. Strategies for displaying anatomy have, then, often deliberately blurred distinctions between the dead and the living, the inanimate and the animate. Gazing back at viewers, the exploded skull might, furthermore, seem to offer a memento mori message about the transience of life and the certainty of eventual death; a message that has historically prompted a search for self-knowledge in the face of mortality.

The exploded skull's articulation, its tailored armature, enables the display of its intricate, separated components. In anatomical terminology, as Lockhart explained, 'articulation' refers to 'any union between adjacent bones'.[23] Articulations are therefore relations – shown in the exploded skull by its brass system, which makes connections and linkages, helping viewers to see and understand the shape, scale and relative position of bones.[24] To articulate in anatomical practices, then, is to display relations between parts of the body. This book expands out from these bodily relations to encompass the material, visual, social and spatial relations involved in displays of anatomy.

If anatomical practices take bodies apart to analyse the internal relations between those parts, this book offers a social and cultural anatomy of one museum – the Anatomy Museum at Marischal College, with its rich collections that have developed over the last two centuries, and its associated surviving archives.[25] From perspectives in anthropology and history, the museum's internal composition is examined – its spaces, displays, preserved body parts, personnel and visitors – showing how its anatomy (and hence its display of human anatomy) has changed over time. Informing its shifting composition are the articulations of the museum's interior with adjacent rooms in its immediate architectural complex as well as with other local and geographically distant sites where bodies have been collected, displayed, anatomized, buried and memorialized. Here in-depth analysis of one particular anatomy museum proceeds through detailed exploration of that site, not as an isolated entity but, rather, within a network of museums in Britain and elsewhere. In practice – through the work, communications and social connections of the people involved with it as well as its holdings and displays – one museum relates to many museums, not only of medicine but of anthropology and zoology, as well as to sites of display such as fairs, menageries, circuses, shop windows and art galleries. As such, processes of anatomical display have often cut across distinctions between the popular and the learned. So while displays emerge within particular localities – in this case in the northernmost anatomy museum in Britain, which has received very little academic attention to date compared with other sites of anatomical knowledge-making, such as London medical schools – those localities are very much interconnected with the wider world.[26]

Just as anatomical knowledge of *the* human body has been constituted through the study of *many* bodies, so *one* anatomy museum can be seen to have emerged and changed in relation to *many* museums.[27] The Anatomy Museum, like the other displays and institutional exhibitions with which it articulates, has formed and transformed through the collection, making and use of visual images and material objects, including those that incorporate human remains.[28] Analysing this formation reveals how bodies after death have been variously shown or concealed, how what is preserved of the deceased crucially shapes perceptions of the living.

OPEN OBJECTS

The material objects currently held in museums and collections of anatomy are wide-ranging, from preserved body parts and three-dimensional models to photographs, drawings, paintings, printed atlases and textbooks. These entities are not static; they have varying degrees of stability and flux in terms of both their material and conceptual definition as they are caught up in changing medical teaching methods, technologies, exhibition schemes and institutional agendas. Despite attempts to materially stabilize

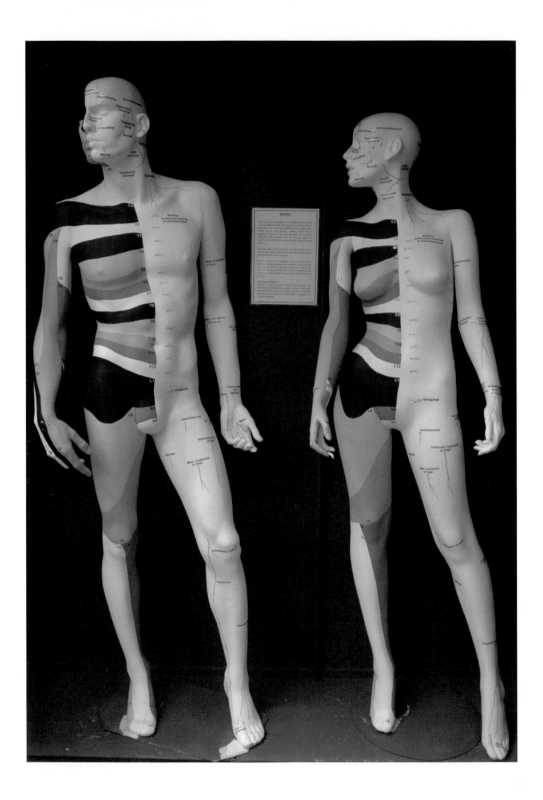

them and to guide their interpretation, these entities have an indeterminacy and fluidity – an openness – that becomes especially apparent over time. Analysing material objects within processes of production, transaction and use elucidates how they are perceived and manipulated by their makers, users and viewers. As Nicholas Thomas has noted, objects are always 'historically refigured'; they 'are not what they were made to be but what they have become'; they are constituted and reworked through time.[29] Studies of the many ways in which human remains have been collected suggest not only that parts of bodies can come to be regarded as both objects and (fragments of) persons, but that reactions to them are modulated by their wider contexts, for example, colonial expansion and war.[30]

Deceased bodies and parts thereof in anatomical displays – where physical matter becomes especially salient – have been defined as 'cadavers', 'specimens' and 'material', terms with historically and culturally specific connotations. How the very matter of bodies, alive or dead, is apprehended, described and shaped in anatomical practices is of central interest in this book.[31] Although past medical practices and contemporary biomedicine have treated bodies as material, the perceived nature of that material requires contextual analysis.[32] As anthropological studies of material culture suggest, the perceived properties of materials in the lived world – including human bodily substance – and the forms those materials come to take, are emergent within dynamic environments.[33] Material objects are thus open in that they are enmeshed in processes of physical and conceptual making, modification and re-making; objects, and indeed subjects, along with their attendant attributes (including apparently stable boundaries), are in formation rather than already given.[34]

Gathering and exhibiting human remains in anatomy museums has required, for instance, considerable work of maintenance and protection against decay; techniques of preservation, such as drying, varnishing, immersion in fluids and sealing in containers, have been crucial in the display of bodily parts.[35] Rather than viewing these as finished or completed objects, the focus here is instead on how these entities are variously created, manipulated and dissolved. Similarly, anatomical models of the human body, rendered in many materials using as many different techniques, are also in process. For example, they have been produced by recycling other objects – as in the Museum of Anatomy at the University of Glasgow during the late 1980s, when professor of anatomy Anthony Payne and medical artist Caroline Morris obtained two mannequins to convert into models of anatomy (illus. 3). The life-size male and female figures were originally used to display clothing in shops, and were later acquired by the People's Palace, a museum of Glasgow's social history. From there Payne selected the figures, and Morris painted them to show

3
Models showing
dermatomes, 1980s,
in the Museum of
Anatomy, University
of Glasgow, 2007.

dermatomes (areas of skin each with sensory nerves derived from a single spinal nerve root), aided by Payne's sketches and illustrations in anatomy textbooks.[36] The models are still used to teach medical students, and they can be viewed by members of the public, who are allowed entry when the Museum of Anatomy is not booked for university classes and other events.

Many anatomical models are also open in that they are designed to be put into action; they are deliberately endowed with features and properties that prompt visual and tactile interaction with them, and by these means they enhance understandings of anatomy. Such models often explicitly rely on users' interactions with them to reach their potential. For instance, two anatomical models at the Hunterian Museum of the Royal College of Surgeons of England (RCS) in London are made to be tried on by visitors, including the general public. In contrast to the majority of exhibits, which are behind glass, the 'Skeleton Jacket' and the 'Organ Waistcoat' were made by designer Jo Sheffield in 2005 as anatomical garments that invited hands-on exploration (illus. 1). Sheffield constructed the models in fabrics that are suggestive of anatomical parts in look and feel, such as deep-red velvet for the liver, beige corduroy for the large intestine and pink seersucker for the small intestine. The model can be regarded as an instance of an 'open work' whose form and materials purposefully invite the viewer/wearer's interaction for its fuller realization.[37]

Attending to material objects within social and cultural processes, rather than just considering them as 'end products', is necessary, as Martin Kemp suggests with regard to historical analysis of art and science.[38] Exploring process, the unfolding material practices in which people engage, brings us closer to the perspectives and experiences of those involved with anatomical displays. For the lives of material objects are entwined with those of the persons who produce and interact with them. By creating, modifying, using or disposing of an object, a person is influenced or in varying degrees shaped by those actions – they learn skills, express their identities, modulate their emotions, attune and educate their senses.[39] The lives of objects and persons, living and deceased, are entwined – open to one another – in anatomy museums where material interactions facilitate learning and generate knowledge while giving rise to valued collections and authoritative displays.

Important aspects of the openness of material objects are the relations that develop, and are posited, between them in processes of anatomical display.[40] Objects rendered in different materials – from flesh and bone to paper, wax and plastics – are produced and utilized in relation to one another. So, for example, bodies have been dissected and examined in relation to museum specimens and those specimens, such as preserved human organs, have been displayed in relation to relevant three-dimensional

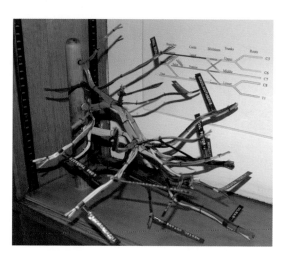

4
Model of the brachial
plexus, c. 2004,
displayed with a
diagram, in the
Anatomy Museum,
Marischal College,
University of Aberdeen,
2008.

models. Deceased bodies and models, constituted as media for the generation and communication of anatomical knowledge, have been made to articulate with – to relate to – further media, including photographs, radiographs (X-rays), slides, films, drawings, printed illustrations and other two-dimensional images as well as anatomy textbooks and manuals (all of which have their own specific material aspects).[41] Relations between these entities, realized in anatomical practices, are intermedial; they work across different media even as they register distinctions between those media.[42] In the contexts of collecting and display analysed throughout this book, then, relations between material objects, images and texts can be understood as emerging patterns of anatomical intermediality.[43] Within practices of anatomy, objects, images and texts refer to and reiterate, build upon and modify one another; they variously quote, echo, augment, answer, modify or work against one another over time.

The concept of anatomical intermediality thus refers to the manifold connections and interactions between diverse media used in the exploration and display of anatomy. In Marischal College's Anatomy Museum around 2008, for example, there were visual linkages between a preserved dissection of the head and a photograph of the same specimen with labelled anatomical parts: the latter was displayed beside the former to offer visual clarification when viewers observed each in turn (see illus. 136). A model of the brachial plexus (a network of nerves running from the spine, through the neck, and into the arm), made in the Anatomy Department, was displayed with a simplified diagram so that one was viewed to elucidate the other (illus. 4). When anatomists and their assistants construct and exhibit such objects they do so with awareness of previous display techniques, while utilizing the current resources available to them. Material, visual and textual renderings of anatomy are thus linked, juxtaposed and enmeshed, the precise combinations and permutations of which are contextually configured. Anatomical intermediality is historically shifting as media and the relations between them develop and alter, as when new visual imaging technologies emerge, for instance. Intermediality in anatomical practices can also operate in different ways; some relations between objects, images and texts might remain only as latent implicit traces, while other relations are deliberately pronounced and made more explicit. Furthermore, some intermedial connections might be obvious to trained anatomists, but not so apparent to medical students still developing their competence in this field.

Just as bodies of the dead are drawn into intermedial relations, so are those of the living. Performative work involved in displaying anatomy, for instance, has brought the bodies of both teachers and learners into intermedial processes. One teacher's performance of 'flowing moving diagrams' in Marischal College's Anatomy Department during the 1950s, for example, made lasting impressions on students. Illustrating the development of human embryos from fertilized egg to fully-grown foetus, the teacher drew with chalk from one end of a blackboard to the other, erasing parts and adding more as he formed this diagrammatic flow.[44] His moving body, in the action of teaching by drawing, became a medium for anatomical demonstration, creating a bodily/diagrammatic display that students watched and heard, then later related to relevant models and textbooks.[45]

From a student's point of view, these embryo diagrams were 'multi-sensory images'; produced in the performance of anatomical display, they appealed to sight and hearing.[46] When students recalled the diagrams in subsequent learning situations, as when handling a related dissection, for example, the diagrams could also have been reimagined through touch. As this example suggests, teaching and learning anatomy are practices that co-opt and direct bodies of the living, relative to deployments of the dead, in the production and reception of intermedial displays. The dynamics of such displays, within their changing historical contexts, are traced in this book through analysis of bodies and material objects that – enmeshed in processes of anatomical intermediality – are always open to remaking and reinterpretation.

MUSEUMS IN MOTION

Despite notions that museums are institutions of preservation, they are always in motion. They have their own distinctive dynamics, changing in their architectures, spatial arrangements, staff, collections of objects, exhibitions and audiences.[47] That museums are subject to substantial alteration is evident in, but by no means confined to, their displays. See, for instance, striking alterations made at Marischal College's Anatomy Museum (see illus. 35, 87, 124) and at the University of Edinburgh's Anatomical Museum (see illus. 37, 74) which took place in the twentieth century.[48]

Exhibitions are mounted, dismantled and replaced by numerous participants 'behind the scenes', including curators, technicians and many other people involved in museums as functioning organizations.[49] Beyond the immediate museum sites themselves, there are the people who made, used, traded and collected material objects before they entered museum collections. Analysing the Pitt Rivers Museum at the University of Oxford, with its ethnographic and archaeological objects from all over the world, Chris Gosden, Frances Larson and Alison Petch describe the myriad social relationships entailed in forming that museum's collections, from the mid-1880s to 1945. Approaching the museum as a complex compound of a building, people and objects, they reconstruct the manifold connections – between museum personnel, collectors, researchers, students, dealers, travellers and object makers within a 'huge galaxy of people' – that have formed this shifting 'relational museum'.[50] Turning to anatomy museums, this book develops a relational approach, analysing the diverse social relationships that have facilitated the acquisition and collecting of bodies, objects and images for display.

Collecting, combined with practices of preservation and display, were referred to as 'museum-making' by John Struthers (1823–1899) – an activity that was central to his role as professor of anatomy at Marischal College during the second half of the nineteenth century.[51] So while museum-making has been enabled by extensive social relationships reaching from museum institutions into the wider world, it has also entailed intensive cultural practices within museum settings. What displays are and how displaying is enacted are questions to be posed with regard to these historical and contemporary settings. Methods of anatomical display have involved dissecting, modelling, drawing, painting, plaster casting and photographing as well as demonstrating, lecturing, labelling, describing and narrating. These practices, some with distinctive performative dimensions, have produced anatomical exhibits along with conventions and expectations regarding their reception and use. Important here are the spaces utilized for the display of anatomy; these include exhibition galleries within anatomy museums as well as further rooms in museums' wider architectural surroundings. The curator Hans Ulrich Obrist proposes that museum spaces are 'always in contact with other oscillating spaces'.[52] Certainly anatomy museums in medical schools have developed in relation to other adjacent or proximate spaces, including dissecting rooms, museum stores, workshops, mortuaries, laboratories and dark rooms for photographic processing. Practices within these changing spatial arrangements intimately shape the display of bodies for anatomical purposes. Tracking museums in motion, then, involves tracing the movement of bodies and material objects within and across these shifting spaces, situating anatomy museums within their spatial contexts of associated rooms, corridors and staircases.

Relationships emerging between museums and further display sites locally, nationally and internationally are also significant. Historians have noted that nineteenth-century museums, for instance, developed within a 'larger museological world' embracing botanical gardens, libraries, lecture halls and laboratories; this expanding 'exhibitionary complex' encompassed display sites such as public museums, international exhibitions, zoos and theatres.[53] Similarly, anatomy museums have formed and transformed among related sites of display and knowledge production, between which there has been traffic in people, material objects, techniques, exhibition styles and strategies. Anatomists' curatorial work, for instance, has involved visiting other museums to gather inspiration for displays in their own institutions. As Peter Galison points out, 'scientists are always in the process of appropriating fragmentary bits of concepts, "cannibalized" pieces of apparatus, admixtures of bench practices', and this applies to anatomists' museum practices.[54] Transactions between sites of display, then, create relationships between anatomy museums and further material settings over time. These relations can be understood as a dynamic intermuseality – a process of multiple, shifting links, references and allusions that reverberate between museums, collections and displays in different settings, including those that are geographically and/or temporally distant.[55] Thus the Anatomy Museum at Marischal College was reconfigured, during the twentieth century, in relation to museums of anthropology and zoology, and it operated in connection with memorial displays in a cemetery and in a crematorium's garden of remembrance.

Museums are subject to societal, cultural and technological changes while also participating in those changes. Anatomy museums are necessarily caught up in local and global systems that have their various effects in patterns of collecting and modes of display. Industries and manufacturing, the supply of electric lighting and the accessibility of X-ray machines, the availability of formaldehyde and the cost of glass and modes of transport from tricycles to trains and ships are just a few of the factors influencing museums of anatomy, some more directly than others. Wider social and political relations, in which these museums are embedded, inform the treatment of human and animal remains as well as other related material objects. The nineteenth- and early twentieth-century expansion of European trade and of colonial and imperial contacts and interests – including those extending through practices of science and medicine – facilitated large-scale museum collecting, including the acquisition of human and animal remains, living people and their artefacts.[56] During the second half of the twentieth century, however, many preserved body parts obtained from overseas for anatomical study were redefined and relocated, and their previous modes of display were questioned. For example, plaster body casts of living people from South Africa, acquired for Marischal College's Anatomy Museum in 1880 (see illus. 85), were redisplayed in the Anthropological Museum at the same college with a notice: 'We protest at being exhibited so. Are we curiosities or human beings? Is science more important than compassion? You have cast us in a role that we would not choose.'[57] Since 1995 they have remained in storage. Again, nine Maori *toi moko* (preserved tattooed heads) – some held at Marischal College since the 1820s and some shown in the Anatomy Museum through the twentieth century until the late 1970s (see illus. 87) then during that decade in anthropological displays (see illus. 160) – were no longer exhibited from 1988 onwards following representations by the New Zealand High Commission which stated that to exhibit *toi moko* was disrespectful. In January 2007 they were given to the Museum of New Zealand Te Papa Tongarewa after formal request for repatriation. With this return the *toi moko* shed their status as museum objects, receiving ritualized treatment as ancestral remains.[58] Some preserved bodies in anatomy museums have thus been invested with particular meanings by social groups concerned with the past treatment and disposal of their deceased members.[59]

Anatomy museums are constituted over time by geographical and spatial (re)locations of bodies after death, each involving specific social, cultural and power dimensions that guide their post-mortem journeys. Human and animal bodies from local and distant places have been transferred in and out of museum collections, within and between displays – movements that inform the visual and material qualities of those entities as well as their cultural associations and social relationships. This study therefore charts the motions of anatomy museums, detecting patterns of change and continuity in how bodies are anatomized and how these anatomies – some ephemeral, some longer-lasting – come to be differently produced, treated and perceived.[60] From small beginnings to massive expansion, from rearrangement to transformation, from consolidation to contraction, and from dispersal and disposal to revitalization, this book follows some of the intersecting histories of one and many museums of anatomy.

ILLUMINATED BODIES

Debates in Britain about collections of human remains in museums and hospitals have intensified over the last two decades; they highlight the varied personal, cultural and medical meanings that bodies after death accrue, and point to a wide spectrum of educational, legal and ethical issues associated with displays of the dead.[61] At the same time, there has been great interest in public exhibitions of anatomy, and artists' work concerned with the (deceased) body, featuring in galleries beyond the confines of established medical schools and colleges.[62] So while this book focuses on anatomy as displayed in medical schools, and other related sites, the wider contemporary context for those displays is characterized by an expansion in the exhibition of bodies for public viewing.

Gunther von Hagens's *Body Worlds* exhibitions, opening in cities in Asia, Europe and America from 1995 to date, have attracted around 38 million visitors and according to the official website they are 'the most successful travelling exhibitions of all time'.[63] Temporarily housed in venues such as art galleries, science museums and entertainment complexes, the commercial *Body Worlds* project displays preserved human bodies and has apparently become 'the most visited show on earth'.[64] Some of the show's exhibits reached even wider audiences in cinemas when they featured in the James Bond film *Casino Royale* (2006). *Body Worlds* is controversial, subject to rave reviews as well as protests and attempts to ban it.[65] Von Hagens attributes the intense fascination with his anatomical constructions to their 'authenticity', their status as real bodies or body parts, while at the same time showing how the exhibited bodies have been transformed through labour-intensive processes.[66]

The dissected bodies in *Body Worlds* exhibitions are preserved through plastination. In his shows' catalogues von Hagens explains that plastination removes fluid, amounting to around 70 per cent of a human body, then replaces it with liquid plastics that either harden when dry or retain a durable flexibility to create 'beautiful specimens . . . frozen at a point between death and decay'.[67] Deceased bodies (of consenting donors, according to *Body Worlds*' publicity) are embalmed, dissected to remove skin, fatty and connective tissues and then plastinated to become, von Hagens asserts, highly valuable in educating medical students and for 'enlightening interested lay persons'. Their 'three-dimensional complexity' is more apparent than in books, as is the anatomical variation inside the bodies of individuals, or their unique 'internal face' – details which are not shown in artificial, 'schematized' anatomical models. The *Body Worlds* plastinates are highly crafted and preserved against decay and odour so that they become, it is claimed, attractive and 'aesthetically pleasing'.[68]

In *Body Worlds* exhibitions many bodies are staged in 'life-like' poses, compositions that develop the 'tradition of the Renaissance', as von Hagens professes (see illus. 49). He explains that the corpse as corpse is not of interest but, rather, how 'through it we can study the anatomy of living beings to a certain degree'.[69] The active postures of plastinates make deliberate visual references to historical illustrations of anatomy. One standing plastinate holds a swathe of skin, for instance, a position that alludes to an illustration in Juan Valverde de Hamusco's anatomy book of 1556 showing a flayed man gazing towards his own skin, which he grasps in his right hand.[70] Plastinates are also made to gesture towards recent works of art.

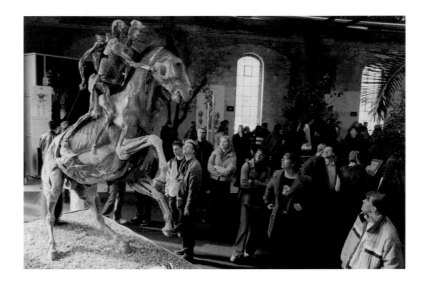

The Runner, with muscles expanded out from bones, seems to reference Umberto Boccioni's 1913 Futurist sculpture of a figure in striding movement, *Unique Forms of Continuity in Space*. The *Fragmented Plastinate*, whose torso and limbs open up with 'doors', resembles the figure in Salvador Dalí's Surrealist painting *The Anthropomorphic Chest of Drawers* of 1936.[71]

Plastinates are also modelled on exhibits constructed by other anatomists; *The Rearing Horse with Rider* (illus. 5) adopts a similar pose to an eighteenth-century preparation by Honoré Fragonard, for instance.[72] The plastinated man, exploded to open up musculature and organs for viewing, rides a horse with its anatomy similarly exposed. Their composition gives the impression of live action, and to reinforce this look of life both rider and horse have open glass eyes. Further plastinates in active arrangements appear not as translations of historical anatomical images or of art works, but instead derive familiarity through reference to sport, performing arts and games. Among the numerous 'real human specimens' exhibited in *Body Worlds*, whole-body plastinates can be seen fencing, swimming, walking, performing ballet and gymnastics and playing football, a saxophone, a guitar, poker and chess.[73]

Gunther von Hagens claims that his shows provide health education for a lay audience, democratizing anatomy by allowing access to the subject beyond professional or expert circles.[74] With this aim, *Body Worlds* employs display strategies that differ from those in current museums dedicated to medical education where whole preserved bodies are not staged in action or choreographed as are plastinates with their particular forms of 'simulated vitality'.[75] Anatomy in *Body Worlds* is intended to be 'visually arresting'; strikingly vivid bodies in theatrical, energetic and playful postures are infused with intense colour and dramatized with the strategic use of light. The exhibitions' official publicity claims that plastinates 'illuminate' the anatomy of living bodies and this metaphor of light as conveyer of knowledge is visually reinforced by brightly lit display schemes.[76] Anatomy exhibitions presented as large-scale spectacular events contrasts with current approaches to body display in medical schools. Von Hagens sharpens this contrast, emphasizing the difference between bodies as shown in *Body Worlds* and the deathly appearance of corpses laid out on tables in dissecting rooms for medical students.[77] Some anatomists' responses to *Body Worlds* have also underlined the difference between these exhibitions and ones they approve of for teaching; plastination as a *technique* for preserving body parts can be very useful in medical-school education, they argue, but von Hagens's plastinates styled for a commercially driven public show can tip the balance of anatomy and art too far towards the latter so that these bodies are positioned to entertain more than to educate.[78]

Visually arresting displays of anatomy are not, however, confined to *Body Worlds* exhibitions. In the past decade in Britain high-profile redisplays of medical collections in the museum galleries of academic institutions that are open to the public have attracted wider audiences beyond medical professionals and students. The Hunterian Museum at the RCS – whose collections are very different to those in *Body Worlds* in terms of institutional history, educational functions and status – reopened in February 2005 with a public gallery designed for spectacular effect. At the centre of the museum, the Crystal Gallery was reported in the press as 'astonishing' and 'hauntingly beautiful' – exhibiting many preparations of human and animal anatomy and pathology once belonging to Scottish-born surgeon and anatomist John Hunter (1728–1793; illus. 6).[79]

Two storeys of steel and glass cases glisten with preserved body parts in glass jars, dried or suspended in fluid. Simon Chaplin, senior curator at the time, explained that the gallery was 'designed to recapture the "scale and spectacle" of Hunter's work'.[80] During the late eighteenth century Hunter accrued over 13,000 items, including anatomical preparations enough to fill the museum at his residence in London's Leicester Square. Hunter's collection was purchased by the Government and transferred to the RCS in 1799; the Crystal Gallery is a contemporary translation of Hunter's display.[81] A staggering array of body fragments are viewed through so many glass containers and transparent shelves that they seem to surround visitors, almost like a hall of mirrors. To view exhibits in this way is to always catch glimpses of many others; reflective surfaces compound the impression that something staggering and endless is being offered for contemplation.

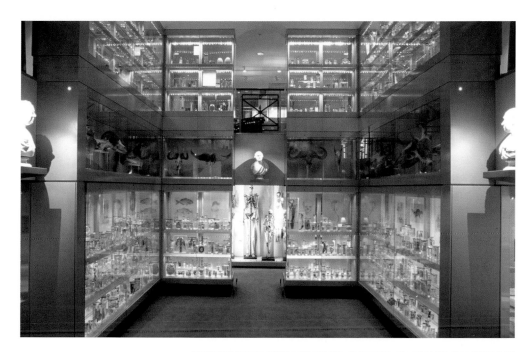

6
The Crystal Gallery
at the Hunterian
Museum, Royal
College of Surgeons
of England, London,
2007.

7
Selection of William
Hunter's anatomical
and pathological
preparations, in
*A Healing Passion:
Medicine in Glasgow
Past and Present*,
exhibition at the
Hunterian Museum,
University of
Glasgow, 2007.

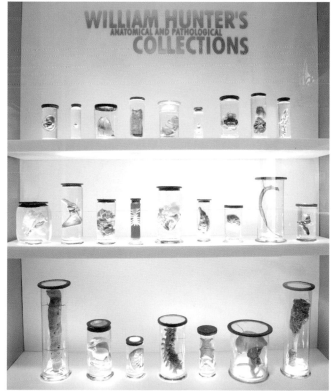

The Crystal Gallery's lighting scheme is essential in achieving this effect. The cases are fitted with fibre-optic lighting supplying myriad points of bright light to illuminate the preparations and enhance their visual clarity. Soft tissue and bone are lit to attract viewers and focus their attention. Over 600,000 visitors have seen the displays since the reopening, and, with reactions ranging from awe to disgust and horror, many viewers have been 'transfixed'.[82] Visitors to recent displays at the University of Glasgow's Hunterian Museum, launched in 2007, can view a selection of anatomical and pathological preparations from the collection of William Hunter (1718–1783), John Hunter's brother (illus. 7). While William's collection from his medical work is exhibited in the Museum of Anatomy at the same university (see illus. 36), the preparations selected for redisplay have been granted upgraded aesthetic appeal, again with the use of lighting: each glass jar is spot-lit from underneath to highlight the contours and textures of body parts.

Observations of specimens in the Surgeons' Hall Museum at the Royal College of Surgeons of Edinburgh (RCSEd) – whose emphasis is currently reported to be shifting from surgical teaching to public display – indicate the affective potential of these preserved bodily remains from visitors' points of view. [83] 'This is a world turned inside-out, / a republic of the flesh / both strange and strangely familiar', writes Anna Crowe of specimens such as nerves and blood vessels, in which she sees the forms of lace and seaweed.[84] In the same museum the poet Kathleen Jamie sees a foetal skeleton with finger bones 'as fine as dressmaker's pins'.[85] She is attuned to the museum's atmosphere in which she moves: 'The hall is illuminated by a soft daylight, which falls evenly from frosted glass roof lights and the windows, which are screened by pale blinds. Beyond the windows is a world, where it is autumn.'[86] In the quiet of the museum, the writer can hear her own breathing, her slow footsteps on the polished floor and then, 'Leaning over the white banister, I look down at the hall below with its jars of stilled disasters and diseases, its fixedness. But nothing is truly fixed. The world changes . . .'.[87] Of the preserved parts of bodies, Jamie writes: 'I wonder what they are becoming, even as they stay the same.' Then later, she finds: 'The conjoined twins make me weep and I turn away.'[88]

Exhibitions of anatomy and of death in Britain since the late 1990s have tested the limits of comfortable viewing, from *Spectacular Bodies: The Art and Science of the Human Body from Leonardo to Now* (2000–2001) at London's Hayward Gallery to *Exquisite Bodies: Or the Curious and Grotesque Story of the Anatomical Model* (2009) at the Wellcome Collection, and from *Doctor Death: Medicine at the End of Life* (1997) to *Death: A Self-portrait* (2012–13), both also at Wellcome's London galleries.[89] Characteristic of these exhibitions was the juxtaposition of visual images and material objects from science with works by contemporary artists. *Spectacular Bodies* probed connections between anatomical drawings, prints, paintings and models from the fifteenth to the nineteenth century and artists' photography, sculpture, video and installations from the late twentieth century. Life-size wax anatomical models, such as a dissected female head and torso from the early 1800s (for an example see illus. 58), could be viewed in relation to John Isaacs's *A Necessary Change of Heart* (2000), for instance. Making this wax piece in response to models of anatomy at the University of Florence's museum 'La Specola', he cast parts from his own body to create a flayed corpse, with muscles and bones revealed, lying on a slab 'with the suggestion of fresh blood – in contrast to the "blood-less" historical waxes'.[90] In the exhibition were 'wondrous and awful things', according to one review which described Isaacs's contribution as 'a work about what is fit to be seen and about how much one can bear'.[91]

Adopting a similar exhibition strategy, *Anatomy Acts: How We Come to Know Ourselves* at Edinburgh's City Art Centre in 2006 also displayed contemporary art works with anatomical and medical objects and images – in this case items, spanning the past 500 years, which were borrowed from collections in educational and medical institutions throughout Scotland. Here, for example, Christine Borland's *Black, White and Shades of Grey* (2006), a cut tree sapling blackened by fungus and resting horizontally on supports, resembled the branch-like bronchial structures often depicted in anatomical images of human lungs. Using medical museums and collections – including the Museum of Anatomy in Glasgow – Borland investigates matters associated with the body, growth, destruction and viewers' 'sense of self' through sculpture and mixed-media installation.[92] The form of her tree sapling echoes that of the glass blown into subdivided branches – like the bronchi in lungs, the passageways of respiration – in her *Bullet Proof Breath* (2001), which is wound with spiders' silk and highlights the human body's fragility and strength (illus. 8).[93]

The prominence in themes of the body and mortality in contemporary art in Britain is perhaps nowhere more visible than in Damien Hirst's media-exposed work. Referring to the glass-encased tiger shark in *The Impossibility of Death in the Mind of Someone Living* (1991), anthropologist Alfred Gell observed that 'as dead as a dead thing can be, [it] is still residually alive, watching and thinking, or seems to be, because it keeps its eyes open and stares at us.'[94] The cycle of life and death, decay, preservation and metamorphosis are repeatedly explored by Hirst through the display of animal and insect bodies, some still alive, as in his fly and butterfly installations. One of his stated aims is to make the gallery a 'focus for amazement'.[95] The artist describes his *For the Love of God* (2007) – a human skull cast in platinum (retaining the real teeth), set with 8,601

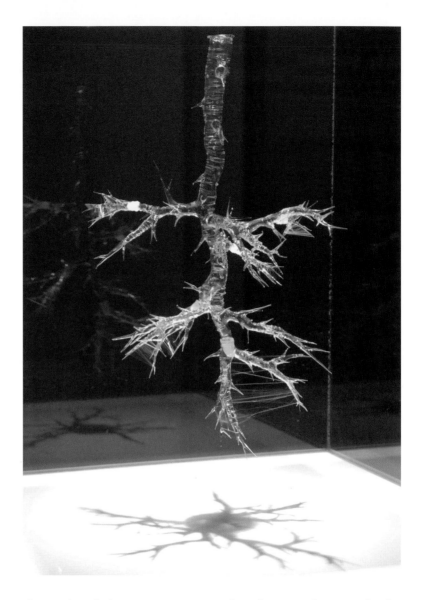

diamonds including one 52-carat pear-shaped stone and estimated to be worth £50 million – as the 'ultimate symbol of death' covered in the 'ultimate symbol of luxury' which sticks 'the ultimate two fingers up to death'; 'I want people to see it and be astounded. I want them to gasp', Hirst declared.[96] Surrounded by heavy security, the piece was exhibited in London in 2007 and 2012. In a blacked-out room visitors were attracted by the skull's dazzle; to one journalist it appeared to be 'the only source of light, a macabre glitter ball which casts a planetarium sparkle on the awed faces of those who have come to gaze at it'.[97]

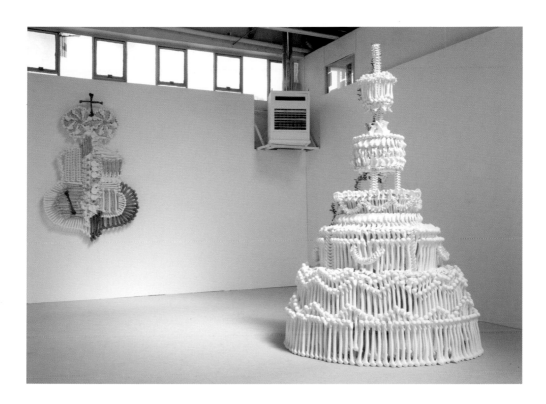

Art works that cast body parts as memento mori for public display are
also created by Jodie Carey, whose compositions are concerned with 'ritual,
artifice and mortality in contemporary Western society'.[98] Her *Untitled
(Monument)* comprises some 2,000 human bones cast in plaster and
assembled into a structure like a giant white wedding cake (illus. 9, right).
Decorated with icing (sugarpaste) flowers and leaves, these 'bones' are both
celebratory and commemorative; they are made to carry associations with
both marriage and mourning. Cary's *Untitled (Shield)* (illus. 9, left) appears
as an iced plaster translation of the human bones in elaborate arrangements
at the Sedlec Ossuary in Kutná Hora (Czech Republic; illus. 10).[99] Exhibited
in *Death: A Self-portrait* (2012–13), her one-tonne, 4-m chandelier *In the
Eyes of Others*, composed of plaster bones, appeared as a further reiteration
of her labour-intensive works with these cast body parts; it again alluded
to the ossuary's compositions with its famed chandeliers built from human
bone. In Cary's pieces there is the suggestion that while transient flesh
disappears, the treatment of resilient bony remains with intricate and time-
consuming craft work is evocative of repeated acts of remembrance that
attempt to counter loss through death.

10
Postcard of a display
of human bones at
the Sedlec Ossuary
in Kutná Hora, Czech
Republic, *c.* 1950,
postcard collected
by Robert Lockhart.

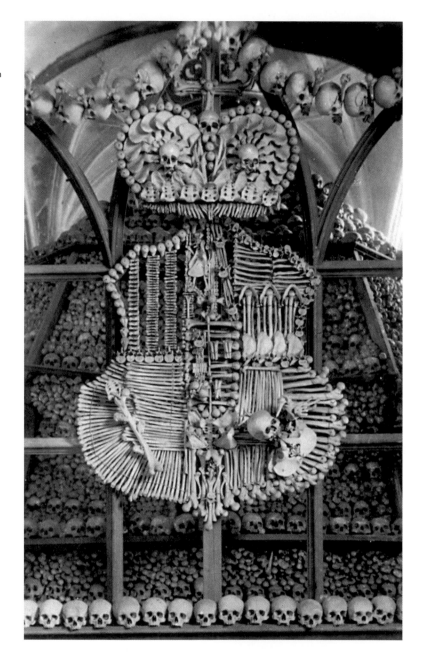

MEMORIAL BODIES

Anatomy museums operate in social and cultural contexts where prevalent cultural conventions and regulations guide the treatment of bodies after death, their ritualized disposal and memorialization.[100] Anatomical displays in medical education have tended to define deceased bodies and their parts primarily as resources for instruction and learning, although specimens have potential to acquire memorial significance – as when they are viewed as reminders of the anatomists who dissected them in the past. Preserved bodily remains and images of the deceased have, however, been displayed in further contexts specifically to memorialize the dead. The historical development of memorial displays of the body is located in sacred and domestic spaces. In these settings physical remainders of persons are retained in rituals of disposal and memory-making that invest bodies after death with high degrees of personal and social significance. Thus a part of a person – such as a bone or lock of hair – can become a focus of emotional attachment, and can come to form a 'social nexus', a materialization of social relatedness especially among family, kin and wider communities.[101]

Ossuaries have acted as repositories of bones since the thirteenth century in Catholic Europe (see illus. 116).[102] The dead are given a temporary burial for several years until the flesh decomposes; then the skeleton is exhumed and placed in a building that communally houses the remains, in a graveyard or near a church. At the crypt beneath the church of Santa Maria della Concezione dei Cappuccini in Rome the bones of Capuchin friars, who died between the 1520s and the 1870s, are arranged in patterns

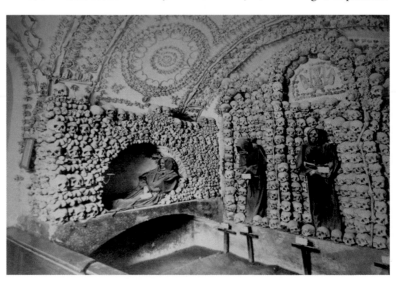

11
Photograph of displays at the Capuchin Crypt in Rome, kept in an album (anonymous), 1882–5.

and as full skeletons wearing hooded robes and holding crucifixes.[103] The memento mori message of this ossuary was to remind visitors that all flesh withers but the spirit endures. In ossuaries' 'calcified exhibition[s]' the bones of particular individuals often lose their previous identity, becoming anonymous when incorporated into ensembles of repeated motifs and when singular bones are subsumed by densely packed compositions.[104] Some nineteenth-century ossuaries, however, in Brittany, Austria and Greece, afforded skulls a distinctive identity when they were painted with the deceased's name and date of death, as well as flowers, leaves and crosses, allowing those skulls to function as memorials for particular persons.[105]

During the nineteenth century photographs of ossuaries were collected in albums, so that images of bodies in sacred spaces could be kept and viewed within domestic settings. One such image of the Capuchin Crypt in Rome was mounted in an anonymous woman's album in Aberdeen, along with her treasured letters, photographs, paper souvenirs and autographs (illus. 11).[106] Here bones, albeit in image form, were assembled with watercolours of people, places and plants, as well as pressed flowers, that documented and acted as reminders of this woman's travels in France, Italy and Algeria (illus. 12). The combination of bones and flowers was a common pairing in European reliquaries, where the skeletal remains of

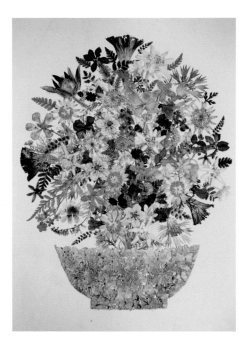

12
Pressed flowers arranged in an album (anonymous), 1882–5.

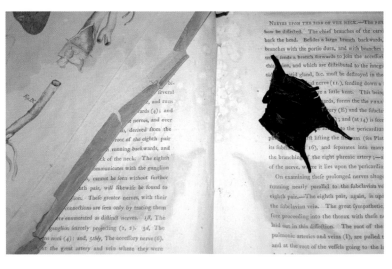

13
A 'mermaid's purse' dried and pressed in detached pages from Charles Bell, *A System of Dissections, Explaining the Anatomy of the Human Body*, vol. I (Edinburgh, 1798).

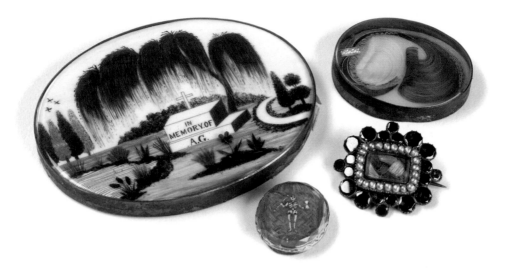

14
Mourning brooches
containing the hair
of deceased persons,
dating from the 17th
to the 19th century.

saints could be framed with flowers fashioned in various materials (see illus. 47).[107] If this album had reliquary associations it also partly resembled a natural history compilation of preserved botanical specimens including seaweed. Perhaps living in a household with medical interests, the woman who compiled this album used pages from *A System of Dissections* (1798), by the anatomist and surgeon Charles Bell, to press leaves, grasses and a 'mermaid's purse' (egg case of a fish) washed up by the sea (illus. 13).[108] Albums of this sort were produced to record and evoke memories, and within this format a photograph of an extraordinary ossuary might be viewed in drawing rooms, reflected upon by the album's compiler and narrated for her family and friends.[109]

Pages of albums also became dedicated memorials to departed loved ones, enclosing within their pages photographs and sometimes locks of hair framed with pressed flowers and paint.[110] Hair was used as a potent reminder of the deceased in Europe from the seventeenth to the nineteenth century, worked into brooches, lockets, rings, pendants and bracelets to powerfully evoke memories of persons through this enduring bodily remainder.[111] Seventeenth-century brooches holding plaited hair under crystal incorporated memento mori imagery, such as a skeleton holding an arrow and hourglass (illus. 14). Finely crafted late eighteenth-century brooches displayed hair in curls and weavings set with pearls, which signified tears and thereby incorporated the bereaved's emotional response to a death. Mourning jewellery might also contain the hair of more than one person, with locks of different shades repeatedly entwined, keeping together the bodily substance of departed relatives and carrying family connections over several generations. Mourning jewellery of the nineteenth century was produced with miniature scenes composed from hair arranged as, for instance, a weeping willow, an inscribed memorial stone, shrubbery, grass and flowers.[112] Here (see illus. 14, left) initials on the depicted memorial stone link the piece specifically to the departed while the brooch's scene links the jewellery with the place of burial, reinforcing the connection between the body of the wearer and that of the deceased. For the memorial meanings and emotive qualities of hair as jewellery were amplified when worn by those in grief.

Nineteenth-century mourning adornment included lockets and brooches that combined the deceased's hair and a portrait photograph, so that the body part was joined with an image of the dead taken during their lifetime.[113] Photographs of the dead taken in the immediate aftermath of a death, in Europe and the United States, were also used to display and remember loved ones. Like European deathbed portraits painted since the fifteenth century, post-mortem photographs provided memorial images of the deceased from around 1840 onwards and into the twentieth century. Widespread among most social classes in the United States, they were probably less common in Britain but, again, were obtained by the wealthy as well as those with modest incomes.[114] Keen to keep reminders of their last moments with deceased family members, people commissioned professional photographers to produce images of their dead. These were composed in ways that were culturally acceptable and personally meaningful to the bereaved.

Common conventions of post-mortem photography presented the deceased as though asleep, clothed and with signs of physical damage minimized, and often laid in domestic settings indicated by furniture, wallpaper, curtains and bed linen. The 'sleeping' dead might be made to appear almost alive in these photographs – as were many babies and young children, held in parents' arms and seated upright. But from the 1880s these images, still set mainly in domestic spaces, often showed the deceased in a casket with funerary wreaths and bouquets, making their death unambiguously visible.[115] In *Sleeping Beauty under Canopy in Slumber Room* (*c.* 1915), a woman in a gown is laid beneath lace drapes, the white fabric and flowers marking not her wedding but her death (illus. 15). Here she is posed in a space furnished in the manner of a private sitting room with a table, vases, a rug and chair.[116] Masking physical deterioration and emphasizing beauty, these photographs belonged to an emotional domain; they represented the continued love and affection felt for the departed, perhaps easing the pain of loss, and prompting relatives and friends to recall a life and death when viewed in albums or framed in sitting rooms.[117]

The production and consumption of post-mortem photographs during the nineteenth century in Britain was part of ritualized burial and mourning practices in which familiarity with deceased bodies was maintained. The

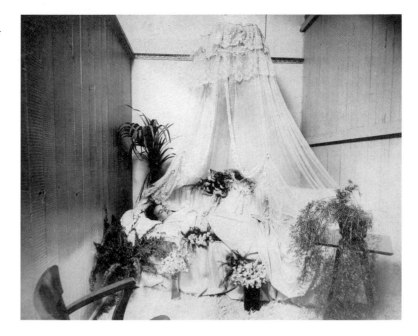

dying were nursed at home, where they were also laid out before burial and viewed by family, kin, neighbours and friends.[118] Post-mortem photographs were, however, increasingly stored or disposed of rather than displayed when, during the twentieth century, a certain distancing from the physicality of the dead occurred with the institutionalization and professionalization of dying and death; dying was to take place in hospitals, and (later) hospices, and the preparation of deceased bodies for disposal became the work of undertakers/funeral directors.[119] These shifts were accompanied by changing attitudes to post-mortem photographs that, after the Second World War, came to be regarded as inappropriate for domestic display, especially in a context where restraint rather than open expression of grief came to be positively valued.

This does not, however, necessarily suggest a decline in the significance of deceased bodies for family and kin involved in ritualized funerary and memorial practices during the second half of the twentieth century.[120] Controversies in Britain during the late 1990s surrounding the treatment of human remains in medical contexts indicated the perceived importance of bodies after death in personal and familial mourning and remembrance. Public concerns intensified when it emerged that at Alder Hay Children's Hospital in Liverpool and Bristol Royal Infirmary organs from children undergoing post-mortem examinations had been retained without the parents' consent. Inquiries were launched and the legislative response was the Human Tissue Act 2004 (for England, Wales and Northern Ireland), strengthening provision on informed consent for the medical collection and use of human bodily materials, and the Human Tissue (Scotland) Act 2006.[121] Publicly reported reactions to, and debates around, the 'organ scandal' highlighted the extent to which bodies after death can be invested with intense emotional meanings, especially when those bodies are considered to have been violated.[122]

Different meanings assigned to bodies become apparent when people actively choose to donate themselves to medical science – a practice that, in Britain, has developed especially from the mid-twentieth century onwards.[123] In such cases people give explicit permission for their bodies to be used in medical education and training. Such donations are, however, still enmeshed within cultural and legal processes of ritualized body disposal and memorializing. Bodies are kept in medical schools for a limited time, after which they are buried or cremated according to the donor's wishes. Furthermore, anatomists and professionals involved in medical education, along with medical students, have taken an increasingly active part – from the 1950s onwards – in memorial practices for body donors by organizing dedicated events for remembrance, and by instituting memorial books and monuments (see illus. 165, 166).[124]

That people currently opt for whole-body donation is perhaps a manifestation of the wider tendency in Western societies where, from the late twentieth century onwards, people have generally preferred more individual choice and personalization in their funerary arrangements.[125] Still the deceased's body often remains highly significant in practices of memorialization that maintain the close proximity of bodies not through preserved physical fragments or post-mortem photographs but through material replacements such as personalized headstones at graves, or specially chosen trees that mark interments in natural burial grounds.[126] A headstone provides an enduring and stable site of contact for the living and dead, while a tree beside an interment might be perceived as a transformed and growing manifestation of the deceased, a living memorial.[127] Cremation has become the most common mode of disposal in Britain, and relatives of the deceased now deal with bodily remains – ashes – in personally meaningful ways, such as scattering in special places associated with the deceased during their lives, burying ashes in gardens or retaining them at home.[128]

MATERIAL AND VISUAL CULTURE OF ANATOMY

While some bodies are illuminated for spectacular effect in public galleries, and others are made integral to the intimacies of memorializing, this study explores how bodies are incorporated into the material and visual culture of anatomy in museums and related display sites. This changing field embraces anatomized bodies alongside sculpture, models, printed and illustrated books, glass slides, tools and equipment, furniture, drawings, paintings, photographs – the list goes on. This is not an isolated material domain even when defined as the specialized territory of experts – rather, objects and images within it shift and are mobilized so that there are interfaces and appropriations as anatomical practices draw upon and feed into their wider social and cultural contexts. The material and visual culture of anatomy also encompasses the verbal and the textual; anatomists' working practices have developed extensive terminologies, descriptions and vernacular turns of phrase so that words spoken and written have often been integral to the exploration, display and communication of anatomy.[129]

Human anatomy is historically and contextually defined, so that what is known about bodies, how it comes to be known and by whom changes over time, as extensive histories of this subject in Europe since the thirteenth century suggest.[130] In contemporary Britain the work involved in anatomy is regarded by its practitioners as an 'ever-changing environment'.[131] University anatomy departments in Scotland, for instance, have seen a decline in teaching staff, rising numbers of students and a reduction in the number of hours dedicated to anatomy in the medical curriculum since the 1980s. More generally anatomists and medical educators draw attention to a decline in human dissection during this period, a rise in the use of plastic models and computer-based anatomical images, and divergence in teaching methods in different medical schools. Questions regarding the best methods and materials to deepen students' understanding of complex three-dimensional anatomy remain open to debate.[132] Depending on the (intertwined) history of each medical school, an anatomy department might have collections of materials acquired since the nineteenth century which are redisplayed (or consigned to storage) in relation to more recent imaging technologies used in medical diagnosis such as computerized tomography (CT) and magnetic resonance imaging (MRI).[133]

Anatomists and those involved in medical practices have been especially active in amassing collections and in forming museums. During the sixteenth and seventeenth centuries in Europe physicians, apothecaries and surgeons were keen to acquire, preserve and display items of natural history as well as anatomical rarities, and in the eighteenth century anatomists expanded their collections of body parts through their dissecting activities.[134] As the example of the exploded skull earlier in this chapter suggested, assembling collections was and still is conducted through social relationships and transactions, so that the material and the social are very much entangled. One further example illustrates the material, visual and

16
Pair of stereoscopic
photographs in an
album, compiled by
Alexander Ogston
in Aberdeen,
c. 1900–1928.

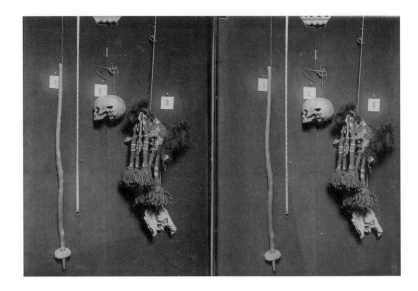

16
Pair of stereoscopic
photographs in an
album, compiled by
Alexander Ogston
in Aberdeen,
c. 1900–1928.

textual aspects of these relations: a photograph album compiled by Alexander Ogston (1844–1929), professor of surgery at the University of Aberdeen from the early 1880s to 1909, who had trained and held posts at Marischal College since the 1860s. Ogston's collection of 'ethnological objects, weapons and other curiosities', kept at his residence, included 'A skull from a Borneo Head-hunter's hut'.[135] This he recorded along with the rest of his collection in three volumes of stereoscopic photographs – that is, photographs in pairs where each of the two is taken from a slightly differing angle and the pair converge when viewed through a stereoscope to provide the illusion of looking in depth at a three-dimensional image (illus. 16).

Ogston labelled the photographs, stating from whom and where the objects were obtained, and thus the skull was linked to a Dr James Walker in Borneo – one of Ogston's many medical friends and contacts working abroad, mostly in colonial territories, who contributed to his collection. Ogston's father and sons also gave items so that his collection, and its albums, materialized family relationships too. Ogston was part of the extended social relations of the Anatomy Museum at Marischal College: he contributed an animal skeleton in the 1890s, and his collecting network overlapped with that of the Anatomy Museum as the latter and Ogston's collection both received items from, for instance, Dr Francis Walker Moir, a colonial medical officer based in West Africa, and Dr William Middleton, Medical Officer of Health for Singapore – both men having previously studied medicine at Marischal College.[136] These are just a few of the multiple social relations, and connections between collections, in which the Anatomy Museum has been enmeshed through its history.

17
Dr Gray and a
nurse (anonymous),
both holding a
surgical mask, at
Aberdeen Royal
Infirmary, c. 1900,
photograph by
George Washington
Wilson & Co.

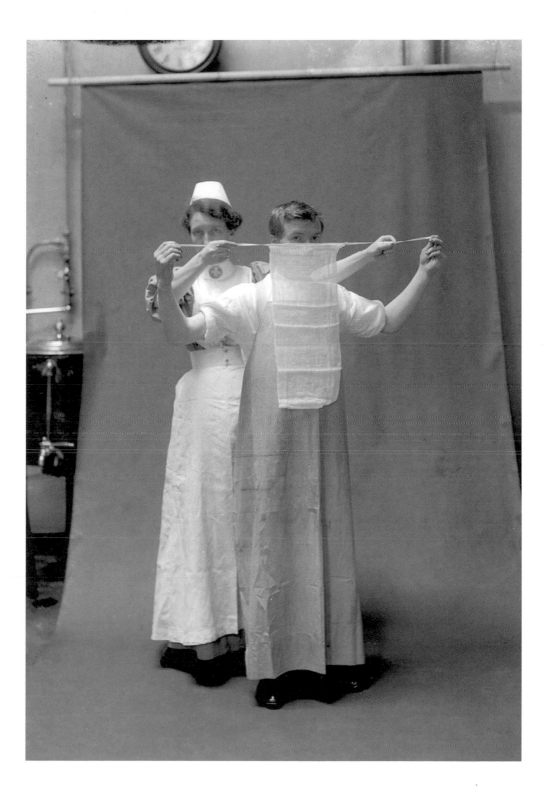

The material and visual culture of anatomy embraces not only bodies of the dead but those of the living who have created and engaged with displays in museums, dissecting rooms and other related spaces. There are crucial embodied dimensions involved in making and using displays of anatomy played out through the physicality of anatomical work, the changing actions, interactions and performances involved in knowledge generation that have entailed appropriate action, comportment, conduct and dress. Anatomists' sartorial habits, for instance, have been significant in the constitution of their social identities, status and professional standing.[137] While the human body has been described as fabric and anatomists' work likened to tailoring, putting anatomy into practice involves appropriate clothing in which to do so. Anatomist Robert Knox, teaching in Edinburgh during the 1820s and '30s, for example, 'in the highest style of fashion, with spotless linen, frill and lace, and jewellery . . . standing in a class-room amid osseous forms, *cadavera*, and decaying mortalities, was a sight to behold, and one assuredly never to be forgotten'. Knox's apparel – dark puce or black coat, embroidered vest, striped cravat, gold chains, a diamond ring on a pointing forefinger – were considered elegant and suitably attention-grabbing in lectures at the time.[138]

An image from around 1900, on the other hand, indicates the importance of plain uniform, not just for reasons of health but for projecting medical authority (illus. 17). Dr Gray at Aberdeen Royal Infirmary, in a photograph by George Washington Wilson's company based in the same city, was shown as though preparing for surgery, wearing a long apron, shirt sleeves rolled up and with a nurse assisting by lifting a gauze mask to his face. Early twentieth-century medical students' dress was considered part of their disciplined training; their clothing should be 'business-like', observed one anatomist in the 1920s, and by the 1940s white laboratory coats were worn by both male and female students (see illus. 119).[139] The material culture of anatomy, including fabrics, furnishings and apparatus of all kinds, is explored in this book with regard to the bodies of the deceased as well as the bodies of those teaching, learning and undertaking work associated with this shifting field of knowledge.

Within museums, the material culture of anatomy has emerged in significant ways, and here the focus is on the changing social lives of those museums as they have developed through processes of collecting and display.[140] In Alexander Ogston's photographs there are glimpses of the house where his collection was kept – slivers of bookshelves are just about visible behind the screens on which items are arranged in illus. 16. In other photographs throughout his albums, velvet-lined display cases or household furniture used as supports for objects appear, despite attempts to mask this domestic setting. When Ogston's collection was subsequently bequeathed to the Anthropological Museum at Marischal College in the 1920s, it followed a common path where collections, including anatomical ones, were transferred from private ownership to institutional settings, especially during the nineteenth century.[141]

When human body parts enter anatomy museums' social lives, their post-mortem existence becomes entwined with the lives of people involved in those museums. This entwining varies in intensity, entailing differing degrees of proximity and distance perceived between museum objects and those who interact with them. During the nineteenth and early twentieth centuries, museum employees would often reside in the buildings where they worked. This was the case at Marischal College and at the RCS where, for instance, the articulator (person who prepares and mounts skeletons as specimens), with 43 years of service, lived in residential rooms until his death in 1913.[142] For Robert Lockhart, in the late 1940s, his anatomical

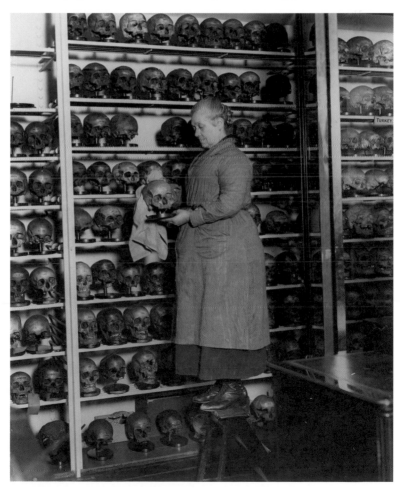

18
A cleaner
(anonymous) at the
Royal College of
Surgeons of England,
London, early 20th
century, photograph.

work at Marischal College intersected with domestic concerns and family relationships when his mother, Elizabeth Lockhart, died and he requested the artist Alberto Morrocco – who was preparing illustrations of dissected bodies for Lockhart's co-authored anatomical textbook (see illus. 132) – to draw his mother's deathbed portrait.[143] Marking her death and his grief, the anatomist would go to work in a dark mourning suit, his familial and professional roles combined.[144]

Family relationships have been significant in the formation of anatomical collections, just as they have in the workings of museums that house them. For example, Arthur Keith (1866–1955), conservator of the Hunterian Museum at the RCS from 1908 to 1933, characterized his workplace as a 'museum of living men as well as of dead things', describing three generations of men – grandfather (Edward Pearson), son (Thomas) and grandson (William) – who served this institution, the first as a porter from 1804 and the last as a dissector of specimens until 1914.[145] Keith recalled the men connected with the museum, from pathologist-curators and medically trained volunteers to cleaners, dusters and messenger boys, alluding to the

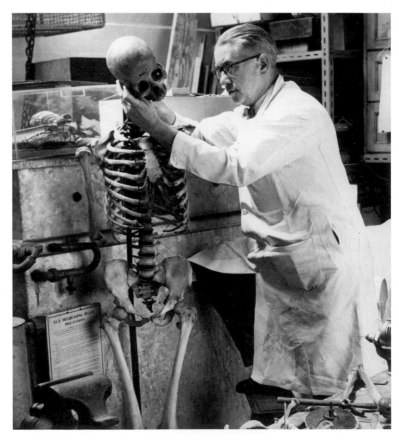

19
Charles Bush, museum articulator at the Royal College of Surgeons of England, London, c. 1960, photograph.

'patriarchal family feeling' of the museum in his early years there, even as
he sensed change with the emergence of a 'modern business atmosphere'.[146] Exploring the social life of anatomy museums reveals the
involvement and participation of many men and women, including
people whose contributions and perspectives have tended to remain 'invisible' in historical studies of anatomy and science more generally.[147] For the
material and visual culture of anatomy has been produced and maintained
not by isolated individuals, but by anatomists with, and supported by,
many other workers: the now anonymous cleaner at the RCS's Hunterian
Museum in the early twentieth century (illus. 18), for example, and
Charles Bush, photographed in one of his main roles from the late 1940s
to the early 1960s – as an articulator of osteological specimens (illus. 19).
Both participated in the 'backroom work' that makes museum display
possible, labour that is of course conducted in relation to the bodies of
those acquired for museum purposes.[148]

Family connections for some staff in the Anatomy Museum at
Marischal College were still pertinent at the beginning of the twenty-first
century: the junior technician's decision to train in this role was influenced
by her mother, who was previously employed as a technician at the university; the cleaner remembered her aunt, who had been employed at
Marischal College's Anthropological Museum.[149] These and the many
other people have who have contributed to the Anatomy Museum have
lived it and perceived it in very different ways. While, for instance, students
have used it to see into bodily interiors, the cleaner, entering the building
alone in the quiet of daybreak, was especially alert to the sound of the
place. When first working there, a little nervous and aware of the covered
bodies on tables in the adjacent dissecting room, she would often hear a
loud, alarming noise that she later realized was the sound of birds' wings
beating against the high glass roofs as they landed on the building.[150] She
became familiar with the Anatomy Museum by interpreting its distinctive
and, to her, eerie sounds. It is with attention to perceptions of the varied
and changing sights, textures, smells and sounds of material anatomy in
practice that this book explores the body, death and display.

SYNOPTIC MAZE

Museums have been described as 'synoptic mazes' – synoptic in providing
a summary view of their subject, yet maze-like in their labyrinthine
pathways that are difficult to navigate.[151] The metaphor of the maze has
also been applied to the study of human anatomy, and as the following
chapters suggest, the material and the metaphorical are closely enmeshed

20
Detached pages,
with cuttings, from
an edition of Andreas
Vesalius' *De humani
corporis fabrica*, in
the archive room,
Anatomy Department,
University of
Aberdeen, 2007.

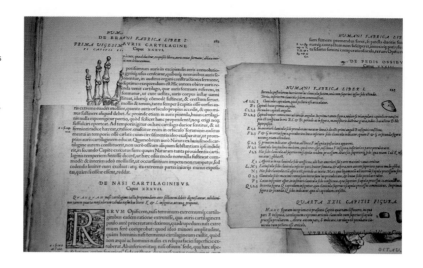

in the constitution and perception of both bodies and museums.[152] To find ways through the Anatomy Museum, and its network of interconnected museums, this study combines archival research with fieldwork including in-depth observation on site, interviews and conversations. During the time of my research in Marischal College's Anatomy Department, which began in 1999, an old office – near the Anatomy Museum – had come to form something of an archive room (see illus. 21), a room that opened up so many historical perspectives. Here were accumulations of texts, images and objects relating to anatomy over the previous two centuries: manuscripts written in distinctive hands; fading photographs; aged anatomical atlases, textbooks and dissecting manuals. All bore marks of use and reuse over time; a copy of Andreas Vesalius' *De humani corporis fabrica* (*On the Fabric of the Human Body*), first published in 1543, for instance, had had cuttings taken from it for a now unknown purpose (illus. 20).[153] Sifting through this accumulation provided glimpses of the Anatomy Museum as an unavoidably changing entity, a place where dismantled bodies have been remade and rearranged as anatomists reworked the ground formed by their predecessors. I came to see the Anatomy Museum of the (then) present day as just one manifestation among the many forms it had taken in its still unfolding history.

Chapter One explores twenty-first-century anatomical display, focusing on how it has been put to work in generating knowledge of the living body via the dead. Subsequent chapters then offer deeper historical interpretation of this process. Chapter Two traces the figure of the 'live' or animated corpse in displays of bodies from medieval relics to eighteenth-century anatomical preparations. Chapters Three and Four examine anatomy museum formation during the nineteenth century through social relations that extended from the local to the farthest reaches of empire to create vast collections of preserved body parts for medical education. How displays of anatomy were reconfigured in the twentieth century is explored in chapters Five and Six, especially in the aftermath of two world wars and in relation to drawing, photography and further techniques for studying deceased and living bodies. Chapter Seven probes the significance of substance and form in the constitution of anatomical knowledge, focusing on materials such as paper, wax and plastics that were variously utilized to engage medical students' own living bodies in practices of learning. The last chapter analyses anatomy museum transformation in the 1960s and '70s, alongside the increasing involvement of anatomists in memorializing the dissected dead from the mid-twentieth century onwards.

In August 2009 the Anatomy Museum underwent the most radical change since its foundation when the Anatomy Department vacated its nineteenth-century accommodation at Marischal College for newly built facilities, alongside the rest of the medical school, at the site of the city's Aberdeen Royal Infirmary.[154] Here the museum's collection is again redisplayed within spaces designed for the future of anatomy. Since the 1930s there had been plans to move to this site, and other medical subjects, such as pathology, had long been relocated to it.[155] By the late twentieth century only the Anatomy Department and the Anthropological Museum (renamed the Marischal Museum) remained in the neo-gothic architecture of the college, surrounded by cavernous vacated rooms, dilapidated laboratories and empty basements in one of the world's largest granite buildings (see illus. 92).[156] One onlooker observed, in 2005, that the windows of the grey granite building looked like closed eyes.[157] During 2009 the building's inner architectural structure was demolished – and countless tonnes of stone, plaster, wood and electrical wiring were removed – leaving the towering facades in place so that the college could be internally reconfigured and the external granite cleaned for its new purpose as Aberdeen City Council's headquarters. Prior to this destruction and rebuilding, archaeological excavations uncovered the ruins of a Franciscan friary over which the college had been built following its foundation in the late sixteenth century.[158] In the front quadrangle the skeletons of seven men, believed to have been friars, were unearthed from their 500-year-old grave. Their hands were clasped together as if in prayer, a position held over centuries by hands bound in cloth that had eventually rotted away.[159]

One
HAND AND EYE:
DYNAMICS OF TACTILE DISPLAY

'Anatomy is the people around you, alive and moving . . . Remember our anatomy is alive and moving, not dead and static.'[1] Anatomists currently define their subject with reference to the living body even as they highlight the value of the deceased in revealing the internal complexity of the human body. In the anatomy museums and dissecting rooms of medical schools in Britain displays of the body are created and used to teach and learn anatomy, and they are usually closed to the general public.[2] These displays are intended for the hands as well as the eyes, as vision and touch are intimately related in the generation and communication of anatomical knowledge. Such displays are also mobile and changing, not static: they are regularly constructed, modified, dismantled and redesigned to render human bodies comprehensible from anatomical perspectives. The dynamics of tactile display, involving practices of making, use, storage, sorting and disposal, inform perceptions of bodies, living and deceased. To explore these issues, this chapter focuses on the Anatomy Museum in the Anatomy Department at Marischal College, Aberdeen, from 1999 to 2009, with comparative reference to further anatomy museums and medical schools in Britain and the USA. The material and visual dimensions of anatomical displays are central to this analysis of how such displays are mobilized when they are made and used by anatomy teachers, technicians and students.[3]

Museums of anatomy are not isolated entities since they are crucially related to their adjacent spaces. Indeed, understanding how the Anatomy Museum has operated at Marischal College requires appreciation of the practices undertaken in its surrounding rooms within the department: here the movement of people and materials within and between spaces was fundamental to the functioning of anatomical display. In particular there was a reciprocal shaping of displays in the Anatomy Museum and the dissecting room (referred to as the DR), which were connected by a doorway.

And as these displays required concerted efforts of preservation and maintenance, so they were dependent on several antechambers and adjacent rooms – a mortuary, workshop and museum store, kept strictly out of sight – where the work of embalming, repairs, model construction and storage took place. 'Invisible' practices (that is, those kept strictly out of sight for people unauthorized to see them) conducted at the embalming table and the workshop bench were crucial in sustaining displays at the dissecting table and the museum table.[4] How students' senses, especially of touch and vision, were engaged and trained through interactions with these displays is explored in what follows, with attention to enactments and perceptions of work with anatomical 'material', including that constituted from human bodies.[5]

Anatomical material, which composes displays of the body, is produced and defined in specific contexts. In the Anatomy Department at Marischal College, staff used the term 'material' to refer to a wide range of artefacts and preserved human remains acquired since the mid-nineteenth century for anatomical purposes. While 'embalmed subject' was the term for recently deceased bodies prepared for dissection, parts of those bodies were referred to as 'human cadaveric material'. Anatomical material also included preserved, fleshy 'specimens' in jars or 'pots', bones (osteological material), plastic models, diagrams, a variety of paper-based and digital images and texts and, significantly, the bodies of students, which were regarded as 'living models'.[6] The variety of this material was important because no *single* medium for exploring anatomy was considered sufficient in the successful teaching and learning of anatomical knowledge. Indeed combinations of materials were made to connect and converge – to enter into patterns of anatomical intermediality through which the human bodily interior was rendered visible and tangible in this setting (see Introduction). The treatment of human remains, however, unlike work with other anatomical material, was guided by a 'code of behaviour and practice'. These remains required particular kinds of 'care', and donated bodies were also subject to ritualized practices of disposal through cremation or burial. The 'layout' of anatomical material – its spatial positioning – and its utilization depended on temporal distinctions made between, on the one hand, recently embalmed bodies of donors and, on the other, skeletal and soft tissue specimens preserved between the 1860s and the 1960s.[7] Here there were varying degrees to which this material was associated with deceased persons. Its designation as 'material' did not necessarily extinguish the awareness that preserved human remains were once persons, but this awareness fluctuated.

Through the dynamics of tactile display in the Anatomy Museum and associated spaces, a present-centred orientation became predominant.

Anatomy, 'alive and moving', was taught in the present tense and recently acquired anatomical material, open to extensive handling, was activated in preference to material defined as 'old' or 'historical', which remained, stilled, on shelves or behind protective glass.[8] As this chapter shows, signs of decay and ageing could be problematic, while resilient durability and bright newness were qualities especially appreciated. Although anatomical materials sometimes prompted reflection on the past, especially the personal pasts imagined for the recently deceased body donors in the dissecting room, and historical aspects of the Anatomy Museum were also occasionally glimpsed in its exhibits, these forms of historical awareness tended to remain peripheral to the embodied learning of anatomical knowledge. To analyse the processes of display involved in this constitution of knowledge, with their tactile, visual and imaginative dimensions, this chapter tracks movements of people and materials through the complex of interconnected spaces in which the Anatomy Museum was enmeshed during the first decade of the twenty-first century.

VISION AND TOUCH

Sensory histories of museums in Britain point to an elevation of the sense of sight, especially from the mid-nineteenth century onwards when exhibits open to the public were presented primarily for the eyes. Touching objects has been largely denied, except to an elite or expert few, to help preserve collections and to encourage modes of 'bodily discipline'.[9] However, in contemporary museums of anatomy, usually inaccessible to the public, there is a different orientation towards touch and its relation to knowledge as tactile engagement is required for displays to properly function in facilitating the visualization of anatomy. Anthropological studies of medical education have foregrounded dissecting rooms as sites either of intensive visual training or of multi-sensory learning involving sight, touch and hearing, but the role of museums and the material dimensions involved in learning anatomy are under-researched and deserve further exploration.[10] At Marischal College *both* the dissecting room and the Anatomy Museum were key sites in which teaching staff encouraged students to learn by 'doing', through active and engrossing 'hands-on' participation.[11]

Focusing on both their tactile and visual capabilities, students were required to develop 'anatomical skills' through 'practical experience', especially the skills of 'being able to visualise in the mind's eye and feel with an examining hand the body structures as they lie beneath the skin'.[12] This explicit linking of the student's mind's eye and their tactile sensations was important. For although it reinforced the notion of anatomical knowledge as consisting of an image that resides in the mind – the very concept of the mind's eye having a deep history in Western epistemology, and one that has been variously formulated in past anatomical practices – it also related this knowledge to bodily experience.[13] Thus the intensive reciprocal training of eyes and hands was seen as necessary action that would enhance students' capacity to visualize in three dimensions and to remember 'how parts of the body are put together and how these components work'.[14]

From this perspective, skilful mental visualization of a generalized human anatomy was achieved through particular modes of visual and manual exploration involving many deceased bodies, preserved parts and models. However rooted it was in examination of the tangible, it also entailed imaginative work, especially the extrapolation from the dead to the living body and from the bodily exterior to the interior – so much so that these distinctions were somewhat destabilized. Faced with the task of intimate exploration of the dead, students were reminded that 'anatomy is the people around you, alive and moving, from the vigorous flexing of muscles to the gentle peristaltic movements of the intestines.'[15] Anatomical visualization was therefore intended to transform inert fragments into animated flows, disjointed dead fractions into a complete living body. *The body* referred to in anatomical practices was taken to embrace *all* human bodies, while physical differences, especially those relating to age and sex, were highlighted, as was the 'spectrum of usual variation of normal human structure and function' beyond which is 'abnormality'.[16] Anatomical practices in medical schools – which are materially situated and institutionally validated – thus participate in the very definition of the (normal) human body; moreover they are influential in constituting this body, even as they purport simply to reveal it as an already empirically present entity.[17]

In the department's three main rooms assigned for practical learning, all located near the lecture theatre, particular kinds of 'human material' were deployed: mainly embalmed bodies in the dissecting room, preserved specimens in the Anatomy Museum and bones in the science laboratory (illus. 21). The 'moist' human material in the first two rooms was displayed alongside anatomical models, radiographs (referred to as X-rays), diagrams and texts. The 'dry' human material in the latter room was also accompanied by these materials, as well as MRI and CT scans and histological and embryology images.[18] Histology, the study of microscopic anatomy, was dealt with only briefly, as was embryology, the study of the development of embryos, as teaching focused mostly on the gross anatomy (anatomy visible with the 'naked eye') of adult bodies.[19] Attention was directed to living human material in the form of students' own bodies when, in smaller tutorial rooms, they were asked to volunteer as models for surface anatomy classes. Here the aim was to 'teach what lies under the skin by examining

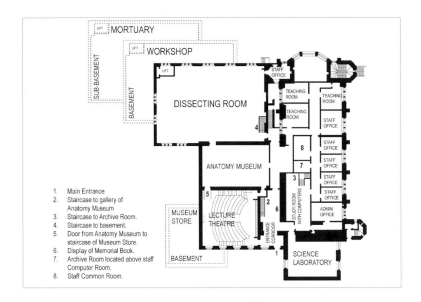

21
Floor plan, Anatomy
Department,
Marischal College,
University of
Aberdeen, as
in 2009.

the shape and contour of the body surface'. Students were told: 'One of
the advantages to studying human anatomy is that you possess a working
model in yourself – do not underestimate the value of using that gift!'[20] In
these interrelated spaces of display visualization of anatomy was therefore
developed through tactile exploration not only of the deceased inanimate
bodies of others but of the living, moving self.

Visualization in science involves diverse practices that render objects
'observable and intelligible', as Michael Lynch argues, and through these
practices images become enmeshed in a 'nexus of activities' such as
observing, demonstrating and displaying.[21] Anatomical visualization, in
the dissecting room and Anatomy Museum at Marischal College, was
understood as a process that creates a three-dimensional image of the human
body in the mind through extended periods of close visual investigation
coordinated with the work of the hands. Staff instructed students on how
to approach 'cadaveric material' in the dissecting room:

> do not be satisfied with examining it from a distance. You must pick the
> material up, and look under the muscles or other structures to see what
> lies deep to the more superficial structures. Unless you do this you will
> not be able to build up a complete 3D image in your mind.

Although students learned anatomy in 'pieces', these had to be fitted
together so that the relations between them could be visualized and the
body understood, in terms of structure and function, as a 'single unit'.[22]
And although the mind/brain was envisaged as the location where

anatomical knowledge builds up, the embodied participation of students in practical activity was seen as necessary in acquiring the skills that gave rise to this knowledge.[23] Hands were particularly subject to discipline – when studying preserved bodies by, for instance, moving muscles and blood vessels, students were told that they must work with care and also respect both body donors and staff who prepared those bodies for anatomical study.[24] The practice of touch, which enabled visualization, was thus guided by codes of conduct and students' awareness of their social position in relation to others, whether donors, authoritative teachers or, indeed, fellow students.

If anatomical visualization developed through disciplined embodied learning, it also entailed imaginative entry into the body so that it could be seen from the inside, as the interior required observation from 'all angles'. To help students understand the spatial nature of anatomy, they were asked to imagine their bedroom at the university's halls of residence, to imagine themselves on top of the wardrobe and then to describe the position of all the furniture in the room – the window, cupboards, bed and so on. This was the kind of imaginative exercise that they would be doing when learning anatomy, they were told by a teacher, except they would be visualizing a body rather than a room.[25] The analogy worked to place the student imaginatively within the body, looking at it from the inside, from an elevated vantage point so that all of the body's parts, like furniture in a room, were visible in their particular spatial locations. Such analogies, relating aspects of human anatomy to everyday sensory experiences of familiar situations or material objects, were commonly used by teaching staff to develop students' capacity for three dimensional visualization.

Learning how to describe human anatomy was important in visualizing it: during the training of students' eyes and hands they also acquired an extensive vocabulary. There are currently over 150,000 anatomical terms for bodily structures in Latin and English (this terminology having been periodically revised since the late nineteenth century).[26] In addition the location and relationships between parts are given in precise terms, be they 'anterior' (nearer to front), 'posterior' (nearer to back), 'superior' (nearer to head), 'inferior' (nearer to feet), 'superficial' (nearer surface) or 'deep' (further from surface).[27] With this terminology the positions of parts are identified, and spatial orientation through the body is facilitated, with terms also given for the body's movements at the joints of bones.[28] Staff advised students that

> anatomy learning involves coming to grips with a very large number
> of terms and names of structures. This can only be achieved by work-
> ing continuously and constantly revisiting material to embed it
> within your brain.[29]

This language learning was achieved not by simply reading anatomy textbooks, and hearing and speaking words, but through embodied modes of study where students repeatedly explored anatomical materials, looked at and drew diagrams, made notes and sought explanations from teaching staff. As anatomical terms often indicate the shape or position or action performed by bodily parts, students were told that learning the language of anatomy is 'half the battle', that once they could 'grasp the terminology' they would be able to 'read into' the names of parts to understand their form, location and function.[30] Furthermore this 'international vocabulary' of anatomy was necessary for communicating with health professionals in students' future medical work.[31]

When learning anatomy, then, students developed interrelated skills of looking, dissecting, handling, drawing, writing and reading by interacting with anatomical material. This was intended to generate a three-dimensional image of the body's interior in the student's mind's eye that was not regarded as static, or finished, but was rather conceived as a dynamic image to be augmented and honed as the student engaged with further material during their training. As such this image was neither entirely derived from that material, nor entirely imagined, but emergent somewhere in between. Suggesting ways in which this might work as an embodied observational and imaginative process, Stefan Hirschauer discusses the unfolding relationships between pictures of anatomy, the bodies of medical patients and those of surgeons in the late twentieth century. A surgeon will undergo training of her/his own body, developing specialized manual skills, and will also acquire a second body in their mind learned from anatomical texts and illustrations. This mental image both guides surgery and is further refined by impressions gained from the surgeon's ongoing visual and manual work on the concrete bodies of patients. So there is a continuous 'cross-fading of experience and representation', where the concrete body and the mental image of the body form 'models for one another'.[32]

Similarly, in Marischal College's Anatomy Museum and dissecting room learning to visualize anatomy was to become fluent in moving between external anatomical materials and an internalized image of these (retained but continually augmented and modified) in the mind's eye. But although Hirschauer's account refers to corpses and anatomical textbooks as 'dead substitutes' for the living body that bear little resemblance to it,[33] in the Anatomy Museum and dissecting room this material was 'animated' in processes of learning. Central to this was students' active correlation – their careful comparison – of the dead and the living, the organic and the fabricated, through which they came to recognize and understand similarities and differences. If distinctions between the living and the dead body were sometimes starkly apparent, they could also fade and become less marked when students traced relationships between anatomical materials, finding intermedial connections – connections between anatomical parts rendered in different media including preserved specimens, plastic models, printed illustrations, diagrams and photographs. Learning how to see and feel intermedial relationships aided in translating the bodies of the dead into an anatomy which was 'alive and moving'.[34] While tracing (finding and following) intermedial relationships was crucial in generating knowledge of relationships between anatomical structures, these relationships were of different orders – becoming adept at identifying intermedial relationships was not regarded as an end in itself but as a necessary route to knowledge of relationships between anatomical parts.

The discussion to follow explores the dynamics of tactile display – the emerging interactions and relations, the movements and impressions, that are integral to anatomical displays in their making, modification and use. Given the significance afforded to touch as a mode of knowledge acquisition, what was out of reach or not to be handled tended also to be largely excluded from anatomical visualization. This directed attention to material deemed to be of the present rather than that defined as belonging to the past, and these temporal distinctions had implications: the histories of bodies, with their social, cultural and power dimensions, remained predominantly out of focus, even though an institutionally approved history of anatomy in Aberdeen, and references to historically influential anatomists elsewhere, were displayed. Such a focusing of attention on the anatomical present reinforces claims to the naturalness and seemingly obvious facticity of the human body as presented through this disciplinary framework.

ENTERING

The complex of rooms and facilities including the Anatomy Museum at Marischal College, like many anatomy and pathology museums in Britain, was a tightly controlled zone. Although listed on the University of Aberdeen's website, only those with legitimate interests were permitted to enter with the permission of the honorary curator, a position held by the senior anatomy lecturer (who was also the licensed teacher of anatomy). Thus a sign at the front entrance to the Anatomy Department alerted anyone passing through the small back quadrangle of the college that access was restricted to 'authorised personnel only'. These included the senior anatomy lecturer, the secretary/anatomy bequest administrator, teaching staff (four core members and additional medical professionals), technicians

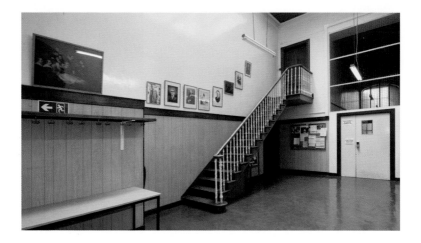

(three during the period studied) and, each year, over 200 medical and science students in the early years of their studies. On entering, the main corridor led to the lecture theatre, science laboratory, a study room and staff offices (illus. 22). Movement beyond the entrance corridor into the museum and dissecting room was restricted by inner doors with security code locks, the codes known only by those allowed to enter. The corridor was a display space leading to the museum and just as the museum has changed over time so has the corridor, conveying different impressions of the scope of anatomy (see illus. 89, 159).

Built into one wall, a locked glass-fronted case contained a memorial book enclosing the names of, and expressing gratitude to, the people who have donated their bodies to medical science (see illus. 165). On the opposite wall, beside the main entrance to the lecture theatre, hung a print of a painting after Rembrandt's renowned group portrait *The Anatomy Lesson of Dr Nicolaes Tulp* (1632; illus. 23). Tulp, elected praelector, or reader-demonstrator, of the Amsterdam surgeons' guild, attends to a

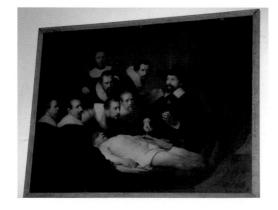

corpse's dissected hand and forearm, closely observed by members of the guild. He demonstrates the mechanism of the hand by holding tendons with an instrument in his right hand while showing the hand's movement in life by gesturing with his left.[35] In the corridor, this image – of corpse, observers' sustained visual attention and praelector's dextrous hands – linked current students' own lessons at Marischal College with an established tradition of anatomical work. Reiterating references to anatomy in Amsterdam as a prestigious seat of learning, this print was the first in a series of reproduced versions of seventeenth- and eighteenth-century 'Anatomy Lesson' paintings displayed in the Anatomy Museum since the 1960s.

To the right of this print, a series of eight photographs of portraits ascended in parallel with the stairs, representing anatomy in terms of its professors at Marischal College. Beginning with the professor who retired in the early 1990s, it charted the dates of their service, moving back in time with Edward J. Clegg (1977–93), David C. Sinclair (1965–77), Robert Douglas Lockhart (1939–65), Alexander Low (1925–38), Robert William Reid (1889–1925), John Struthers (1863–89), Alexander Jardine Lizars (1841–63) and Allen Thomson (1839–41). This reverse chronology extended deeper into the past as it worked its way up the staircase, suggesting connection through time, institutional continuity and authority. It projected a particular view of anatomy – as a domain of knowledge with a history conceived as a succession of established (male) anatomists. This figuring of the history of anatomy is not uncommon. Historians of science note that the natural sciences are 'amnesiac disciplines' that tend to erase their past, and 'in so far as they have a history of their own making, it is an epic history of titanic (and quirky) individuals.'[36] Allusions to the history of anatomy through the display of likenesses of its leading figures was also evident elsewhere in the Anatomy Department: in the dissecting room, where portrait busts were kept, for example, and in a display (from the 1960s) on the gallery of the Anatomy Museum. The latter was reached via the stairs in the corridor but, seldom used by staff, the door leading to it had long been locked.

Similarly, the framed images in the corridor were largely inactive in that they did not usually command attention. They were rarely viewed by staff and left unobserved by students. Remaining in position for at least the last decade, it was as though these images, routinely unnoticed, had merged with the fabric of the walls. They became 'invisible' in that they could be seen in passing but were not actively looked at. In this way such images had passed into the category of the historical, offering only a visual backdrop to anatomical material defined as current and directly relevant in present-day teaching. The corridor's framed displays, historical and memorial, were kept behind glass, not to be touched in contrast to anatomical material presented for tactile exploration. This differentiation of material – current or historical, amenable to touch or distanced from it – was also operative in the spaces to which the corridor led, with various implications for how anatomical displays were composed and used.

ANTECHAMBERS AND ADJACENT ROOMS

Tactile displays in the Anatomy Museum and adjoining dissecting room were dependent on practices in the mortuary, the workshop and the museum store. Behind locked doors, these facilities were invisible in that they were strictly inaccessible to anyone except staff in the Anatomy Department – they formed the composite inner sanctum of anatomical practices at Marischal College. The unseen work (that is, work seen by only an expert few) in these antechambers sustained displays and enabled their handling. The necessary movement of human remains and material objects between these spaces required substantial equipment, especially trolleys for moving bodies and heavy material. Furniture, such as dissecting tables, and large models, for example those of male and female articulated skeletons, had castors to facilitate mobility within the display spaces of the dissecting room and Anatomy Museum. The ongoing transit and repositioning of material was closely monitored by staff to guarantee security – they were 'required by law to know the location of all material', especially as human remains, again by law, could only occupy particular rooms in the department licensed for this purpose.[37] In the dissecting room and Anatomy Museum, although students were required to handle material, there were restrictions regarding the degree to which students were permitted to move this, especially preserved body parts, within each room and only staff transported materials between rooms.[38] The transit of anatomical material, integral to the process of display, within this complex of rooms was thus a matter of authority and expertise.

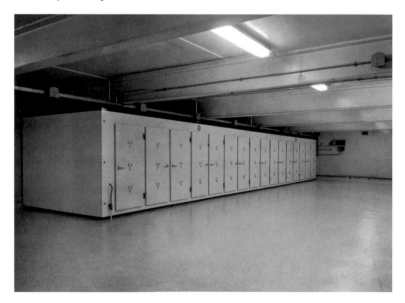

24
Mortuary, Anatomy Department, Marischal College, University of Aberdeen, mid-20th century, photograph.

Mortuary

The mortuary was located in the Anatomy Department's sub-basement, two floors below the dissecting room to which it was connected by a lift (see illus. 21). Here technicians conducted the difficult work of preserving and storing bodies donated to the department for dissection. Bodies were embalmed, to arrest decay so that they could sustain extensive visual and manual exploration in the dissecting room, then kept in individual storage compartments until needed (illus. 24).[39]

Once a donated body had been accepted, with the consent of the person in lawful possession of it (usually the next of kin), the funeral director delivered it discreetly, in a coffin and hearse, from the place of death to the department, where it was directly transferred to the mortuary. Donors, ranging in age from their late fifties to over 100, were mostly people living in the north of Scotland, including Aberdeenshire, the Highlands, the Western Isles, Orkney and Shetland. For a donor to be admitted upon death a number of conditions had to be met – no 'history' of certain diseases, recent major surgery or autopsy – and they had to be delivered within 48 hours of death to avoid deterioration.[40] It was lawful for the body to remain on licensed premises for up to three years, but preserved parts of a body could be kept for longer if the donor and next of kin had granted written permission.[41] The preparation of the body in the mortuary ensured its durability over this period of time, after which it was removed from the department, again by the funeral director, for cremation or burial. Mortuary practices for anatomical purposes refashioned a donated body so that a dead person also became a 'cadaver', subsequently referred to in the dissecting room as such but also defined as an 'embalmed subject', as 'human material' and 'cadaveric material'.[42]

Duties in the mortuary were undertaken by two technicians, including one junior who began in 2004 as a young trainee. There had also been a chief technician, previously employed in the department from 1985 to 2004. From his perspective, embalming bodies for anatomical purposes was different to embalming performed by undertakers for a funeral: technicians' work was to preserve the body, whereas undertakers embalmed for presentation, to prepare a body for viewing by bereaved relatives and friends.[43] When morticians embalm at funeral homes, as Glennys Howarth argues with regard to this work in Britain, the aim is to enhance the 'human-likeness' or the 'physical presence of the individual' as he or she appeared in life.[44] The mortician will give colour and elasticity to skin, position limbs and face, repair damage, apply cosmetics, comb and style hair, and dress the body in clothes selected by relatives, either the deceased's own or a burial gown. When restored, as far as possible, to a lifelike appearance, as though asleep, the deceased person is considered ready for viewing in a chapel of rest at a funeral director's premises. Thus displayed, the body provides a last 'memory picture' for the bereaved. The head and hands, regarded as particularly expressive of personal identity, are made visible but the body's veneer of life is unprobed beyond the gentle touching of its surface.[45]

By contrast, embalming for anatomical purposes takes place in a context where the deceased becomes an anonymous body, made robust enough to withstand extensive intervention and manipulation. Anatomists explain to students that 'embalming is necessary to preserve the tissues for examination, prevent decomposition and the growth of microorganisms'.[46] It entails physical changes in the deceased's body and shifts in how that body is perceived. Donated bodies were depersonalized in the mortuary, but they were nevertheless treated with care and respect.[47] The junior technician described (to me) her work in the mortuary, which was learned partly by observing her more senior technician colleague. Upon delivery she recorded the donor in the logbook, noting the person's name and wishes regarding burial or cremation, and assigning a unique number to them (each donor received a consecutive number). Thereafter, in the department, the person was not referred to by their name – though when later transferred out of the department to be buried or cremated their number was removed and their name was reattached to the person.[48] Once the body was laid out on the embalming table, clothing was removed and any jewellery reserved for the next of kin. After washing, disinfecting the body and shaving off hair, the body was moved into position for embalming, with face and palms of hands upwards. Bodily fluids, including blood, were drained and a pump used to distribute litres of embalming fluid, containing the preservative formaldehyde, through the body's blood vessels. Then metal tags engraved with the body's unique number were attached with string to the hands, feet and ears.

During this initial phase of accession and preparation in the mortuary the two technicians were the only people in sustained contact with the 20–30 women and men whose donated bodies were accepted each year. The junior technician described how her perceptions of the body changed during this process. When the deceased donor first arrived and was laid on the embalming table still in their clothing, usually nightwear or hospital wear, she was very aware of them as a person whom, she imagined, had relatives 'now left behind'. She was careful in her procedures, treating the body as a person almost as though they were still alive. However, through embalming she saw the body's changing appearance – previously loose skin, for example, became taut as the body was enlarged or 'bulked' and also hardened by the embalming fluid. To her the physicality of the dead body became more pronounced than the deceased person, who seemed to have receded.[49] Having undergone the technicians' transformative practices of embalming, the body was regarded as appropriate for display and examination in the dissecting room.

In the mortuary the transition from deceased person to (primarily) a body or a cadaver occurred and socially recognized markers of personhood and individuality, especially names, were removed. With these removals a person's previous relationships and life history were displaced by their new designation as a current instance of human anatomy, as anatomical material of the here and now. However, the link between person and body was never entirely severed. With number tags a body was displayed in the dissecting room without disclosing that person's name, thereby preserving their privacy while also allowing the body, or parts of it, to be identified by staff. In addition to this numerical device for the linkage of body to name, material traces of a person and their previous life were also seen to remain on and within the embalmed body. An indication of this persistence was evident, for example, in perceptions of the deceased's hands. For instance, a teaching fellow regarded nail polish on the hands of embalmed donors as a sign that those women had been cared for at the end of life.[50] The presence of nail polish triggered an association of the deceased body with the person as imagined prior to their death.[51] This visibility of living persons, and aspects of their former lives, on/in their deceased body remained a mostly latent possibility, sometimes glimpsed in the dissecting room, where embalmed bodies became visual and tactile learning resources for students of anatomy.

Workshop

Just as in the mortuary bodies were prepared for the dissecting room, so in the workshop anatomical specimens, many preserved in fluid-filled

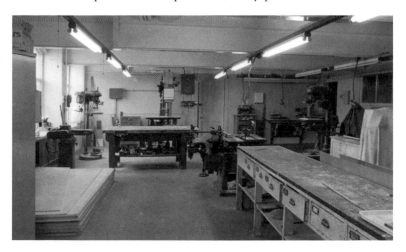

25
Workshop, Anatomy Department, Marischal College, University of Aberdeen, mid-20th century, photograph.

transparent Perspex cases or 'pots', were restored and models constructed and maintained by the department's technicians for display in the Anatomy Museum. In the basement – one floor above the mortuary, immediately below the dissecting room and again connected to it by the lift – the workshop provided facilities for technicians' work with wood, metal, acrylic and other materials (illus. 25). Parallel with the mortuary, where bodily decay was arrested, in the workshop the wear and tear endured by objects was counteracted or at least repaired as far as possible. This work of preservation ensured that body parts on display were stabilized and signs of decomposition minimized. Here were attempts to counter disintegration, to hold anatomical parts in a state of suspension.

Unlike in the mortuary, where the focus was on the preservation of whole bodies not yet anatomized, in the workshop the technicians' work focused on anatomical parts in soft tissue or skeletal form, or as models thereof. As the technician continually monitored the condition of specimens in the Anatomy Museum, any that were noticeably ageing – with parts dissolving or falling away, for instance, or whose pot was leaking – were identified. He carried out the necessary repairs, sometimes topping up or replacing preserving fluid or making replacement cases to 're-pot' specimens. In this way each specimen was maintained within its transparent enclosure. Further workshop activity included making tags for embalmed bodies prepared for dissection. At least six metal tags for each body were engraved with the body's unique number. Once attached, these tags ensured that dissected parts, when they became separated from one another, could be identified by staff and linked back together when it was time for the body to be removed from the department for cremation or burial.

Practices in the workshop sustained and renewed anatomical displays, but university investment in this area appeared to have declined, especially since the 1980s.[52] The chief technician emphasized this in 2003 when he was about to retire and wanted to pass on his knowledge to another technician. He pointed out (to me) that not only were few people prepared to become technicians of this sort, given the demanding tasks and specialist skills involved in work with deceased bodies, but there had also been a decline in resources so that the number of technicians employed in the department had fallen, in his recollection, from six to two. He had also noticed a contraction in the range of technicians' duties. For instance, although he would repair existing anatomical models, he was not asked to construct new ones as frequently as in the past, when, for example, he had made such models as a spinal column, in wood with internal springs, to show how vertebrae fit and move together.[53]

A diminishing personnel count and the diminution of tasks carried out in the workshop was materially evident in this space. Three wall clocks had stopped at different times and much of the once active mechanical equipment – saws and drills – was dormant or covered with dustsheets. Rows of tools were testimony to past industry and a wooden carpenter's workbench bore years of marks. Extensive joinery, including the construction of display cabinets, had taken place there. Coffins for the burial or cremation of donated bodies had previously been made by technicians but by 2003 coffins were supplied by an Aberdeen funeral director. As the workshop's machinery, tools and furniture had reached redundancy, this room had partly become a storage area. Thus in the workshop anatomical material was updated with repairs and some new models were also made (see illus. 4), but with the reduction in technicians and their role, much of the once functional equipment had gradually become deactivated historical objects.

Museum store

More overtly articulated than the slow drift into obsolescence in the workshop was the deliberate consignment of material to the past in the museum store. Many disused objects of diminished relevance, and those that were excessively worn, fragile or broken, had accumulated in the store by the late 1990s. The store, located beneath the lecture theatre in the residual space created by ascending tiers of seats, was only accessible to staff, like the mortuary and workshop, and it was entered through a discreet door in the Anatomy Museum. Material removed from display had been packed away, with some kept in storage since the late 1960s when

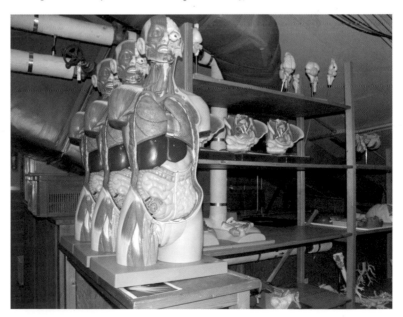

26
Anatomy Museum store, containing Somso models from Adam,Rouilly, 2007, in the Anatomy Department, Marischal College, University of Aberdeen.

there were substantial changes in the museum. As the store was not static (it had, for instance, been reorganized in the early 1980s),[54] from an anthropological perspective it was a shifting palimpsest where material accumulations could reveal historical aspects of anatomy, past collecting practices and traces of dismantled displays that were no longer visible in the current museum. Nineteenth- and early twentieth-century anatomical models of comparative (non-human) anatomy by Dr Louis Auzoux's firm and of the development of embryos by the Ziegler studio had settled into deeper regions of the store, packed in boxes for decades (see chapters Four, Five and Seven). By contrast, on open shelving for easy access were recently purchased plastic models regularly used in short phases of teaching (lasting approximately two weeks each) when they were displayed in the dissecting room. These models were thus periodically held in temporary storage only to be taken out again later when required, so that they were caught in alternating cycles of use and dormancy (illus. 26).

The spatial arrangement of the museum store separated material defined as historical from that in regular use. One area accommodated shelves of skulls, no longer used in teaching, which had been inscribed with classifications such as 'European', 'African' and 'Melanesian', their handwritten labels carrying dates between 1835 and 1938.[55] Adjacent to, but differentiated from, the historical skulls were further preserved bones defined as 'old', some derived from the dissecting room in the 1890s.[56] But as these were robust and unmarked by obsolete labels they were still used in teaching. They were grouped so that those from the same part of the body, resembling one another morphologically, were kept together in boxes, for example, of 'half skulls', of 'femora' (thigh bones) and of 'tibia and fibula' (bones of the lower leg).

27
Wax model of the heart, late 19th–early 20th century.

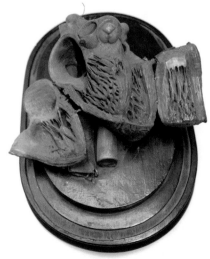

This morphological ordering of osteological material was reiterated in the arrangement of current plastic models in a different area of the store. On shelves were neat rows of model skulls, brains, ears, arms, hands, feet, hearts, pelves (male and female), lungs and torsos. These multiples of anatomical parts had a certain uniformity of design, having been recently purchased from the same German manufacturer – Somso, whose models are distributed to medical schools in Britain by the highly reputed company Adam, Rouilly. Similarly, in another area of the store redundant instruments were also grouped according to their form: there were clusters of stereoscopic viewing devices, microscopes and microtomes (used to slice tissues to be mounted and viewed on

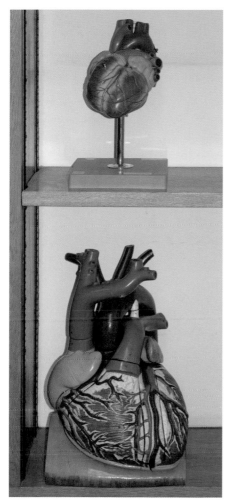

28
Plastic models of
the heart by the
Deutsches Hygiene-
Museum, Dresden,
c. 1960s (bottom),
and by Somso
from Adam,Rouilly,
c. 2000 (top), in the
Anatomy Museum,
Marischal College,
University of
Aberdeen, 2007.

microscope slides). However, this ordering did not work with those historical models kept open on shelves (rather than packed in boxes) but seldom used in teaching, for these were single instances of different body parts rendered in a variety of styles and materials by various makers over at least the last century. A plaster-cast eye, a pair of papier mâché lungs and a wax inner ear appeared among the miscellany of remainders from past anatomy teaching practices, contrasting with the uniform sets of apparently identical new models (see illus. 26).

However, despite their aged and sometimes broken condition, these historical models were not entirely detached from current anatomical material, as anatomists saw connections between what they regarded as 'generations' of models, where antecedents had given way to more recent versions of the same bodily part.[57] A wax heart from the late nineteenth or early twentieth century, for instance, held in storage and dusty with age (illus. 27), had been superseded by later models, on display in the Anatomy Museum and still in use; the latter were rendered in more robust materials and positioned vertically on minimal stands rather than fixed horizontally to a wooden platform (illus. 28). But while old anatomical materials were displaced by new ones, a previous anatomical form was still discerned in its successors.

The three predominant categories of material in the museum store — human skeletal remains, anatomical models and redundant scientific instruments — each occupying a distinct space, were thus, where possible, subdivided by temporal and morphological distinctions. This order was established in 2003 when the entire contents of the store were emptied into the dissecting room and sorted, with some material removed and the remainder reinstalled, so that the museum store, like the museum itself, has been selectively shaped by curatorial decisions and practices.

Prior to the store's 2003 reorganization, staff regarded its holdings as a miscellaneous mix of things among which it was difficult to see and to extract items deemed useful and relevant in current teaching practice. Decades of accruals defied complete description but they included dissected specimens once used to teach comparative anatomy (the study of anatomy in different species), such as the heart of a mute swan preserved in 1892 and the head of a dog from 1923; devices and callipers previously used in anthropometric studies; a case of glass lantern slides projected in anatomy lectures during the early twentieth century; and a framed photograph of two late nineteenth-century plaster casts of African people, labelled 'Bushman' and 'Bushwoman' (see illus. 85). Regarded as residual material from past anatomical practices, the accumulation in the store seemed a daunting mass for staff in the department, a difficult inheritance from previous anatomists, but still one for which they recognized a continued responsibility of care.

Sorting the store's holdings in June 2003 was explicitly guided by contemporary understandings of human anatomy and how this knowledge should be learned. Technicians moved the store's contents to the dissecting room, assigning items to specific groupings: new and old models; human skeletal material; disused instruments and equipment; photographs, X-rays and posters (see illus. 100). The latter two groupings were particularly varied, encompassing, for instance, a 1937 formal photograph of dinner-jacketed medical students, a North Borneo cigar box recycled to store microscope lenses, and a canister of film and projector (see Chapter Six). The store's eclectic contents were disentangled and laid out for inspection: a row of chairs, empty specimen jars, a pile of metal nuts and bolts, an old leather suitcase. Some items had reached a dead end, as had a heavy bunch of keys, wired together but disconnected from their long-gone locks. Other items were unidentifiable, such as a contraption made from blue strips of metal Meccano (manufactured as a mechanical construction toy) whose function remained elusive; a teaching fellow observed that such 'home-made' devices had often been constructed in the past by technicians and their intended purpose was now indecipherable. Some unfamiliar items, again no longer anchored in current anatomical practices, were associated with more familiar objects, the teaching fellow remarking that a microtome in its wooden case reminded her of an old sewing machine.[58]

Anything irretrievable for current use, and not of historical interest, was regarded as 'rubbish' to be disposed of – mainly old equipment (test-tube holders, old lamps and so on) and broken furniture. All of the human skeletal material was returned, sorted, to the store, the bones evaluated by a teaching fellow who decided which were suitable for teaching purposes. Those deemed inappropriate to use included skulls collected from different parts of the world in the nineteenth and early twentieth centuries with old inscriptions and labels still attached (accompanied by a newly discovered box of letters from men who originally presented some of the skulls to the Anatomy Museum). Bones that had acquired 'messy' surface markings in previous anatomy classes, such as handwritten names of anatomical parts and lines drawn to represent veins, were also problematic. Such tangible traces of past use rendered human bones awkward to use in present teaching: bones with discernable post-mortem histories were diverted away from students' attention as too potentially distracting from their present task. By contrast those bones without visibly evident post-mortem histories were to remain available for study in present teaching. Further separations occurred when the human remains in the store were distanced from those of other animals. The majority of non-human specimens had been transferred from the Anatomy Museum to the university's Zoology Museum during the late 1960s (see illus. 157). But some had been kept in the store until 2003 when these, along with a crocodile skeleton from the Anatomy Museum's gallery (see illus. 71), were also transported to the Zoology Museum. Far from the inert repository often assumed of storage spaces, the museum store had altered over time in content and internal organization, the recent modifications synchronized with those in the Anatomy Museum, as discussed later in this chapter.[59]

Practices, materials and facilities in the three antechambers made possible the displays in the Anatomy Museum and dissecting room such that bodies exhibited were always already modified and selected, while efforts of preservation in this context also entailed alterations, removals and disposals. To sustain anatomical materials for present-day usage they were subject to embalming, restoring and sorting. These processes enacted temporal differentiation and separation even though traces of the past were still discerned in material designated as current, and certain persistent traces sometimes surfaced for particular attention and overt interpretation.

DISSECTING ROOM

Located on the ground floor, the dissecting room had the largest teaching area and was the location of displays that were, in practice, attributed status as the most significant in the Anatomy Department at Marischal College. It had been built and equipped to maximize light and maintain cleanliness, with its nineteenth-century high glass roof, large frosted-glass windows to let in daylight while ensuring privacy, walls glazed with off-white tiles, and a row of sinks running the length of the room. The numerous stainless-steel dissecting tables were brightly lit from above. The distinctive, often disliked, odour of formaldehyde used in embalming fluid, which many medical students never forget, was diffused throughout this space, sometimes spreading down the interconnecting corridors of the college.[60] Dissecting rooms have been variously described as scenes of initiation and emotional rites of passage, sites of fear and identity formation.[61] Here students might be reminded of friends or family who have died, be provoked into self-reflection and become more sharply aware of their own mortality.[62] Dissecting-room displays of the dead are, however, made to generate anatomical knowledge of the living body, even as they act as reminders of death and of the deceased. At Marischal College disciplined interaction with tactile displays in the dissecting room informed students' engagements with displays in the adjoining Anatomy Museum – and, as discussed later, patterns of anatomical study in the museum also in turn fed back into dissecting-room learning.

Entry into the dissecting room was restricted to staff and students of anatomy, the latter only allowed access under supervision and provided they acted according to a strict 'code of behaviour and practice'. Students were taught to appreciate the examination and dissection of 'human subjects' as a 'privileged opportunity' dependent on the 'generosity of local people' who donated their bodies. They were required to 'respect that generosity and to behave accordingly', also showing respect by attending a dedicated memorial service at the end of the course for those donors.[63] Body displays in the dissecting room were thus synchronized with the required timing of donors' ritualized cremation or burial and formal memorialization, performed no longer than three years after donation, unlike the museum's displays of long-preserved body parts which were kept indefinitely rather than being subject to requirements of ritualized disposal at particular times.

To reinforce the code of behaviour in the dissecting room, students were notified that 'the use of human cadaveric material is carried out under the Anatomy Act 1984 as amended by the Human Tissue (Scotland) Act 2006 and its regulations.' Within this legal framework, alongside 'local rules', studying deceased bodies was confined to licensed premises and students were not allowed to escort friends or relatives into the department or to take photographs ('or other forms of image capture') in any area where 'anatomical specimens may be located'.[64] In this way the viewing of deceased bodies, either in the flesh or in photographic form, was strictly guarded and controlled. The code of behaviour also required all students to wear clean white laboratory coats in the dissecting room and to avoid wearing 'casual headwear', such as baseball caps or 'hoods', as they were 'considered disrespectful'.[65] White coats protected clothing from embalming fluids and other residues while also distinguishing the numerous students in the room from several teaching staff in green coats and two technicians in blue coats. Eating, smoking and drinking were not permitted and mobile phones had to be switched off.

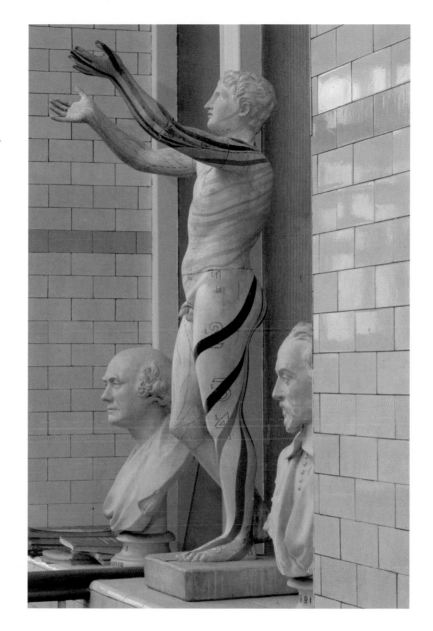

29
Plaster-cast busts
of John Hunter,
1873 (left), and
William Harvey,
1881 (right), with
the Berlin Adorante
(cast *c.* 1880) used
as a model to show
dermatomes (centre),
in the dissecting
room, Anatomy
Department,
Marischal College,
University of
Aberdeen, 2005.

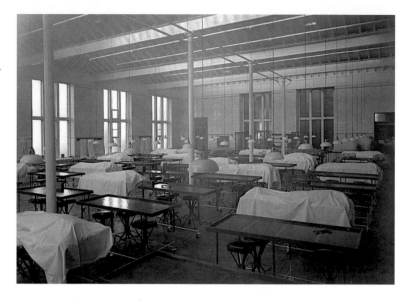

Remnants

In alcoves around the periphery of the dissecting room were several plaster casts – portrait busts of anatomists John Barclay, John Hunter and Georges Cuvier, dated 1863, 1873 and 1881 respectively, and of the physician William Harvey, also dated 1881. While the busts commemorated figures often celebrated in histories of Western medicine, their inscribed dates in this context referred not to their own lifetimes but to years once considered important in the development of anatomy at Marischal College. But in the twenty-first century these casts seemed to have sunk into their architectural surrounds so that once significant likenesses had become 'invisible faces'.[66] A further plaster cast figure showed the body's dermatomes – sections of skin each supplied by the same spinal nerves (illus. 29).

This dermatome figure was a copy of the classical bronze statue the Berlin Adorante, a life-size nude boy, cast by Domenico Brucciani's prominent London-based firm in the late nineteenth century. The cast had been adapted for anatomical instruction, during the 1950s, with the application of coloured paint to indicate the distribution of nerves on the body's surface (see illus. 154), but years of exposure to sunlight had bleached the fading paint. An aged label, probably by Aberdeen anatomist Robert Lockhart, invited observers to compare the figure with illustrations in his 1959 co-authored textbook *Anatomy of the Human Body*. By 1999 these plaster casts stood as reduced remainders of the reproduction classical sculpture that would have commanded a prominent place in medical schools during the second half of the nineteenth and into the early twentieth century (see illus. 95). Once positioned as important focal points, the plaster casts in the dissecting room at Marischal College no longer attracted attention. Instead they merged with the architecture, gazing outwards towards the main activity in the room.

Embalmed subject

For students learning anatomy old plaster casts of historical figures and faded allusions to the classical human form were of little import. Their interest was in the recently preserved cadavers and most up-to-date models that were displayed and demonstrated – that is, actively shown, pointed out, described – by their current teachers. Here patterns of work at dissecting tables guided the visual and tactile exploration of bodies. Rows of dissecting tables (in varying numbers) were a prominent feature of the dissecting room throughout the twentieth century (illus. 30) and until 2002, when changes in teaching methods involved adjustments as described later.[67] Every academic year from 1999 to 2002, approximately 30 tables each accommodated an embalmed body. Groups of about eight students would each be assigned a body to dissect from October to March, focusing on this intensive work for a total of around 100 hours.[68] During this time students shared some of the responsibility for maintaining the preservation of the body they progressively dismantled, keeping it moist with preserving fluid and covering it with a white cloth at the end of each session.[69]

In the dissecting room body donors remained anonymous and, with a number rather than their name, the deceased person was disconnected from their previous social identity and relationships.[70] Only the information deemed relevant for understanding a donor's anatomy was disclosed to students, namely their age and cause of death. Embalmed subjects were expected to be those of strangers, socially unknown to the students who dissected them. These subjects were detached from their life histories, dehistoricized – rendered 'biography-less', as Ruth Richardson argues has routinely happened to corpses in medical education.[71] Their physical appearance also reinforced the disjuncture between their present bodies and once living persons: naked and without hair, the effects of embalming were evident in the lack of blood, loss of elasticity and hardening of tissues and organs, and changes in body colour to muted shades of beige and grey.[72] In colour, texture and malleability, embalmed subjects lacked resemblance to the living body, yet they provided the foundation for students' visualization of living anatomy. Students were shown how to recognize (in order to see through) the effects of embalming so that they might imagine the body as though alive. Although students could identify traces of technicians' work of preserving and preparing bodies, these traces would routinely in effect disappear, or become transparent, for students approached embalmed bodies as if viewing them at first hand.

From the start students were reminded that all the bodies they were about to dissect were those of donors, but the perception of the embalmed subject as a person tended to diminish as the dissection progressed, as bodies came to be seen anatomically.[73] Students said they could not regard the body as a person while they were engaged in dissecting, so body was detached from person as students focused on tasks of cutting and exploring. Heidi Lempp's study of another medical school in Britain notes a similar reaction from students who said that when cutting 'you don't let yourself think that this was a person who had lived and loved.'[74] However, body and person were not completely separated, as students at Marischal College pointed out that during dissections they could also see traces of a person's former life in, for example, scars, marks of childbirth and internal evidence of surgical operations. These were viewed as indicators of a person's previous experiences, their life lived in emotional and social as well as physical terms.[75] Thus students were aware of the deceased as a body *and* as a person, as dead *and* as once living. These shifting positions concur with nurses' treatment of the recently deceased in hospital settings where they 'oscillate between poles of nearness and distance to the dead patient, experienced alternately as a sentient person or an inanimate body'.[76] In the dissecting room students had to manage this oscillation and, although these swings tended to lessen as the body was dismantled and the anatomical exploration deepened, deceased bodies remained 'ambiguous entities',[77] with an 'ontological duality', as Rachel Prentice points out, a state of being which is both 'person and thing', both subject and object.[78]

First cut

At the very beginning of dissection students tended to be anxious about their first incision into the skin of the embalmed subject but this anxiety subsided as they worked, though they continued to encounter various difficulties in their ongoing learning.[79] At their table, each group of students shared dissecting instruments – scalpels, scissors and forceps – which they purchased, borrowing larger tools, such as chisels and saws, from the supply in the dissecting room. At first unsure how to hold the scalpel and what to look for as they dissected, they often sought guidance from staff who supervised the sessions and acted as demonstrators. Holding the scalpel like a pencil and also using their fingers, like instruments, to dissect, students took turns to separate, define and feel anatomical parts while others in their group read directions from instruction manuals, observed and discussed the dissection or studied relevant X-rays and diagrams.[80]

Dissection proceeded according to established divisions of the whole body into anatomical regions: 'Upper Limb', 'Lower Limb', 'Back', 'Thorax', 'Abdomen', 'Pelvis and Perineum', 'Head' and 'Neck'.[81] Diagrams in anatomy textbooks outlined these regions and students mapped them onto the embalmed subject, dissecting each in order so that they began with the upper limb and ended with the head and neck. Areas of the cadaver were only uncovered when worked on; the rest remained concealed to prevent damage through drying. This practice of covering also focused attention on the body part rather than the whole, the concealment of the head perhaps masking the deceased person in a way that made dissection of their body easier to countenance.[82]

Moving from the 'surface' to deep within the body, dissecting helped students to understand the body's internal 'three-dimensional configuration'.[83] According to contemporary anatomy textbooks, the 'essence of a good dissection is to display each structure fully, clearly and cleanly', allowing a 'mental picture' to be obtained of that structure, such as a muscle or a blood vessel, by cleaning and defining it rather than just recognizing its existence.[84] Skin was either detached or folded into a 'flap' to recover or 'wrap' the dissection when not being worked on, thereby helping maintain its moistness.[85] Thus the skin, which is regarded as expressive of the person, was separated from the body so that the anatomical interior could emerge.[86] Fat was cleaned away and tissues teased apart so that students could see and feel distinct muscles, tendons, organs, nerves, blood vessels and bones. They located and named these parts using anatomical terminology, also identifying 'layers', 'fibres', 'tissues', 'bundles', 'tubes', 'levers', 'compartments' and 'cavities'.[87]

Finding their way through the body and coming to understand the relations between anatomical parts, students learned how to organize a 'forest of detail'.[88] They also studied 'functional systems', which are 'distributed' throughout anatomical regions but often predominantly associated with one particular region. For example, when dissecting the thorax they learned about the cardiovascular system, with attention to the heart, and the respiratory system, attending to the lungs, focusing on how such 'structures . . . enable function'. Displays in the dissecting room also drew students' attention to the 'normal variation' of anatomical structures in different bodies. They were advised that variation in 'surface features', such as hair colour, height, weight and posture, is 'paralleled beneath the skin by variation between individuals'.[89] Textbooks reinforced this principle, stating that 'all bodies have the same basic architectural plan but no two bodies are identical'.[90] To see this for themselves, students were required to 'tour other groups' cadavers to examine these variations as well as differences in male and female bodies.[91] Beyond the range of normal variation, students were also shown commonly encountered 'anomalies' and 'deformities', which could be either harmless or physically damaging, thus heightening students' awareness of possible internal anatomical differences.[92]

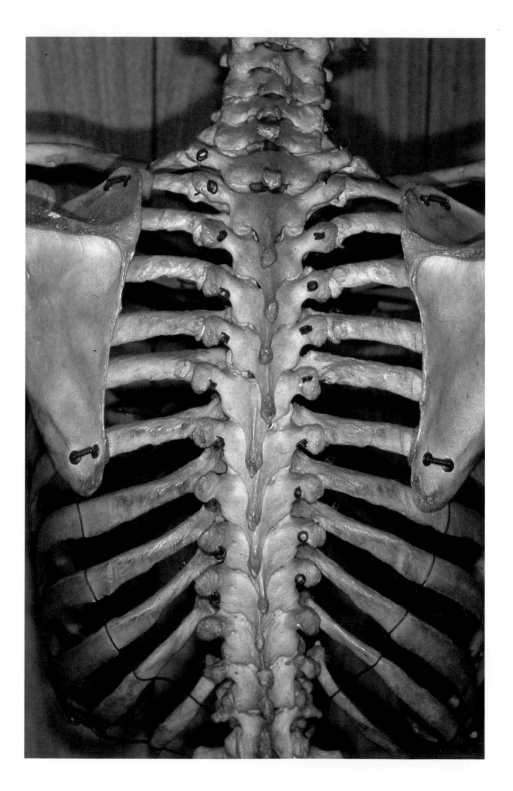

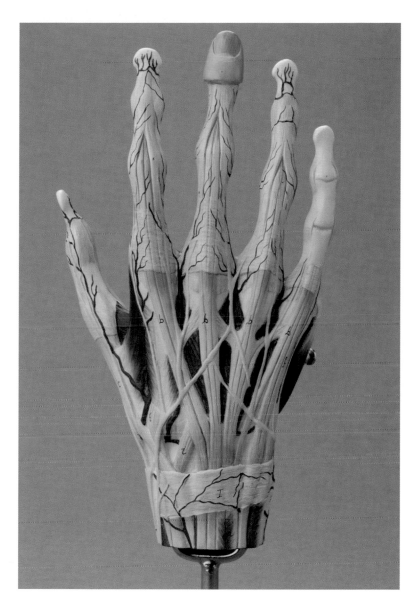

32
Plastic model of
the hand, 2005,
by Somso from
Adam,Rouilly.

31
Articulated human
skeleton (detail
showing the spine),
undated, on display
in the Anatomy
Department,
Marischal College,
University of
Aberdeen, 2003.

Patterns of reference

Dissection required coordinated action: excavating the embalmed subject, reading, observing images and examining models. Students learned, from teaching staff, how to refer to relevant sections of anatomical textbooks, a dissection manual and plastic models, such as those of skeletons which were regularly wheeled into the dissecting room (see illus. 42). They handled preserved osteological specimens, such as separate skulls and limb bones, and studied a fully articulated human skeleton (illus. 31). X-rays displayed on illuminated light boxes were compared with equivalent parts of bodies undergoing dissection. In this mobilization of anatomical material, patterns of reference were instigated and regularized, creating links or relations between textual descriptions, visual images, material objects and bodies. Students traced these intermedial relations, developing skill in visualization and thereby building their anatomical knowledge.

For guidance in what to look for when dissecting, students referred to prosections – parts of embalmed bodies previously dissected by staff. This enabled them, one student said, 'to look at and see what you are supposed to be seeing' as structures, such as nerves or blood vessels, had already been identified, separated and made distinct.[93] The finely crafted expert prosections were viewed as exemplary, as guides to students' own novice dissections. One student described a prosection as a 'good copy', skilfully produced by experienced staff with more time to dedicate to it.[94] By comparison students saw awkwardness and errors in their own dissections. Some cut through the very structure they were seeking, or mistakenly dissected what they recognized as 'the wrong thing'.[95] One student described her dissections as 'messy' – after taking off fat she had realized that, by mistake, she had also removed some muscle. Making mistakes was, though, she said, a way of learning – reviewing her error had helped her to better understand that anatomical part.[96] When dissecting, students tried to reproduce a 'good copy', to reveal in their own dissections what they could see in expert prosections, while also recognizing the anatomical variations they encountered in so doing and developing their competence with all of the blunders and messiness this entailed along the way.

Students were also encouraged to relate their dissections to models featured in the dissecting room's sequence of temporary displays. Models relevant to each region undergoing dissection were brought from the museum store and arranged on tables. For example, during the two weeks assigned to the dissection of the upper limb, models of the arm and the hand were displayed for students to examine (illus. 32). Staff returned these to storage when the dissections moved on to the next region, for example the back, during which time models of the vertebral column were displayed, and so on until each region had been explored. Students regarded plastic models, with their simplified and clearly defined parts, as easier to learn from than dissected bodies. Models have 'perfect' parts, said one student, and 'everything is where it should be'. But then, he explained, you have to look at the 'real thing', the dissection, to find those same anatomical parts. The notion of the deceased body as more real than other material used to learn anatomy was reiterated when another student declared, while he was dissecting, that 'this is as real as it gets'.[97] Nevertheless anatomical structures, such as ligaments, fine nerves and blood vessels, were difficult for students to identify through dissection, especially as, in their embalmed condition, they all tended to be the same brown-grey colour. So students looked to models, with anatomical parts distinguished in different colours and with distinct labels, to 'correlate' (to link and compare) with, and thereby clarify, their dissections.[98]

This correlation was conducted with awareness of the limitations of current plastic models, drawbacks that were highlighted by staff when they taught students how to use and interpret models. For instance, models of any given anatomical part, such as those of arm muscles, are identical and lacking the variation apparent in all living bodies, which differ and change as they grow. Also, models cannot adequately show how living bodies move, especially as they permit movements impossible in human action. Articulated models of hand bones with rubber ligaments, for instance, can be manipulated into extreme positions beyond the capacity of living bodies. The senior anatomy lecturer demonstrated this (to me) by moving a model of the hand, then comparing this with the movement of his own hand. The plastic model was a 'compromise', he said, 'something between movement as in life and the possibilities that the model's design permits'.[99]

Living model
Given the emphasis on living bodies in the study of anatomy, students were taught how to observe their own bodies, and those of fellow students, to identify anatomical structures and to deepen their understanding of function and movement. In surface anatomy classes, held in tutorial rooms, students acted as 'living' or 'working' models, focusing on those anatomical regions under exploration in the dissecting room but this time learning to visualize the bodily interior by examining the surface.[100] Students volunteering as models wore sportswear, or T-shirts and shorts, so that the relevant parts of the limbs and trunk could be examined in groups of two to four. The skeleton, muscles and internal organs were identified and examined via their 'surface anatomy'; they were observed and palpated, or felt.[101] To aid in this students drew anatomical parts on the models' skin using coloured face-paint crayons, the cosmetics in this context, as in other medical schools, used as 'tools' for learning.[102] When drawing on living bodies, students made mistakes and then tried again. To study the abdomen, for instance, kidneys were drawn and redrawn on models to help students learn their size, shape and position.[103] Unlike plastic models, living models also had pulses that were felt, responses that were tested and sounds that were searched for – students would listen, with a stethoscope, to heart sounds 'produced by normal blood flow' and breathing sounds 'from the movement of air through the airways'.[104]

To focus attention on living bodies, full-length mirrors were provided in surface anatomy classes and the dissecting room where students observed the anatomy of their head, neck and limbs in their own clothed reflections. Embalmed bodies undergoing dissection were, then, directly compared with students' own moving bodies so that the anatomy of the deceased could be visualized as though living, or animated. Indeed, medical educators assert that 'surface anatomy is a method of bringing cadaveric dissection to life' as students correlate dissected parts with their equivalents in living bodies.[105]

Thus students' intensive visual and tactile exploration of the deceased through dissection was coupled with an emerging anatomical awareness of their own bodies. This interrelation of dead and living body was described by a medical student at Cornell University, New York:

> The heart that we hold in our hands once beat as strongly as the ones within us. The vessels, now dry and collapsed, are shadows of the bustling highways of blood flowing to the tips of our own fingers . . . After touching the spongy lung . . . we draw deep breaths and picture the dramatic expansion and contraction within our own chest walls. With each muscle, we memorize, flex, and extend our own, noting the range of motion.[106]

During the revelation of the deceased body's anatomy, students' own living anatomy becomes increasingly apparent, so that living and dead enter into a reciprocal shaping. As one psychiatrist recently recalled of his medical training, 'You studied anatomy until it became part of yourself.'[107] And another student reflected on this vivid anatomy of the self: 'Whenever I see my own body now, in my mind, I see what's underneath my skin.'[108]

Manual mnemonics

To visualize anatomy in sufficient depth and detail, students engaged in specialist manual training. They were taught to develop their 'awareness of precisely what lies beneath' their 'examining hands', a skill learned through tactile interactions with bodies which would be necessary in their future medical work with patients.[109] Rules of conduct required clean hands, careful and respectful handling of embalmed bodies and no 'rough' handling of models. But while practical learning placed emphasis on manual skills, students were often initially reluctant to touch the bodies of others, living or dead.[110] Many students also regarded practical learning in the dissecting room as less important than listening to lectures and note-taking.[111] So resistance to learning with the hands had to be overcome and, with guidance, students would usually participate actively. By dissecting they became familiar with cutting, pushing aside and scraping to find and identify anatomical structures, feeling their way through the body. Many preferred to wear surgical gloves, but the texture, tension and thickness of internal parts could still be felt to aid in identification. Having located structures, such as veins, students would trace them and follow their course by means of touch, coming to understand the spatial relationships between parts.

Students displayed some body parts in situ within the body, such as muscles, while others they released and lifted out, such as the heart and intestines, becoming sensitized to their size, shape and weight and rotating them for closer observation from different angles. In this process students' acts of demonstrating and describing anatomical structures were central to learning. Effective demonstration – a mode of tactile display in action that oriented visual attention towards particular aspects of bodies – involved students accurately pointing to and correctly naming particular structures using actions learned from teaching staff. Here the hand operated as an indicating device, performing a conventionalized and authoritative gesture regularly used in anatomical practice, and sometimes also performed with a pen acting as an extension of the finger.

Repeated tactile engagement with embalmed bodies, in concert with visual exploration, generated and consolidated students' knowledge of anatomy during six months of dissection. Their extended navigation of bodily exteriors and interiors was educated into 'skilled movement', facilitating the visualization and remembering of anatomy.[112] The regular, and what became habitual, performance of actions developed students' anatomical skills, and such skills were incorporated as embodied memories. They learned particular techniques, manually revealing and tracing anatomical structures and also performing referential gestures by pointing to and identifying those structures. In doing so students adopted certain proprieties, expressed particularly through the hands, for example the respectful handling of embalmed bodies. Such a process enabled each student to acquire, reflect upon and utilize their own 'mnemonics of the body'.[113] This collective bodily and mental training, which concentrated especially on students' hands and eyes, was conducted at the tactile interfaces between students, embalmed bodies and other anatomical material. Rather than recalling the individual persons who were dissected, students' remembered – through the practice of visualization – an anatomical body, subject to a range of external and internal variations, together with a repertoire of manual and social skills for investigating and demonstrating anatomy.

Incision to inscription

The manual dexterity required of students in the dissecting room was, however, modified at Marischal College with changes in teaching methods from 2002 when, rather than dissecting whole bodies, students studied with prosections.[114] So, instead of actively participating in the display of bodies by dissecting to reveal anatomical structures, students interacted with the displays of body parts produced in advance by staff. This method of learning was considered less time-consuming and more efficient for students than dissecting. As a result, however, students' learning became less 'hands-on' as teaching fellows prepared the prosections 'behind the scenes', on four dissecting tables in a screened-off corner of the dissecting room.[115] Separation of the prosection preparation area from the teaching space was reinforced in 2003 when large wooden wall-mounted cupboards were removed from the science laboratory and assembled, by the chief technician, into an L-shaped partition so that teaching fellows could dissect without interruption from students. The partition had glass-fronted shelving, facing into the dissecting room, to display historical anatomical models, such as a wax torso, for viewing but not handling (illus. 33).[116]

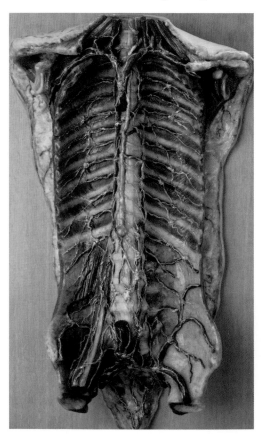

33
Wax model of the torso, with blood vessels and lymphatic vessels (highlighted in a silver-coloured substance), c. 1883, by Maison Tramond, Paris.

Prosections were prepared from embalmed bodies divided into anatomical regions so that the upper and lower limb, head and neck, thorax and so on were dissected, as a teaching fellow explained, to 'show what students need to see'.[117] The teaching fellow likened making prosections to sculpting, working with the best physical qualities of each embalmed body and enhancing these with her dissecting techniques, which followed the body's internal contours. She produced up to five prosections from each body, all with a tag for the body's unique number (to enable staff to link prosected parts with the donor's name). Prosections were stored in the mortuary until required in the dissecting room, where they were displayed on dissecting tables in the same sequence that previous students followed when conducting whole-body dissections – that is, according to anatomical region. Thus, from 2002, students' tactile engagement with embalmed bodies shifted so that they would learn from already divided parts, examining and demonstrating already defined structures such as muscles, tendons and blood vessels. At the beginning of the course one whole male and female would, however, be displayed to emphasize to students the importance of learning the anatomy of an integrated rather than fragmented body.

The prosections were correlated with relevant plastic models (as dissections had been), and with diagrams and textual descriptions displayed on mobile display boards placed next to the dissecting tables. This temporary arrangement of material, on tables and boards, formed approximately eight 'stations' that students were expected to work their way around.[118] The station displays were changed each week by staff, and students moved on to the next anatomical region. Although there was an emphasis on handling cadaveric material as central to learning, students made no incisions into prosections. Instead they traced with their hands those already made by experts, reading descriptions on display boards to facilitate their understanding of that bodily part. Here they replaced scalpel with pen, taking notes as they studied: 'I need to write things down to learn, not just read', explained a student.[119] The anatomical illustrations and diagrams displayed at the stations, which were produced on a computer by the technician, were also often traced by students who held paper over them and redrew the underlying outline in pen.

This shift towards note-taking coincided with changes in surface anatomy classes which reduced students' tactile contact with other students acting as living models. Students' persistent reluctance to touch the living models led to a modification in the classes.[120] Instead of drawing anatomical parts directly onto bare skin with face paint crayons, as described above, staff suggested students wear white disposable plastic aprons over their clothes onto which students used pens to outline anatomical parts, such as the lungs, liver, stomach and pancreas.

Thus, with modifications in tactile learning, making inscriptions became more pronounced in the dissecting room. Yet students continued to examine cadaveric material, visually and manually, to develop their three-dimensional spatial knowledge of anatomy. So tactile learning was coordinated with inscribing, a balancing act that the senior anatomy lecturer suggested students achieve by manipulating prosections with one hand and making notes with the other.[121] In this way the tactile displays in the dissecting room informed embodied memory, in that they were incorporated in practice, while also acting as a site of inscribing practice – noting, tracing and outlining – to facilitate remembering. Indeed these forms of inscription were also incorporated, entailing as they did embodied learning.[122] Students' learning patterns cultivated in the dissecting room, especially the tracing of connections between two- and three-dimensional material, also developed in parallel in the Anatomy Museum, as discussed below. In its relation to the dissecting room, the museum was often considered a subsidiary place for revision – for follow-up learning through repeated observation and tactile examination.[123] And in this museum-based consolidation of knowledge there was, again, a separation of material deemed relevant in present learning from that seen to belong to the past.

ANATOMY MUSEUM

Immediately adjacent to the dissecting room was the Anatomy Museum, the two connected by an inner door for staff to pass rapidly between them and both with their own main entrances used by students. With a ground floor, gallery and glass roof, the museum, like the dissecting room, retained its nineteenth-century architectural structure (illus. 34). A collection of some 300 human 'skeletal specimens', 200 'fluid preserved specimens of human tissues', 200 'modern plastic models' and 200 'historical models' were either displayed in the museum or kept in its store, in addition to approximately 900 anatomical 'works on paper', such as illustrations, and around 40 'non-biological artefacts' relevant to the history of anatomy such as old instruments and equipment.

The museum's ground floor was its main space for learning activities, where open-shelf display cases formed bays, installed in the late 1960s, with tables and chairs for study of the material that covered 'the whole of the human body'.[124] In addition to further study tables in the centre of the museum, eight computers near the entrance were provided for viewing anatomy software.[125] The gallery, locked and only accessible to staff, was

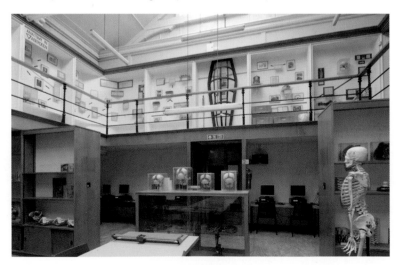

34
Anatomy Museum,
view of ground-floor
displays and gallery,
2007, in the Anatomy
Department,
Marischal College,
University of
Aberdeen.

mainly used as a storage area for an extensive collection of human bones from archaeological excavations in Aberdeenshire. Also in the gallery, an exhibit, *Anatomy in Aberdeen*, again from the late 1960s, narrated a history of the subject in northeast Scotland from the foundation of King's College (1495) and Marischal College (1593) to the mid-twentieth century.[126] Like the display of portraits in the department's entrance corridor, this institutional chronology highlighted leading anatomists, but it also featured issues such as the 'supply' of bodies for anatomy and the Anatomy Act of 1832. Although, from the ground floor, the displayed texts were illegible, and photographs not clearly visible, some larger items were discernable, especially an iron mortsafe with padlock and key – an early nineteenth-century device for protecting fresh graves against robbers who supplied bodies to anatomists. The epistemological status of this exhibit was similar to the dissecting room's portrait busts in that it was regarded as illustrative of anatomy in the past rather than active in the constitution of present anatomical knowledge. As such it remained, for the most part, unnoticed by medical and science students.

Displays of anatomy on the museum's ground floor were related to, yet differed from, those in the dissecting room. Preserved 'specimens' were encased in transparent Perspex pots on open shelves. These dissected human feet, legs, hands, arms, stomachs, intestines, hearts, heads and brains were mainly prepared in the department between the 1860s and the 1960s, although several osteological specimens were purchased from commercial suppliers in the late nineteenth and early twentieth century (see illus. 2).[127] Their unembellished containers were devoid of decoration to allow uninterrupted viewing of specimens, with soft tissues suspended in preserving fluid by transparent threads and bones in sealed dry pots supported by discreet wires (see illus. 162). Here specimens were displayed as examples of 'normal' anatomical structures, except for the select few defined as 'rare anomalies'.[128] All were derived from now unknown bodies and their labels assigned each specimen a position within the museum's organizational scheme – unlike the numbered tags on embalmed bodies in the dissecting room that linked each body and bodily part to a person's name. While bodies temporarily displayed in the dissecting room could only be retained for up to three years from each donor's death to their burial or cremation, museum specimens were intended for longer-term exhibiting. For instance, two vertical sections of a woman's head, neck and torso, displayed beneath the clock in the centre of the museum's end wall, had been maintained for over a century (see illus. 99). Eyes closed, she was displayed alongside the rectangular light boxes used to illuminate X-rays.

Museum preservation was not, however, everlasting as specimens remained subject to the effects of time, despite ongoing maintenance by technicians. Clear preserving liquid tends to discolour to a pale amber described by one pathologist as a 'yellow twilight'.[129] Soft tissues gently dissolve and fade over time. Recognized as fragile, ageing and rare, specimens in the Anatomy Museum were inaccessible to touch, some 'so delicate' that they could not 'withstand normal wear and tear', some too heavy to be easily moved from the shelves, and so students were not allowed to pick them up.[130] This specific denial of tactility contrasted with the emphasis on handling recently embalmed, robust bodies in the dissecting room, so that older specimens not to be touched appeared to students as somewhat remote and of the past. Ageing specimens also differed from the museum's colourful plastic models, which were regularly utilized by students, encouraged by staff who explained that for learning anatomy these models were useful adjuncts to 'cadaveric material and the living body', although 'not as good as the real thing'.[131] This explicit and authoritative evaluation of material produced implicit comparisons of the dissecting room and Anatomy Museum in which the latter acquired subsidiary status, even though staff promoted the museum as an important teaching resource.

Despite the differentiation of museum and dissecting room, however, there were significant continuities between them, reinforced by the regular to-ing and fro-ing of staff, students and anatomical material. There were commonalities in the structuring of, and interactions with, anatomical displays comprising recognizably similar material in both spaces – especially the plastic models, which were actively deployed in both. Selected museum specimens were also temporarily displayed in the dissecting room alongside relevant dissections. Furthermore, there were parallels between the museum's tables and the dissecting tables, as students developed consistent and complementary learning practices at both, following the same code of behaviour, dress and conduct when studying the preserved 'human material' displayed there, except that in the museum there was no need for laboratory coats and surgical gloves to be worn.[132]

Anatomical division

The Anatomy Museum's ground floor was divided into the same anatomical regions as the bodies in the dissecting room, so that its very structure materialized the divisions apparent in dissections, prosections and current anatomy textbooks whose chapters are organized predominantly according to regions (illus. 35). So, like an anatomical body – or a model thereof – the museum comprised, on entering through the main door, three bays to the left with signs announcing the display of the *Upper Limb* and *Lower Limb*, the *Thorax* and the *Abdomen*. To the right, in symmetrical formation, were three further bays housing the *Head and Neck*, *Neuroanatomy*

35
Anatomy Museum,
view of ground-floor
displays, 1999, in the
Anatomy Department,
Marischal College,
University of
Aberdeen.

36
Museum of Anatomy,
University of
Glasgow, view
of ground-floor
displays, 2007.

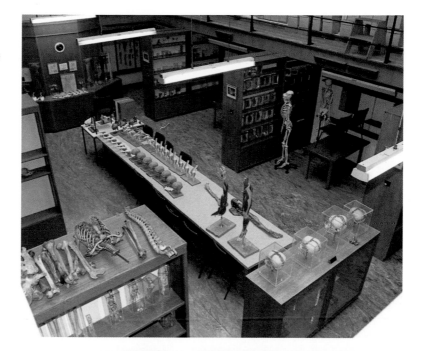

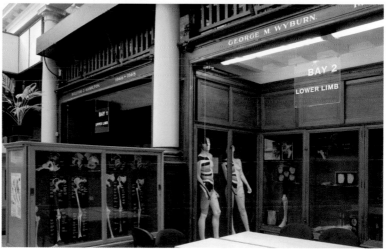

(the study of the nervous system), where specimens of the brain and spinal
cord were displayed, and *Embryology* – the latter two signs highlighting
particular aspects of anatomical study rather than regions.[133]

Displaying anatomy within a regional structure is not uncommon. The
University of Glasgow's Museum of Anatomy has a regional layout on the
ground floor (illus. 36) while the gallery houses specimens and models
from William Hunter's eighteenth-century collection (see illus. 59). The

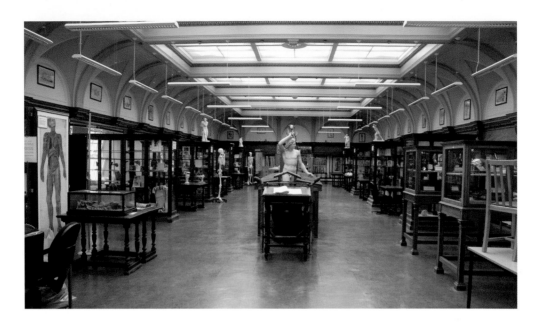

Anatomical Museum at the University of Edinburgh also has regional displays (illus. 37).[134] With a common structure, and all located near dissecting rooms, these medical-school museums also contain similar collections. They all have, for example, nineteenth-century anatomical models by the same eminent makers as well as current plastic models by the same manufacturer.[135] However, local differences are evident in their material, such as in the particular preserved specimens and anatomical images that have been made, over time, at each site. So that while these museums have significant commonalities and connections (past and present), their differences have emerged through historical and local particularities in practices of collecting and preparing anatomical materials, in combining these materials and in their specific patterns of use. Nevertheless, in all of these museums emphasis has been placed on tactile learning, and where there are glass cases, rather than open shelves, they are unlocked for students to closely examine their contents.

A major characteristic of such displays of anatomical regions is their rich composition, as each region features specimens, images and models grouped together and juxtaposed to show, in different media, the main bodily components at varying angles and depths, and in varying degrees of detail. In the Anatomy Museum at Marischal College the regional organization of material, unlike the historical exhibit in the museum's gallery, was not concerned with chronology or numerical sequence, even though some objects were dated and numbered. Instead material was loosely arranged and rearranged on (adjustable) shelves within the appropriate region. The

Head and Neck bay, in 1999, for instance, held preserved skulls, wax models of the inner ear, diagrams and specimens of teeth, a plaster model of the head showing the muscles, brain and eye (illus. 38), and a dissection of the head showing the nerves accompanied by a labelled photograph of the same specimen (see illus. 136). Multiple renderings of the same parts offered elucidation through reiteration and shifts in scale, focus and orientation. Thus when learning to visualize anatomy, students traced intermedial relationships among these materials, studying within and moving between regions of the museum/body: they entered into and engaged with this museum space arranged as an anatomical body.[136]

The museum's six oak bays remained in place from the late 1960s to 2009 and although their holdings were largely preserved over this period, alterations and changing patterns of use were also apparent. Modifications since 1999 saw new signs added to the bays, to highlight the body's functional systems within its anatomical regions – the supplementary sign in the *Abdomen* bay, for example, was the *Digestive System*.[137] The senior anatomy lecturer's curatorial strategy encouraged students to increase their use of the museum; it was redecorated (the ground-floor walls were painted yellow to brighten the room) and, more significantly, the displays were 'de-cluttered' and 'tidied'.[138] From his perspective too many things on the museum's shelves tended to discourage students from engaging with them, and those items most relevant to current teaching were to be kept in prominent positions. Here the aim was to rejuvenate and refocus the museum, to reduce its apparent time lag. Textbooks deemed 'out of date' were disposed of, and selected specimens and old models moved to the museum store. For example, the *Head and Neck* bay was divested of a plaster head dating to *c.* 1887 (see illus. 38), a series of 'mutilated teeth' of Africans presented to the museum in 1911–14 by a doctor in Johannesburg, and an enlarged three-dimensional model of the gasserian ganglion (see illus. 62) made by Robert Lockhart in 1924. Residual animal specimens also went to the store and then to the university's Zoology Museum.

These removals divided current from selected historical material and separated animal from human – distinctions also

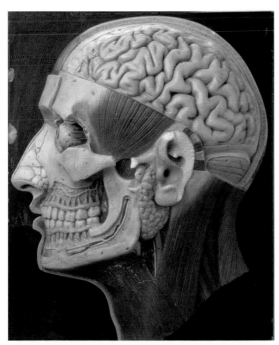

38
Plaster model of the head, c. 1887, by Franz Josef Steger, Leipzig.

evident in the reorganization of the museum store in 2003. From 2001, then, the museum underwent gradual visual simplification, with a slight reduction in objects occupying shelves, and some older anatomical models and specimens replaced by plastic models. Such changes were evident in the *Embryology* bay, where several human foetuses and newborns, preserved as specimens in the early twentieth century, were removed and replaced by plastic models of male and female reproductive organs and pelves, one with a nine-month foetus in the uterus, as well as models of a foetal heart and child's skull. Specimens with no place in the current anatomy curriculum thus gave way to useable models, while ageing models, in chipped plaster or flaking papier mâché, were superseded by the smooth, rubbery bounciness of those in plastic. This material modification of the museum was furnished by influxes of Somso models purchased from Adam,Rouilly, the firm from which the department had periodically ordered models since at least 1985.[139] Thus a large batch of some 90 models in 1999 (see illus. 35) were joined by a further 40 during 2002–4, including multiple skulls, bone joints and parts of the head and spine. By 2006 the museum permanently displayed one example of every plastic model in its collection, as well as several models purpose-designed and made in-house to help students with aspects of anatomy they found particularly difficult (see illus. 4).[140]

Re-vision

In the Anatomy Museum, the 'real' bodies explored in students' previous lessons could be seen again – revised – and further committed to memory. Students used the museum's displays to repeatedly re-view and handle what they recalled of embalmed and dissected bodies, and of living bodies (including their own) examined in surface anatomy classes. Again students traced patterns of reference, as in the dissecting room, moving between and correlating descriptions and illustrations in anatomy textbooks, diagrams, models and preserved specimens. When studying at the museum's computer screens students selected from arrays of digital images of dissected body parts, X-rays, histology slides and videos.[141] Using museum material students clarified vague, ambiguous or insufficiently understood aspects of anatomy to strengthen their skills of visualization. They returned to, and re-engaged with, what were regarded as the same internal anatomical parts as those displayed in the dissecting room, these presented from clearer points of view or from different angles, to help them 'build' their '3D image' of the body in their mind.[142] Rather than working and communicating in small groups, whether to dissect, study prosections or participate in surface anatomy classes, students tended to study alone in the museum. Thus the working together of 'different pairs of eyes/minds' in dissecting-room groups shifted into a more solitary, though no less socially

39
Series of preparations
of the middle and
inner ear, c. 1926.

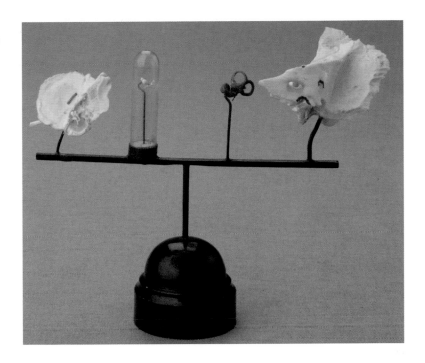

informed, mode of study in the quiet museum.[143] As students' abilities
and interests varied, each one could use the museum to focus on their own
chosen aspects of anatomy, and this would, in turn, further inform their
learning in the dissecting room.

The museum's displays offered opportunities to clarify anatomy
through close observation, and this was particularly useful with regard to
small or delicate parts of the body such as the eye and ear. A 'Series of
preparations of the middle and inner ear' (illus. 39), for example, comprised part of a foetal skull including the tympanic membrane or ear drum
(far left); the auditory ossicles (the malleus/hammer, incus/anvil,
stapes/stirrup) – the smallest bones in the body – inside a protective case
(second from left); and a wax cast of the hollow cavities of the bony
labyrinth (second from right) which corresponded with the dissection of
the adult temporal bone (far right). The latter two preparations were both
painted in green, red and yellow to indicate how they would fit together in
the body. Some models, on the other hand, offered clarification through
enlargement. A large-scale papier mâché kidney, for instance, had anatomical parts made more distinct with pronounced contours and colour
contrasts (illus. 40). However, the protective cases of such museum objects,
these examples dating between the late nineteenth and early twentieth century, rendered them open only to visual inspection, not tactile engagement.
This limitation, in addition to lacking or incomplete labels, tended to

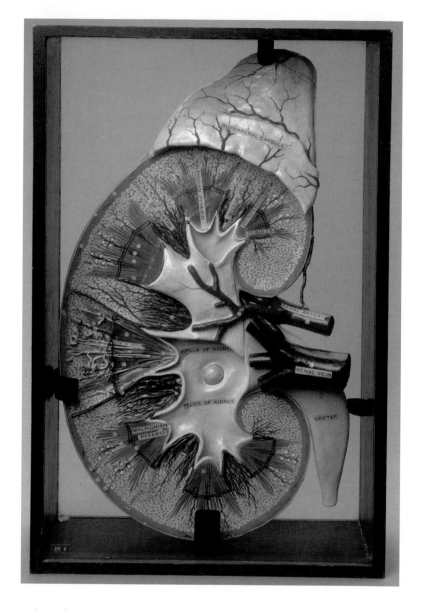

reduce their appeal for students who regularly gravitated towards recently acquired plastic models.

Clear labelling of anatomical parts was crucial to revision in the museum, as revising – which consolidated the capacity to visualize anatomy – entailed focused acts of reading. Just as diagrams in students' textbooks linked outlines of bodily parts to their anatomical terms with plain black line pointers (illus. 41) and, in parallel, the pointing hands of staff and students associated those terms with parts of embalmed bodies

41
Anatomy textbooks,
Keith L. Moore and
Anne M. R. Agur,
*Essential Clinical
Anatomy*, 1st (left)
and 2nd (right)
editions (Philadelphia,
1996 and 2002),
used by students
in the Anatomy
Department,
Marischal College,
University of
Aberdeen, 2007.

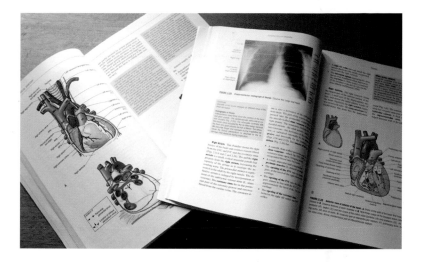

in the dissecting room, on plastic models anatomical terms were linked to parts by means of keys. A model of the hand, for instance, had letters and numerals to relate its parts to their anatomical terms given in a booklet attached to the model's base (see illus. 32). The key avoided cluttering the model with labels that would potentially obscure it with words. Too many labels supplying too much detail was problematic, as the senior anatomy lecturer explained, especially the amount of detail often found in profusion on old models and diagrams. To illustrate this he gave the example of a black-and-white textbook diagram rendered dysfunctional because it had so many black lines to label its parts that those very parts could hardly even be seen.[144]

Potentially confusing density of detail was therefore avoided as students sought the simplicity of labelling on plastic models to help them easily locate and identify anatomical parts. This selective focus meant that other labels on less recent models and specimens, either handwritten or in a variety of fonts and formats – such as those made in the 1960s on a typewriter or with plastic embossing tape (see illus. 164) – were not actively read. Nineteenth- and early twentieth-century labels showing the names of model makers, anatomists and students who prepared specimens, and artists who painted anatomical illustrations, largely remained unread. Just as disadvantaged in attracting and sustaining attention were old models devoid of labels, or whose explanatory keys had gone missing. The museum's preserved body parts were also difficult to read in that their descriptive catalogue, produced in the late 1960s, was consigned to storage (around 2002), regarded as no longer useful in current teaching. To encourage students to observe a series of specimens prepared in the 1890s, a corresponding set of labelled watercolours of those specimens (see illus.

98) were retrieved from the museum store, cleaned, conserved and rehung beside their fleshy counterparts in 2007. But predominant reading practices in the museum tended to draw current models, rather than historical materials, into view.

As in the dissecting room, students were advised to 'always read text/diagram with 3D aid e.g. cadaver or self or plastic model', so that what was read had to be related to what was seen of three-dimensional anatomy.[145] This process of reading was a mode of visual exploration in which students navigated between textual descriptions, diagrams, models and bodies, navigation that was eased by clearly recognizable labels. Lorraine Daston suggests that in anatomists' work 'reading and observing are so tightly integrated as to form a single practice.'[146] Revising anatomy in the museum involved just such an integration: lecture notes were read and reread alongside textbooks and labelled models, and further notes were also taken, consolidating the note-taking or inscribing practices undertaken in the dissecting room.

By working out the relations between textual descriptions and other anatomical materials, students forged their own intermedial routes through museum material, thereby further internalizing anatomical knowledge. A student, for instance, sat at a table in the museum reading a textbook alongside a plastic model of the larynx, drawing from a corresponding diagram in a textbook and then checking this drawing with the model.[147] Students explained that they were able to remember anatomy more effectively when they used plastic models and also drew related diagrams by 'copying' and 'tracing' those in textbooks. Apprehending anatomy by handling and examining the uncomplicated contours of plastic models and by following the unambiguous lines of diagrams sharpened students' visualization of anatomy. When drawing a diagram a student's hand and eyes followed an outline, rendering anatomical parts more distinct and therefore easier to recall. Copying in this way did not exactly replicate the textbook diagram because this drawing by hand also operated as 'creative investigation'.[148] Indeed, the teaching fellow noticed that some students would combine drawing from textbooks with their own 'inventions'. Related to this, according to the teaching fellow, was students' uses of commercially available anatomy colouring books containing anatomical diagrams that students completed and coloured with bright crayons – to aid in distinguishing and remembering relative shapes and locations – sometimes producing striking and 'truly eye-watering' creations.[149]

Revision in the museum was thus a process of reading and note-taking, observation, drawing and colouring, intended to enhance anatomical visualization through repeated exploration of anatomical parts and their relations from various angles, in different scales and media. Anatomical knowledge was augmented through such repetition, which was open to exploration and improvisation yet always concerned with the 'real' body.[150] Revision, as practised with museum displays, was also, significantly, a tactile undertaking which trained students' hands and, as we shall see, allowed them to play.

Jigsaw

One of the main difficulties in anatomical visualization was the ability to relate three-dimensional bodies to two-dimensional illustrations and diagrams that label and thereby identify and help elucidate anatomical parts. Students often found embalmed bodies displayed in the dissecting room difficult to correlate with textbook illustrations, especially as textbooks 'describe the structure of the body in most people' while 'the structure of different people varies considerably in its details'.[151] This skill of correlation, of making connections or discerning relationships, was vital in learning anatomy, and the museum provided materials with which this skill could be honed. As anatomist Debra Patten notes, when students 'move repeatedly between . . . 3D and 2D' renderings of anatomy, this aids their understanding of 'relationships between anatomical structures' and helps them to develop 'a 3D mental map of the body'.[152] Therefore when students practised relating two- and three-dimensional materials in the Anatomy Museum their capacity to visualize and to better comprehend anatomical relationships was enhanced. Here plastic models were used to mediate dissected or prosected bodies and anatomical illustrations, providing an intermediate level of simplification between the absolute detail of the body and schematic textbook diagram. This positioning of models as intermediaries was indicated when they were referred to by teaching staff as a 'stepping stone' towards understanding anatomy; this metaphor captured the notion that this learning requires embodied movement, and imagined transitions, between different renderings of anatomy.[153]

Again, it was durable plastic models, intended for intensive handling, that were used rather than older fragile ones which, like the museum's specimens, were reserved for visual examination only. The senior anatomy lecturer distinguished current and historical models with a crockery analogy, likening the latter to 'best china kept in a cabinet' and seldom used and the former to 'standard teacups' used every day. Teaching staff further articulated the preciousness and value of old anatomical models, referring to them as 'works of art' that are no longer made and are therefore 'irreplaceable'.[154] Thus finely detailed waxes (see illus. 84) and a rare life-size model of the male body constructed during the 1870s in a material much like papier mâché (see illus. 141) – both kept in their original glass cases, the latter untouched for decades despite having been originally designed to be taken apart – were contrasted with recently purchased and regularly used plastic models considered more robust and, though expensive, easier to repair and replace.

The life-size model of the male body, comprising over 90 pieces, was also likened, by the senior anatomy lecturer, to *The Krypton Factor*, a popular television quiz show broadcast in Britain from the 1970s to the 1990s and known for its use of complex three-dimensional puzzles to test mental agility and intelligence. This analogy underlined the perception of this model, although originally built to be repeatedly dismantled and reassembled, as too detailed and difficult to use in current teaching. Plastic models, on the other hand, were regularly sought out and their popularity was expressed when staff and students associated them with toys.[155] This was not a derogatory association but rather one that highlighted the models' advantageous features.[156] Plastic models were seen to invite an element of play or exploratory activity for students, many of whom seemed more comfortable with models than with embalmed bodies, especially during their initial studies. If a model vertebral column seemed, with all of its parts, to resemble a plastic chess set,[157] the jigsaw puzzle was a common metaphor for anatomical models with interlocking pieces of varying shapes that fit together to form a coherent picture.[158]

In the museum students learned how 'parts of the body are put together' by repeatedly taking models apart and reassembling them.[159] This repetition was not possible in students' dissections, as once done a dissection cannot be reversed, and this action of taking apart was not possible with the prosections prepared for students by staff. By rotating and exploring anatomical parts from different points of view students came to more fully understand the approximate shapes of, and relative relations between, anatomical parts, also becoming more accomplished at linking three-dimensional models with two-dimensional labelled diagrams.[160] In this process students did not expect plastic models to perfectly resemble 'real' bodies – they knew that models are substantially different to bodies in colour, texture, weight and sometimes size. Instead they learned how to activate models in order to more clearly visualize, and repeatedly recall, anatomical parts and their relations in three dimensions.

To do this students selected models from the appropriate museum bay's shelves, moving them to a table to study along with textbooks and other models. For example, a student gathered plastic models of the ear, eye, tongue and larynx, exploring them in relation to one another, taking each one apart and clarifying their inner components and relative positions in the body. Another student worked with a cluster of six models relating to the head which, she explained, is particularly difficult to visualize in three dimensions. In this session she studied diagrams with models of the skull

42
Anatomy Museum,
ground floor, 2003,
in the Anatomy
Department,
Marischal College,
University of
Aberdeen.

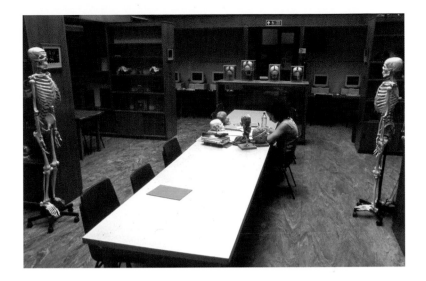

42
Anatomy Museum, ground floor, 2003, in the Anatomy Department, Marischal College, University of Aberdeen.

and the brain showing different sections and views (illus. 42). Although the scales of plastic models selected by students for study were not necessarily consistent, some showing anatomical parts at their 'natural' sizes and others enlarged, the aim was to imaginatively fit them together to 'build a 3D structural image of the whole body'.[161]

This imaginative piecing together, a visualizing of anatomical parts and their relations, entailed coordinated work of hands and eyes. Running hands along parts of models and pointing them out with fingers or writing instruments, the student's 'examining hand' rehearsed the exploratory and gestural repertoire cultivated in the dissecting room, thereby reinforcing those mnemonics of the body in learning anatomy. But in the museum models were explicitly not 'real' bodies so, although students' handling had to be done with clean hands and carefully rather than 'roughly', models were not surrounded by the code of behaviour that guided study with cadavers and interactions with them did not evoke the sense that these were once living persons, nor did they entail contact with fluids and residues from embalmed bodies.[162] Such relative differences made for easier tactile interactions with models. Furthermore, as 'toys', especially 'jigsaws', models when taken to pieces permitted serious play in that students became absorbed in the trial and error of trying out different positions for fitting together three-dimensional anatomical parts.[163] Relations between parts of a single model, between several models, and between models and other anatomical materials were discerned by students engaged in an intermedial process of feeling shapes, seeing colours, interpreting lines and reading labels. Here anatomical intermediality aided the visualization of an integrated anatomical body.

The perceived visual and tactile qualities of plastic models enabled regular and repeated interactions with them, interactions that were seen as inappropriate with old models. Light, resilient plastic was easily handled, its softly moulded surfaces open to manipulation, and simplified parts were accentuated in vivid colours. Bright blues, reds and pinks contrasted with older models' muted and faded wax or papier mâché. The spatial orientation of new models was also aligned with the current emphasis on learning from the living body. Vertically positioned on their (often removable) bases, new models were upright like the living whereas old models in horizontal repose might have appeared dead. Plastic models thus had the capacity to mediate dissected bodies and living models – their interiors were revealed, as were those of embalmed bodies, but unlike dead flesh drained of colour, the interiors of plastic models were vibrant and therefore somewhat 'alive'. In bright plastic, new models were also free of the aged, peeling and cracked surfaces so characteristic of old models that carried evidence of previous use, traces of their own histories in the form of surface markings, inscriptions and old labels.

These glimpses of an old model's past appeared too messy and distracting in current anatomy teaching whereas, by contrast, plastic models seemed to have no history to interrupt or complicate present-day interactions with them. In this respect plastic models were equivalent to embalmed bodies in the dissecting room when constituted as current anatomical material, rather than when perceived as deceased persons with life histories. Under glass domes and protected by locked glass cases, historical models and much other 'old' anatomical material was removed

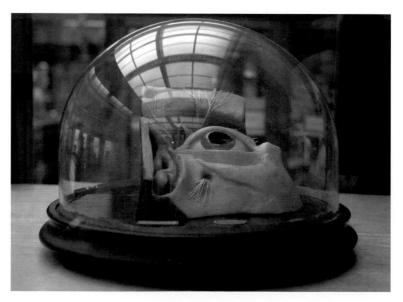

43
Wax model of the eye, late 19th–early 20th century, by Maison Tramond, Paris, displayed in the Anatomical Museum, University of Edinburgh, 2007.

from, and seemingly resistant to, tactile engagement (illus. 43). Such material remained on the periphery of the tactile displays that were central to the generation of anatomical knowledge. This is not to say that current plastic models remained fixed in the present as these too aged through wear and tear, acquiring a patina suggestive of regular use – as on articulated model skeletons whose white plastic bones were smudged with blue ink from the pens used to point out anatomical features. As the senior anatomy lecturer noted, people think that new models are unbreakable but in practice parts come away or screws come out and get lost – it is a matter of constant repair.[164] Nevertheless continuous maintenance kept plastic models active in the present, staged as material of the here and now rather than objects mired in the past.

Contemporary anatomy focuses on the living, moving body even as knowledge of that body is generated though visual and tactile engagement with the dead. At Marischal College embalmed bodies in the dissecting room were animated when visualized with reference to the living bodies of students and in association with vibrant plastic models. It was in students' movement between multiple renderings of the body – in the form of dissections, models, diagrams, descriptions and medical images – that their skills of anatomical visualization developed. This embodied and imaginative process which brought anatomized bodies to life was enacted in display spaces where current materials were differentiated from, and made more pedagogically active than, those from the past. Students were trained to focus on anatomy very much in the present, to become engrossed in the seeming immediacy of observable and handleable bodies and body parts from which they built up a '3D structural image of the whole body' in their 'mind's eye'.[165] This body comprised anatomical parts and their relations abstracted from anatomical materials which were (predominantly but not completely) depersonalized and dehistoricized. Students remembered this generalized anatomical body, along with a range of 'normal' variations and differences, through practices of incorporation, inscription and revision, undertaken in the dissecting room and museum. What was out of touch remained at a distance from this learning process, just as what was 'dead and static' remained on the periphery of concerns within anatomy.

Four exploded human skulls in transparent Perspex cases which faced the door of the Anatomy Museum were accompanied by a significant sign: 'Please do not remove' (see illus. 2, 34). Underpinned by this inscription, they had acquired a fixity that at once anchored them within the museum (they had occupied this position since the late 1960s) and guaranteed they were not handled – only occasionally viewed. This was the fate of anatomical material defined as 'historical'.[166] This material remained, stilled, in the dissecting room, the museum and their supporting chambers. Although kept within these spaces, it was not *actively* displayed and thus not mobilized in the generation of anatomical skills. Through the dynamics of tactile display, intermedial relationships were traced by students, to make anatomical relationships visible and tangible. But what remained invisible, or seldom noticed, were the deeply embedded social relationships through which the Anatomy Museum, and its surrounding display spaces, had formed over its longer-term history. The rest of this book aims to chart and analyse this field of relations, at least in part, so that the thoroughly social and cultural nature of historically changing anatomical display can be better grasped.

While the focus of this chapter was the dynamics of tactile display, involving the movement of people, bodies and materials within and between spaces in the Anatomy Department at Marischal College during the period 1999 to 2009, the following chapters encompass a wider terrain of shifting social relations and changing cultural practices that have shaped and transformed the Anatomy Museum since its foundation in the nineteenth century. This includes geographically distributed anatomists, curators, collectors, donors and unnamed bodies; a diverse range of interconnected museums and sites of display; and practices such as specimen preparation, drawing, film-making and three-dimensional modelling. This previously untold history of the Anatomy Museum is here reconstructed not just from written records but from materials such as anatomical illustrations and photographs, wax and plaster compositions and preserved human remains – materials that provide significant insights with regard to perceptions of bodies alive and deceased.

Two

ANIMATIONS: RELICS, RARITIES AND ANATOMICAL PREPARATIONS

Imagining deceased bodies as though alive – an imagining required in the process of anatomizing – is central to present-day techniques of display and learning in anatomy museums and their related spaces. Yet historically, different kinds of animated corpses have been created through anatomists' work. While Chapter One examined twenty-first-century dynamics of display that produce knowledge of the human body's moving and functioning anatomical structures, as well as an imagining of dead bodies as previously living persons, this chapter explores earlier modes of animation in medieval (and later) saints' relics; early modern theatres of anatomy, cabinets of rarities and memento mori; and eighteenth-century collections of preserved and modelled bodies. In doing so, it traces a history of anatomy museums in Europe, focusing on the changing ways in which the body after death has been sometimes dramatically, sometimes subtly, enlivened.

Aspects of these animated cadavers can be viewed in present-day displays where images designated as 'historical' are deployed more as references to past achievements in anatomical exploration than as material for the current study of bodily interiors. Enlarged copies of famed illustrations from Andreas Vesalius' *De humani corporis fabrica* are exhibited, for example, at the University of Glasgow's Museum of Anatomy and the University of Edinburgh's Anatomical Museum (illus. 44, centre).[1] Muscular male dissected cadavers are depicted moving, in a sequence, rotating and revealing their anatomies from different angles.

At Marischal College, Aberdeen, visual allusions to the history of anatomy placed further animated anatomies on display. Here the Anatomy Museum's bays were, from the late 1960s until 2005, hung with copies of 'Anatomy Lesson' paintings originally commissioned by the Amsterdam surgeons' guild in the seventeenth and eighteenth centuries (see illus. 42,

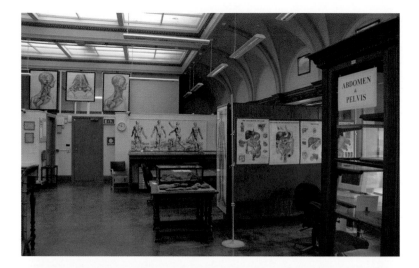

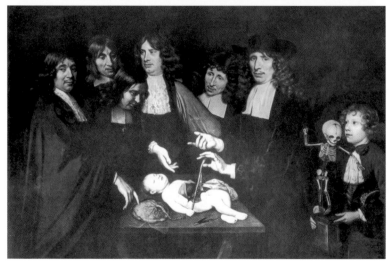

for example, top left). Reduced in size and framed as monochrome photographs, one such copy was of Jan van Neck's 1683 group portrait featuring Frederik Ruysch (1638–1731; illus. 45). Ruysch demonstrates the blood vessels of a newborn's umbilical cord and placenta, his gesturing hands and those of onlookers, drawing attention to – displaying – aspects of the dissection.[2] That the placenta is to be preserved and crafted as an anatomical preparation is perhaps suggested by the painting's composition in that this bodily part's convoluted blood vessels and delicate membranes are visually echoed in the intricately crafted lace shirt worn by the figure immediately above the child.[3] In a further significant echo, the dead child on the table is aligned with a child's skeleton, preserved and articulated in a living posture at the right of the painting. The latter preparation is held by Ruysch's son Hendrik, depicted as a young boy.[4]

From the sixteenth to the eighteenth century, historians note, images of living yet anatomized human figures became particularly striking and culturally salient. As anatomical illustrations in printed books, animated cadavers were inflected with classical, Christian, Dance of Death and still-life imagery to offer lessons in anatomy that could also carry moral and spiritual messages.[5] A deeper and more expansive history of the simultaneously dead and living is discernable if we attend not just to visual images but to interrelated material objects, some of which incorporate human remains. Sacred relics, compelling three-dimensional models of anatomized bodies and carefully wrought anatomical preparations were afforded appearances and qualities that seemingly brought deceased bodies to life in differing and changing ways.

RELIQUARY

In medieval Western Europe human dissection, conducted for the purposes of medical education, developed alongside other modes of body opening and partition, including those associated with holy bodies from which sacred relics were derived. Katharine Park argues that 'dissection like' practices, undertaken in Italy from around 1300, included embalming to preserve bodies for funerary display, autopsy to establish cause of death and the removal of foetuses for baptism when women died in childbirth.[6] The opening of bodies in these ways (cutting the abdomen only) – often at the request of family, kin and others in close social relationships with the deceased and conducted in domestic settings, away from public view, by physicians, surgeons and sometimes by women – was not regarded as violating or dishonouring. Rather, these practices were often part of Christian funerary rituals. Furthermore, within Christian belief holy bodies possessed powers of healing and the cults of new saints focused on the deceased bodies of men and women that were perceived to work miracles. These bodies, especially women's, were opened, their internal organs examined and then displayed as sacred relics. For instance, it is said that when Chiara of Montefalco, abbess of an Umbrian monastery, died in 1308 the nuns embalming her body discovered relics: her heart was cut open to reveal an image of the crucified Christ with the crown of thorns, nails and lance. Soon afterwards the heart began to perform healing miracles and Chiara's dead body remained incorrupt, another sign of her sanctity.[7]

Saints' relics could consist of preserved body parts, such as bones, skin, teeth, umbilical cord and hair, and fluids, such as blood, milk and tears.

They also included materials with which saints had been in contact: shreds of clothing, dust collected at tombs, Christ's shroud and parts of the True Cross.[8] These were displayed in churches and, perceived to be effective in working miracles, they became foci of prayers and devotion. Imbued with divine power and miraculous gifts from God, which could be received for the benefit of the living, relics were far from lifeless or inert matter. Rather, they were seen as active substance: to the devout, relics were alive with the capacity to cause miracles and they were venerated as such. When the relics of St Marcellus were honoured in France, for example, declarations of their animate nature were made: these were not 'dry bones', rather they were 'full of life'.[9] And that physical remains of the holy dead were in some sense animated was apparent when the bodies of holy women secreted oil or milk with powerful healing properties.[10] Saints were regarded as present and sentient in their relics, however fragmented. Thus a relic, as a synecdoche, was both a part of and the whole saint who was both living and deceased, physically present on earth but already received into heaven.[11]

Christian churches throughout Europe required relics in or upon altars but precious relics also circulated as gifts, by theft, through trade and by purchase.[12] The movement of relics was a ritualized undertaking as translations were undertaken, guaranteeing their authenticity when they passed between locations or, indeed, when they were moved from one part of a church to be displayed in another. So the relics of a single saint could, over time, become geographically distributed and dispersed across sacred spaces. Acting as magnets for visitors in large numbers, relics formed centres of pilgrimage where they were approached for help with cures for ailments and suffering or other assistance in exchange for veneration, remembrance and offerings such as candles and ex-votos.[13] Through these exchanges relics actively participated in the social and spiritual life of communities.

Relics were displayed in reliquaries that appealed to sight as well as touch, inspiring awe while inviting intimacy. Through emotionally charged proximity with relics, or even direct contact, pilgrims might receive marvellous visions or benefit from a saint's healing power – though visual and tactile access to relics could be restricted according to social rank and occasion.[14] Richly decorated reliquaries were fashioned from precious metals and jewels, some in the form of body parts such as the head, arm and foot. Shapes of reliquaries often, though not always, corresponded with the body parts they contained, sometimes providing glimpses of the part through small crystal windows. The materials used in the construction of reliquaries were also significant, with precious metals such as gold and silver conveying the importance of their contents when encasing a saint's bodily remains.[15] Framing and embellishing relics with these materials, and sometimes incorporating objects of wonder, such as ostrich eggs, coconut shells,

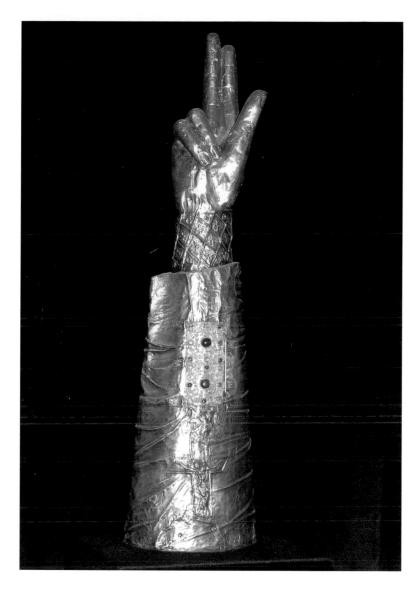

coral and sharks' teeth, reliquaries amplified the sacred charge of body parts.[16] For example, a thirteenth-century silver and gold reliquary of St George (d. 303) in the Abbey Church of St Foy at Conques, southern France, took the shape of the right arm in a sleeve set with semi-precious stones (illus. 46). The shining hand and sleeve masked any decay, displaying the saint's remains as an active arm making a gesture of blessing, the sign of the cross. A hinged plate appears to have provided an opening for the relic to be touched. The relation of an external reliquary and internal relic was not simply one of container and contained, for both were interrelated:

a reliquary's fabric was endowed with special properties, which were enhanced by virtue of contact with the relic, and its form made the saint's remains expressive, renewing them and enhancing their potency.[17]

The settings in which reliquaries were placed in churches contributed to the efficacy of animate relics. They might be stored in special cupboards, or areas of the church, and then revealed at particular times, such as the saint's feast day, when they were displayed and received veneration. While reliquaries were often embellished with visual accounts of the life and death of the relevant saint – such biographies reinforcing the identity of relics necessary in the exercise of their power – their architectural settings might also display narrative scenes, in stained glass windows for example, which similarly enhanced the significance of those same relics.[18] The spatial location and manner in which a reliquary was displayed thus aided in the maintenance of a relic's authenticity, assuring pilgrims that these remains genuinely were those of a particular saint. This was also underlined by inscriptions, and documents kept inside or attached to reliquaries, which linked each relic with a named saint.[19]

Reliquaries containing several saints' relics were also constructed, some for domestic settings, where they could be mounted on walls in glass-fronted cases. Such reliquaries were made by cloistered nuns in Continental Europe from the seventeenth century onwards, and these amplified the impression that sacred relics were animate through the crafting not of precious metals and stones but of more mundane materials. Creating paper

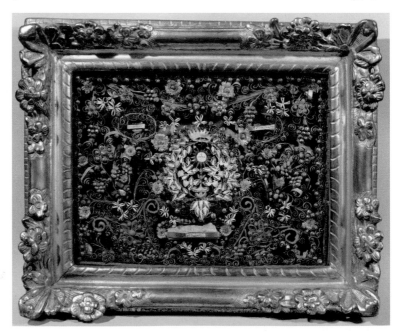

47
Reliquary containing relics of St Euphrosyne of Polotsk and St Boniface, 18th century, mixed media.

filigree from finely worked strips of rolled paper, nuns produced these reliquaries by arranging complex paper compositions around small bones. One particularly elaborate eighteenth-century example contains three labelled bone relics – of St Euphrosyne of Polotsk in Belarus (d. 1173) and St Boniface (d. 754; illus. 47). On a fabric background, intricate paper scrolls – formed as coils and floral shapes, some in blue, some lightly gilded in gold – are arranged around a paper image of a crowned monstrance (a receptacle used to display consecrated hosts, or the body of Christ, and relics), surrounded by red hearts and white leaves.[20] Convents in eastern France, for example, produced reliquaries using this paper technique during the eighteenth and nineteenth centuries; alongside the nuns' needlework and embroidery of liturgical linens and altar cloths, reliquaries were carefully constructed as devotional objects for chapels, altars and convent benefactors as well as nun's families and friends.[21] Because of vows of poverty they chose to work with modest materials – paper, cardboard, fabric scraps, shells and beads.

Within these reliquary compositions the remains of each saint were accompanied by a label bearing their name, and rolled paper embellished the space between relics. The paper filigree in illustration 47 is so densely arranged that it resembles a textile. At the same time the composition seems to have grown and flowered much like a living, fertile garden. Indeed the making of these reliquaries was sometimes regarded as a placing of saints' bones in gardens formed by nuns' hands. Making paper ears of corn, lilies, roses and bunches of grapes, the nuns folded, rolled and shaped paper strips, inspired by their readings of devotional literature from which they derived these plant, floral and fruit motifs. Dedicating hours to patiently intertwining or cultivating their materials, the nuns' work was a devotional act and an expression of humility.[22] These reliquaries engaged the hands of the devout in compositions that visually enlivened relics – saints' bones thrived in intricate 'gardens' that drew viewers' into proximity with the sacred.

THEATRE OF ANATOMY

If the remains of saints displayed in reliquaries were in some ways animated, what of the bodies displayed in theatres of anatomy? Human dissection as a 'pedagogical practice' was conducted in Europe, especially in Italy, from around 1300, but although regulations allowed an annual dissection of a man and woman at the universities of Bologna, Padua and Florence during the 1400s, it was not until around 1500 that dissection was considered significant enough in medical learning to conduct on a regular basis.[23]

Bodies were scarce and usually male – they were mainly those of executed criminals of foreign birth and low status, and dissection in public was deemed shaming for those persons as the naked body was revealed and taken apart before strangers.[24] During the sixteenth and seventeenth centuries public dissections held by institutions in further European cities, such as Amsterdam, Leiden, London, Paris and Zaragoza, became ritualized displays of anatomy, some with processions and music, attracting large audiences including city elites, church officials, professors, students, wealthy travellers and common citizens. In Bologna dissections coinciding with carnival celebrations were attended by masked revellers.[25] The University of Padua's oval anatomy theatre, built in 1595 with steeply rising concentric wooden balconies lit by candle chandeliers, was widely attended by scholars and teachers as well as 'tailors, shoemakers . . . butchers, salted fish dealers, and lower than these, porters [perhaps funereal] and basket-bearers', who were drawn to the spectacular dissection events that had pronounced philosophical, rhetorical and dramatic dimensions.[26] If these annual winter dissections acted as ritualized displays of learned authority, they were also meaningful in religious and legal terms: the human body was considered God's creation, which anatomists dissected to reveal 'the ingenuity and workmanship of the supreme artisan', while this treatment of the criminal corpse was also regarded as an extension of the punishment inflicted through execution, a treatment of the body which might suggest redemption for the deceased's sinful soul.[27]

Printed images of displays in anatomy theatres from the 1540s and the early 1600s represented deceased bodies as though they were, in some ways, alive – whether undergoing dissection or preserved in collections of rarities. Illustrations of human figures that appeared not only animate but to assist in their own dissection had circulated in printed anatomical works since the early 1500s: male figures held up flaps of skin and muscle so that further layers of muscle could be seen, for instance, and female figures revealed their inner reproductive organs. Such images of self-dissection emphasized the truth of anatomical revelation while also responding to the ancient instruction to 'know thyself' – to be aware of human mortality.[28]

The title page of the *Fabrica* (1543), Vesalius' book prepared while he was professor of anatomy at the University of Padua, brought deceased yet animated figures to the centre of an anatomy theatre, where they played a major role in a scene composed to comment on the nature of anatomical knowledge and to show how it was derived (illus. 48). The corpse of a woman is opened and a crowd of male spectators – including physicians, professors, clerics, students and commoners – strain to witness the revelation of the bodily interior, elevated on a platform like those erected as temporary anatomy theatres.[29] Gazing out of the frame towards the viewer,

48
Title page, woodcut from Andreas Vesalius, *De humani corporis fabrica* (Basel, 1543).

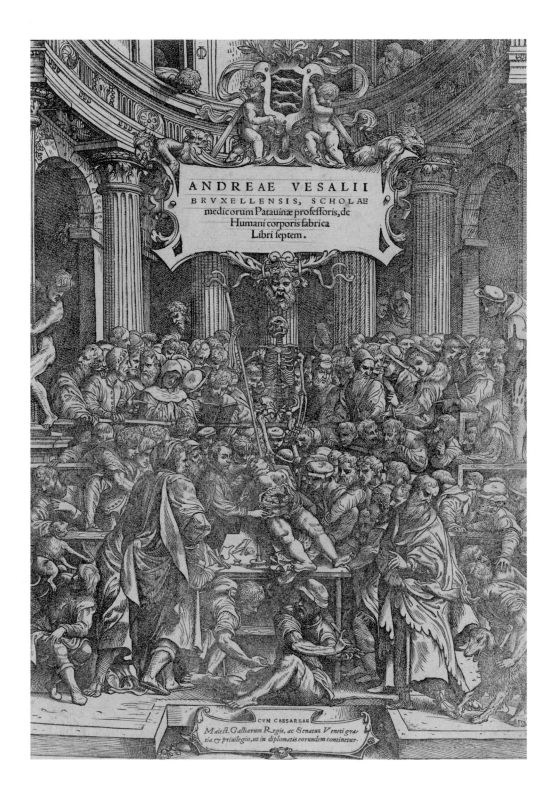

Vesalius places his right hand upon the body undergoing dissection and with his left hand gestures upwards as if towards the skeleton standing above the corpse. A monkey and a dog, at the lower left and right of the scene, perhaps represent animals that were vivisected during anatomy demonstrations to show organs in action or following human dissection for comparative purposes.[30] They may also have signalled a critique of ancient anatomy, especially the work of Greek physician Galen, which relied on animal rather than human dissection.[31] Here Vesalius himself performs human dissection, a significant departure from the hierarchical division of roles represented on the title pages of previous anatomical works in which, from the 1490s, the lector read from classical anatomical texts while the demonstrator indicated with a pointer, or his hand, which bodily parts should be dissected and displayed by the sector, usually a surgeon or barber. Instead Vesalius was depicted both lecturing *and* demonstrating while two barbers (the sectors) were shown at the base of the dissecting table not cutting the body but sharpening blades for the anatomist to wield.[32]

The importance of dissecting and observing human corpses in knowledge-producing anatomical labour was thus accentuated, and the authoritative books of earlier authors were read, enlarged upon and amended in new works committed to 'knowing through direct experience'.[33] The book as a form through which to communicate knowledge was not rejected, but there was a significant focusing of attention on the anatomized body. Vesalius' title page dramatizes this: immediately above the anatomist one figure reads a book while, at the far right of the image, another holds a book but points towards the dissection. In this circuit an open book contrasts with one that is closed and leads back, via a pointing hand, to the opened body. Furthermore, the placement of instruments both of dissection and inscription (a scalpel, razor, inkwell, quill and paper) on the table beside the corpse and candle suggests that as the scalpel dissects so the quill inscribes, dissection giving rise to text in a reversal of previous images of anatomy lessons where text led dissector.[34] Here the female body under dissection is dead but also seemingly alert: her face is turned towards that of the anatomist as though to acquiesce and to acknowledge his actions. Unlike the male bodies lying horizontal and inert in previous images of dissection scenes, the woman is nearly vertical, providing visual access to her opened abdomen but also perhaps enlivening her body or at least partially aligning it with the spectators' living bodies.[35] Given that public dissection of women was rare – the male body being defined as the 'generic human body' and the female probed for the innermost secrets of the reproductive organs – Vesalius could have expected his title page to have a dramatic, and perhaps erotic, appeal to its audience.[36] But the significance of the corpse's gender lay also in its potential allusion

49
Illustration of the
anatomy of the
skeleton and muscles,
woodcut from
Andreas Vesalius,
*De humani corporis
fabrica* (Basel, 1543).

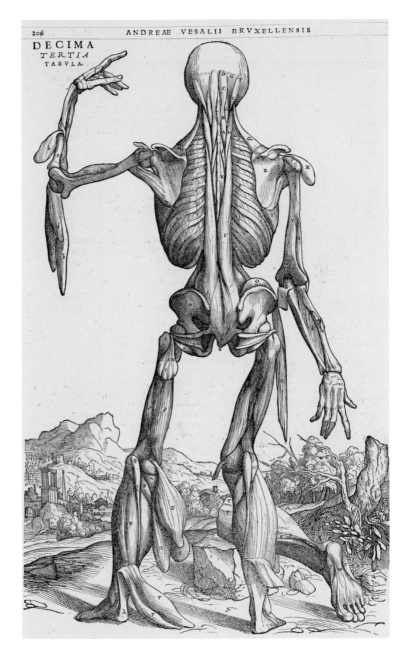

to life: as Katharine Park argues, this image of the anatomist dissecting the
uterus recalled classical scenes of birth through the cut womb, such as the
birth of Asclepius, the Greek god of medicine, and this visual reference to
childbirth underlined Vesalius' claims that his book advanced a 'reborn art
of dissection'.[37]

Further illustrations in the *Fabrica* develop the theme of the animated corpse that aids in its own anatomical display.[38] A sequence of fourteen male figures with finely delineated muscles, carefully labelled with a key, are depicted as though walking in a landscape (illus. 49). Each figure sheds layers of tissue to reveal deeper structures while moving into different postures, demonstrating relationships between parts and showing how they work in action. Sequential alterations in the positioning of the figures' limbs set them in motion and the alert gestures of their hands also serve to guide the viewer's eyes. In illustration 49 muscles have been stripped to the bone but the figure maintains its stance, pointing with its right hand to offer a supplementary view of a further, detached, leg. This additional dissected limb is supported by an architectural fragment so that the foot's muscular base is revealed. The animated figure thus invites the viewer to look at the same body part – the foot – from different angles. By gesturing in this way, assisting the display of its own anatomy, the figure partakes in Vesalius' programme, which was to provide anatomical descriptions not of individual bodies but of a 'human anatomical norm' based on 'reiterated observation' of many dissections.[39] Anatomized bodies in the *Fabrica* were idealized and their postures alluded to classical statuary, just as other sixteenth-century printed anatomical figures drew on famed paintings – one cadaver, for instance, in Juan Valverde de Hamusco's book of 1556 held up his own skin like a flayed version of Michelangelo's St Bartholomew in the Sistine Chapel.[40] If the body's illustration in the manner of heroes or martyrs was deemed fitting for the display of God's 'workmanship', this did not detract from the anatomist's claims, pronounced in image and text, that its anatomy was depicted directly from what was seen.[41]

Throughout its dissection as shown on paper, the body in the *Fabrica* continued to live in so much as it was capable of action and exhibited no signs of decay. Even when withered to the bone, the living body as skeleton adopted expressive postures in this book – printed equivalents of the human bones Vesalius articulated with wire so that they held together as they would in life and which he used in his teaching.[42] The title page's similarly animated skeletal figure forms a memento mori positioned above the female corpse in the anatomy theatre. While the deceased woman undergoing dissection alludes to birth, the living skeleton with which she is visually aligned is a vigorous reminder of death.

LIVELY CABINET

The anatomized yet animate dead also appeared in collections of preserved human and animal remains that were exhibited in theatres of anatomy during the seventeenth century. William Harvey, who had studied at Padua and performed public dissections at the Royal College of Physicians in London from 1616, defined anatomy as 'that branch of learning which teaches uses and actions of the parts of the body by ocular inspection and dissection' and in which the 'observation of rare things' should also be undertaken.[43] This ocular inspection was facilitated by the accumulation in anatomy theatres of rarities, some of which were made to appear, even in death, possessed of life.

Such rarities were displayed in the University of Leiden's anatomy theatre. In a printed image showing the theatre around 1614 a dissected body was uncovered at the centre of the large circular arena, which had been modelled on Padua's first permanent theatre and erected in 1594 within a former church (illus. 50). Here male and female visitors' attention was drawn to the dissection and to the animated human and animal skeletons positioned around it, including a horse and rider – such skeletons having been installed in the theatre under the direction of anatomist Pieter Pauw.[44] In similar images of the same theatre from *c.* 1610 human skeletons carried banners with messages (in Latin) addressed to the living such as 'know thyself', 'we are dust and shadow' and 'we are born to die', so that the living dead, as in the *Fabrica*, operated as memento mori.[45] Thus these deceased yet animated bodies conveyed moral messages about transitory earthly life. They also encouraged reflection on 'repentance and

50
Johannes Meursius after Crispijn de Passe, engraving of the anatomy theatre in Leiden, *c.* 1614, published 1625.

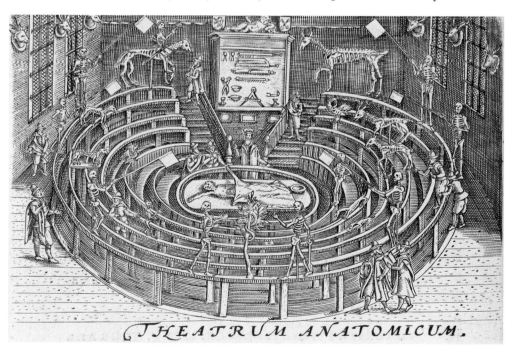

THEATRUM ANATOMICUM.

retribution'.[46] Skeletons of criminals accruing to the collection demonstrated the fate of transgressors, promoting virtue and warning against vice: that of a woman who had killed her daughter was seated on the skeleton of an ass and the bones of a man executed for stealing cattle were posed on an equally bony ox.[47]

During the first half of the seventeenth century, then, Leiden anatomy theatre's collection of rarities was to grow substantially with preserved bodily remains and artefacts. These could be viewed all year round, unlike the public dissections, which lasted only a few days and were usually undertaken in the coldest months, when putrefaction was slower.[48] The animated dead took their place within this collection, an expanding and varied assemblage that was testimony to the world's great diversity understood as God's creation. By 1695 over 300 'cheifest rarities' were on display including, in the entrance, the skins of tigers and leopards, heads of elephants, a 'great oister-schell weighing 150 pound', 'Warlike Arms used in China' and the hide of a seahorse. Hanging high in the anatomy chamber were the 'monstrous bones' and teeth of a whale, and about the circle of the anatomy theatre were numerous skeletons such as those of a cow, wolf, baboon, cat, ape, bear, dog, horse, sheep, ferret and otter, among many others, all skilfully articulated with wire. Amid the skeletons of birds, 'strange sea fishes' and a crocodile were objects notable in their singularity, such as the 'entrailes of a man of which is made a shirt', and cases were filled with items of arresting variety: an Egyptian mummy, 'a corral tree taken out of the East-Indian-sea', a hand of a mermaid, a 100-year-old mushroom, the skeleton of a newborn child, 'a pair of sandles or slippers from the kingdome of Syam', 'a precious stone in Ethiopia', 'a piece of rhubarb grown in shape of a dog's head' and 'a man whole in his miscles and tendrons very curiously set up'.[49]

Just as animal and human skeletons in the anatomy theatre were represented as both living and dead, the rarities with which they were displayed defied easy categorization when they were regarded, for instance, as products of both nature and art. John Evelyn noted in 1641, for example, that Leiden's anatomy theatre was 'very well furnish'd with naturall curiosities; especially with all sorts of Skeletons, from the whale & eliphant, to the fly, and the spider, which last is a very delicat piece of art, as well as nature'.[50] The fine and intricate work demanded in the preservation and arrangement of minute spider's 'bones' brought such an object into the domains of both nature and art, attracting a high degree of admiration.[51] Further collections of skeletons and of rarities accumulating in anatomy theatres by the mid-seventeenth century included, for instance, those at the surgeons' guilds in Delft and Rotterdam, and at the universities of Copenhagen, Altdorf and Oxford.[52] At the last's anatomy school, John

Evelyn noticed 'the skin of a jaccal, a rarely colour'd jacatroo, or prodigious large parot, two humming birds, not much bigger than our humble bee'.[53] Evelyn's eye was attracted by rare colour and, like the spider skeleton in Leiden, displays of unusually small creatures. Rarities could be monstrously large or miniscule, but were always expected to be distinctive and captivating. When rarities refused clear definition either as naturalia or artificialia they provoked intense fascination, such entities forming 'cultural migrators' without stable meanings due to their disruption of or oscillation between categories.[54]

Anatomical rarities were not confined to theatres of anatomy as they were eagerly sought for cabinets of curiosities. The contents of these chambers and elaborate cases, in sixteenth- and seventeenth-century Europe, were akin to anatomy-theatre displays in the profusion and variety of objects they held.[55] While medieval collections of objects prized as miraculous (such as relics) or wonder-inspiring (such as crocodiles) were held by royal families and ecclesiastical institutions, early modern collecting was undertaken by wider social groups including royals but also merchants, military officials, lawyers, scholars, physicians and apothecaries during a period when opportunities for collecting were developing through travel, colonial expansion and commercial and trading links.[56] In the residences of those wealthy and well connected enough to house and maintain them, cabinets were prestigious displays of their owner's learned status and social connections – as shown by objects secured from distant places – and they were admired by visitors from nobles and doctors to gentleman travellers, fellow collectors and sometimes women of high social standing.[57] Among the fossils, dried animals of the land and sea, herbs, plant roots, flowers, seeds and metals that inspired wonder in those who viewed them were human body parts such as mummified heads and stones from kidneys, interest in the latter fuelled by their hybridity as fusions of the human and the mineral.[58]

Diversity and difference characterized the contents of cabinets, and strategies of display tended to accentuate contrasts among the multitudes of items that seemed to condense the universe (made by God) into the space occupied by the collection.[59] For example, the amply filled museum assembled by Ole Worm, anatomist and professor of Greek and then of medicine at the University of Copenhagen, accommodated a huge variety of distinctive items.[60] An engraving in his museum catalogue, published in Leiden in 1655, represents this profusion displayed on walls, ceiling and floor (illus. 51). Worm's museum embraced human remains, including malformed foetuses and mummies, as well as clothing, weapons, antiquities, shells, soil, rocks and dried fish, birds, leaves and parts of mermaids and a crocodile, obtained either locally in Denmark or from Greenland,

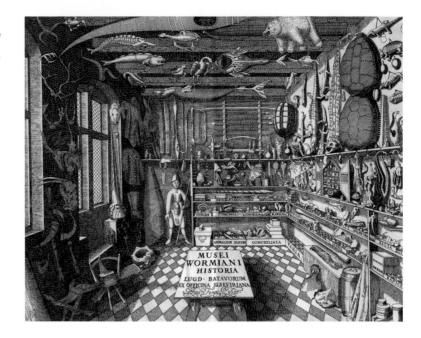

India, Italy, Iceland, Peru, Egypt and other 'remote places', and which Worm intended visitors to 'touch with their own hands and to see with their own eyes'.[61] The riches and intricacy of nature could be explored here alongside human ingenuity in the form of, for example, a mechanical human figure or automaton which, when activated, flexed its limbs in imitation of living movement (see centre left).[62]

At the centre of Worm's catalogue title page is a miniature human skeleton holding a staff, a memento mori that echoes those in images of anatomy theatres. Positioned on the upper shelf of the back wall, this animated figure gazes back at the viewer from within the museum, and a further miniature skull is displayed in a small case on the wall to the right.[63] The dead address the living to emphasize the importance of coming to know the self as a physical, moral and spiritual undertaking. Reference to the acquisition of self-knowledge also featured both in cabinets and in images of anatomy theatres through the device of the mirror. A printed image of Leiden's anatomy theatre from *c.* 1610, for instance, shows a woman holding a mirror, a symbol not of vanity but of self-knowledge gained via anatomy as a 'reflective discipline' – a notion also conveyed by the female figure Anatomia, the emblem of anatomy, who holds a looking glass.[64] If self-knowledge was sought in anatomy theatres, it was also generated in cabinets where the instruction to 'know thyself' was carried out through the collection and study of material objects. Furthermore, the mirror was a metaphor in terms of which collectors thought about their collections (the collection as a mirror of the collector), and actual mirrors were sometimes incorporated into exhibits so that visitors could see themselves reflected among the rarities in a form of living self-display.[65]

MEMENTO MORI

Animated skeletons operating as memento mori were mobilized, as we have seen, in displays rendered in human bone and in printed images where the apparent vitality of the body after it had perished was instrumental in communicating anatomical knowledge with its moral and spiritual dimensions. Memento mori kept death in view for the living, acting as reminders that everyone would inevitably die and that the material world would decay and fade away. The passage of time and its toll upon the human body as well as on flowers, fruit, trees and earthly creatures was a central theme of memento mori, which circulated widely in Europe through printed images, paintings and finely worked objects in diverse materials including wax, ivory and silver. Just as the imagery of memento mori dwelt upon death and decay, so it also brought into play contrasting images of the deceased body as preserved or alive. It was through these tensions and contradictions that memento mori stimulated such fascination as they migrated between popular and learned print, funerary sculpture and decorative ornament, anatomy theatre and museum.[66]

Funerary sculpture, in particular fifteenth- and sixteenth-century transi tombs that displayed the deceased as two bodies – one a likeness of the person shown dead but nevertheless seemingly alert and another in the process of decay – operated as both memento mori and memorials.[67] These double sculptures juxtaposed the body lying in a preserved condition, wearing clothing to show their social status, and, beneath this, a second naked or shrouded body in a state of decomposition – or transition. Erected in cathedrals, these tombs memorialized eminent persons and, by contrasting the body finely dressed as in life with the withered body in death, they offered a commentary, within the Christian spiritual framework, on the transience of material life, urging the living towards self-reflection and moral contemplation.[68] Bodily decay, rendered in sculptures that sometimes interwove worms, snakes and toads, alluded to inner sin and the corruption of the flesh: transi tombs elaborated this decomposition to the extent that the dead body in stone could seem 'alive with vermin'.[69] Gazing upon this was meant to move viewers towards reflexivity, the conception of death as a mirror in which the living see their own mortality reinforcing this process – death was implicit within life and as a mirror it brought self-understanding.[70] The presence of death among the living was also represented in Dance of Death imagery that featured skeletons in energetic dances with those from the richest to the poorest social groups – no one could escape death. Fifteenth-century manuscripts and wall paintings in cemeteries depicted the Dance of Death and, towards the end of that century and into the next, it was widely disseminated in print. Skeletons held hands and danced with figures representing a king, a beggar, an old man, a child, a wise man and a fool, a prisoner, a rich man and a pair of lovers – all were drawn into death's rhythm.[71]

'And as I am so you must be' announced skeletons in printed images that circulated in sixteenth- and seventeenth-century ballads and broadsides.[72] These lively figures addressed viewers, encouraging them to look upon the deceased body reduced to bone and, by seeing in this their own future death, to learn lessons of humility and attend to spiritual rather than material matters. For, as one 1604 broadside emphasized, 'All flesh as grasse doth passe and come to nought. Gods word most pure aye doth endure not chang'd in ought.' The transient earthly world perishes, like grass, in contrast to the permanence of God, so the living must 'In life, for death: in death for life prepare'.[73] In addition to paper memento mori were a plethora of material objects in the shape of skeletons and skulls that reiterated these messages – silver pocket watches, gold pendants, intricately carved ivory miniatures, walking-stick handles and many other trinkets.[74]

Such images and objects were part of the wider visual and material context in which memento mori developed in anatomical books illustrated with animate cadavers and living skeletons offering moral instruction.[75] Vesalius' *Fabrica* teaches the anatomy of bones via images of skeletons

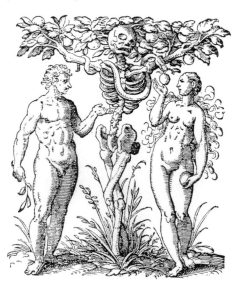

seemingly aware of their mortal condition (either contemplating a skull or weeping), while muscles are displayed by anatomized figures moving in landscapes where crumbling architecture, ruins and withered trees are imbued with memento mori messages. Attention is drawn to dying foliage, for instance, by the pointing hand of one dissected figure, the fading counterpart to the thriving trees seen growing in the distance (see illus. 49). Furthermore, animated skeletons in early seventeenth-century images of Leiden University's anatomy theatre combined memento mori and biblical narrative: a skeletal Adam and Eve, the latter holding an apple, stand at the Tree of Knowledge of good and evil where the Devil, as a serpent, tempts Eve to eat the forbidden fruit, a reference to the Fall in the Garden of Eden (see illus. 50, centre bottom). God's punishment for this transgression was human mortality – the birth of death – and pain in childbirth for women.[76] The combination of memento mori and imagery of the Fall was incorporated into medical books, such as Jakob Rüff's volume on conception, foetal development and birth. The Zurich physician's book was published in several editions from 1554 to 1670, providing instruction for doctors and midwives. In one illustration Adam and Eve stand with the Tree of Knowledge represented as an 'arborescent skeleton' which is both dead and alive, reduced to bone and yet still growing (illus. 52). The serpent coils in the 'branches' of the skeleton's ribs and bony arms blossom into life.[77]

Simultaneously living and deceased figures manifested in eighteenth-century memento mori. One example, a wax tableau comprising a life-size female head and hands, probably Italian from the early 1700s, is vertically divided so that it appears alive on one side and dead on the other (illus. 53). The structure of this memento mori, like many others, echoes the transi tomb's double body – one preserved and one putrefying. But in this instance there are two halves that are united: the alert, fleshy half has an open eye, hair and a hand holding flowers, while the deathly, skeletal side is inhabited by the creatures of decay – worms, toads, a spider, snail, locust and snake. An apple beneath the living hand refers to the forbidden fruit and an inscribed wax label advises: '*Vanitas Vanitatum et omnia Vanitas* Ecc: Chap 1 v 2' ('Vanity of vanities, all is vanity', Ecclesiastes 1:2). Thus the tableau's anatomical aspects, its removed wax skin revealing wax bones, are infused with biblical and vanitas imagery, the latter concerned with the fragility and emptiness of the material world and the transience of beauty. These themes were rendered with extreme clarity and concentrated detail in still-life paintings in which glass shattered, flowers faded, plumes of smoke drifted from extinguished candles, bubbles about to burst floated, hourglasses ran out and human skulls rested on books with aged, flaking pages.[78] The tableau's half living/half dead structure, an often reiterated feature found in printed images as well as miniature paintings and sculptures of male and female figures, also appeared in later anatomical models that presented bodies, especially the head, as though half intact and half dissected (see illus. 84, 156).

Memento mori and vanitas imagery was also invoked in the context of private anatomical collections assembled during the second half of the seventeenth and early eighteenth century. During this period methods for making anatomical preparations developed, along with the investigation of physiological processes such as blood circulation, digestion and the lymphatic system.[79] Syringes were improved for injecting coloured liquids into blood vessels to reveal their course in different organs, and – in addition

53
Wax tableau of a
life-size female head
and hands, half living
and half dead, 18th
century.

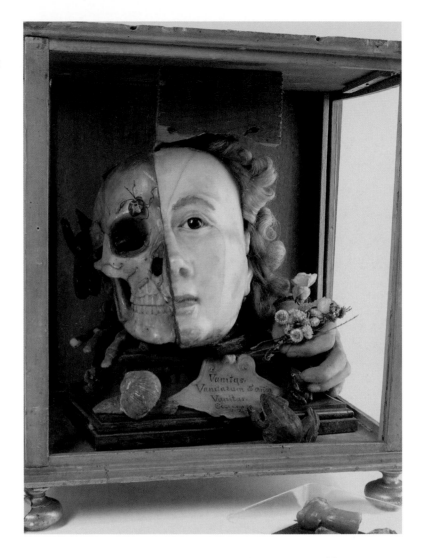

to the preservation of body parts by drying, already practised for some time – further techniques were devised using spirits (alcohol) and oil of turpentine that allowed soft tissues, displayed in glass jars, to resist decay for years.[80]

In Frederik Ruysch's famed cabinet at his Amsterdam residence, which he opened in 1671 and continued to expand, visitors admired his skilled anatomical craft, especially for the life it seemed to impart to preserved human remains.[81] Ruysch, introduced above with reference to the *Anatomy Lesson* of 1683 (see illus. 45), had studied in Leiden and was praelector of anatomy in Amsterdam from 1667 and subsequently professor of botany and supervisor of the botanical garden.[82] He employed a range of techniques to create the contents of his cabinet: blowing air into organs before drying, and injecting substances into vessels such as those that carried air in the lungs, or blood, lymph or other fluids through the body.[83] If filling these with mercury could highlight their branchings like 'silvery trees', Ruysch's secret red wax concoction, which hardened after injection, rendered a profusion of blood vessels visible, even those 'as slender as the threads of a spider's web'.[84] The intricate assemblages of dried anatomical parts composed by Ruysch to impart anatomical knowledge were also replete with memento mori messages conveyed through inscriptions (such as: 'What is life? Transient smoke and perishable bubble') and performed by foetal skeletons in living poses. Displayed in fragile tableaux, these figures wept into handkerchiefs made of fine human membrane, lamented life's sorrows while playing bone violins, held aloft coils of dried viscera and stood on rocks of gallstones and kidney stones where various injected vessels flourished like strange plants in a miniature forest.[85] Life's transience was manifest in perishable anatomies made to be enduring.

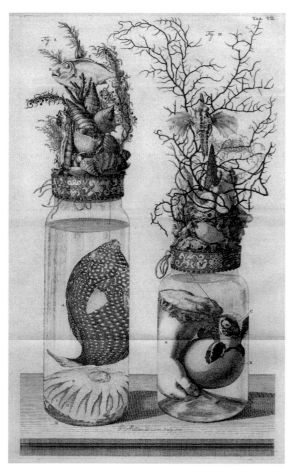

54
Illustration of preparations, engraving from Frederik Ruysch, *Thesaurus animalium primus* (Amsterdam, 1725), Tab. VII.

Ruysch's elaborately worked compositions were striking in their synthesis of the animated and the deathly, the seemingly alive and yet evidently deceased. His preparations of soft tissue – which again included many foetuses and infants, Ruysch having access to stillborn babies via his position as anatomical examiner and lecturer for midwives in Amsterdam – were injected so that they appeared, he asserted, 'full of lively colour'.[86] Some preserved bodies, according to commentators, would 'glow' with a youthful 'lustre' and looked like 'living persons fast asleep'.[87] Engravings of Ruysch's preparations, published with his descriptions of his collection, emphasized their finely wrought qualities and delicate poise. Arranged in fluid-filled glass jars, for example, are a fish with an Urtica Merina ('sea-nettle' or 'animal flower') and an infant's hand holding a hatching turtle – the egg, in Ruysch's view, being the entity from which human and animal life originated (illus. 54).[88] Lids of jars are encrusted with shells, coral and seaweed that seem to grow into marine gardens complete with sea creatures, which are labelled for studying, not mere decoration, along with the jars' contents. Ribbon tied at the tops of jars features shapes that echo both the curves of sea plants above and, below, what might be windings of blood vessels or lace where the arm has been cut. This limb was made to actively participate in its theatrical exposition, aiding its own display – the hand cradles the turtle's egg, offering itself and its oval treasure for view just as, in another of Ruysch's compositions, a child's hand proffers an adult's heart.[89]

The lifelike appearance of anatomical preparations such as heads and arms was enhanced by careful crafting, including the insertion of glass eyes and dressing in fine collars and lace-edged sleeves. Here the function of fabric was to cover severed and stitched flesh but the incorporation of fine

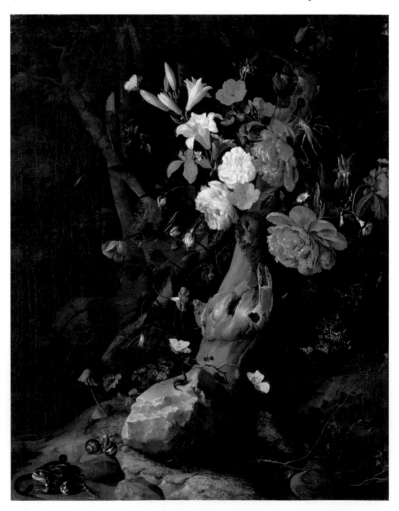

55
Rachel Ruysch,
Still-life of Flowers on Woodland Ground,
c. 1690, oil on canvas.

cloth and lace was also to prompt visual comparison of the body designed by God and material made by human hands: both forms of tissue were fibrous, interwoven, embroidered.[90] Ruysch's son, Hendrik (see illus. 45, bottom right), and his daughter, Rachel, assisted him in making preparations. Rachel Ruysch (1664–1750), with her mother Maria Post, undertook needlework for the fabric components and also helped in the composition of displays.[91] As a painter, Rachel Ruysch produced accomplished still-lifes, especially of flowers, fruit and forest floors, whose motifs and predominant themes intersected with her father's anatomical creations. One of his embalmed foetuses wore a wreath of flowers on its head and held a bouquet.[92] Her cut flowers displayed in glass vases (much like preparations in jars) were inhabited by insects such as caterpillars and a mayfly, the latter representing mortality (or brief life), and also featured in his skeletal tableaux.[93] Her forest floor of *c.* 1690 has flourishing black iris, white lilies and pink roses that attract butterflies, a locust, lizards, snails, a toad and a snake at the mossy base of a broken tree so that blossoming life and purity contrast with decay and corruption (illus. 55).[94] Through these familial relationships, visual exchanges between anatomical cabinet and still-life painting developed, both dealing in the themes of time's passage and of death and life interwoven, both laden with symbols for moral contemplation while also presenting specimens for detailed observation.

LIFE AND DEPTH

A wealth of visual strategies and material techniques bringing 'life' to the anatomized dead had emerged by the early 1700s: bodies in print as well as articulated bones were made to appear capable of movement; fleshy preparations were infused with colour and endowed with gestures and other lifelike features.[95] Subsequently, eighteenth-century animated cadavers and seemingly alive body parts would continue to figure in anatomical practices, both in printed and in sculptural form.[96] The aliveness of wax anatomical models rendered in persuasive detail, and of bodies cast in plaster – materials that long outlasted deceased and decaying bodies – was intimated if not by posture and facial expression then by shape, colour and texture. These, like a multitude of body parts preserved as preparations, made the depths of the 'living' bodily interior compellingly visible in a context where to examine depth was afforded central importance in gaining valued knowledge.[97] Whether as elaborate waxes in museums, or as models, preparations and casts shown in anatomists' own residences, these anatomies (even when protected by glass) could be closely observed by students – much more so than the bodies dissected in public anatomy theatres, which came to be perceived as sites of pomp and institutional ceremonial rather than of effective learning, as attractions drawing spectators from 'the public at large' rather than those seeking deep anatomical knowledge.[98]

Anatomies illustrated, articulated and modelled as though alive became established as approved pedagogical resources, although not without some disapproval. There were alternative moves to advance images of *lifeless* bodies undergoing dissection. For instance, although Frederik Ruysch's cabinet, as both an educational and commercial enterprise, was praised by many visitors, widely utilized in his teaching and admired by anatomists who studied the preparations closely – Alexander Monro (*primus*), for example, doing so prior to working on his own preparations from 1720 as professor of anatomy at the University of Edinburgh[99] – Ruysch's productions were also subject to criticism. In the 1690s the anatomist Govard Bidloo (1649–1713), then professor of anatomy in Leiden, claimed they were misleading and marred by unnecessary decorations. Both anatomists sought to reveal the wonderful craftsmanship of God, but they did so by

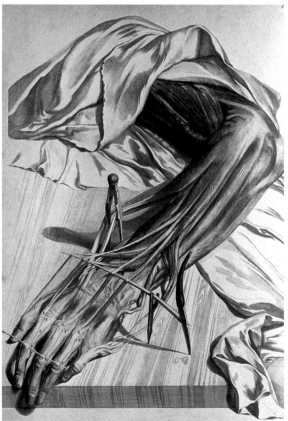

56
Gérard de Lairesse, illustration of the hand and arm, engraving from Govard Bidloo, *Anatomia humani corporis* (Amsterdam, 1685), Tab. 70.

different means – Ruysch enlivening deceased bodies and Bidloo emphasizing their deadness. With this deadening came a critique of the devices and embellishment that had infused life into early modern anatomical bodies.[100]

Prioritizing paper anatomy over preparations made in the flesh, Govard Bidloo asserted that the illustrations in his volume of 1685 were appropriately 'without ornament', claiming that these represented anatomy 'after life' – that is, they depicted what could be seen in a single dissection (rather than an idealized version).[101] Thus many bodies in this book were shown manifestly deceased, with eyes closed, heads covered with cloths, and dissecting apparatus visible in the form of pins, ropes and dissecting tables. The dead weight of limbs and torsos registers in the strained cords used to position bodies for observation; tissues and organs are lifted and suspended by threads, instruments perform balancing acts to display muscles and tendons (illus. 56). Here bodies are evidently worked upon, passive rather than actively auto-anatomizing, their postures dependent upon the anatomist's equipment rather than any self-possessed capacity to hold a pose.

These images have been associated with a 'new anatomical realism' that rejected metaphor and allusion, and sought to document with precision specifically 'what the eye sees'.[102] But realist visual practices, informed as they were by various cultural codes and conventions, produced differing anatomical bodies, some shown dead and others appearing alive, so that across this shifting spectrum signs of death by no means displaced those of life in the display of anatomy.[103] Thus while Bidloo's anatomies looked dead, coloured wax anatomical models of the eighteenth and early nineteenth centuries, also 'trad[ing] on a form of "realism"', were made to closely resemble the living body in form, texture, tone and meticulously detailed internal and external features. They aimed to achieve 'extreme verisimilitude', to open bodies for viewing in depth.[104] Furthermore their very substance seemed endowed with lifelike qualities. Wax that was coloured with pigments supplied the shape, volume and tones of living flesh, unlike dried preparations, for example those made by French anatomist Honoré Fragonard during the 1760s which suffered from shrinkage and distortion of tissues, despite the wax-injected vessels and skilful crafting into elaborate animated postures such as a horse and rider.[105]

Early anatomical waxes were developed by modeller Gaetano Giulio Zumbo (or Zummo, 1656–1701), who also collaborated in the 1690s with Guillaume Desnoues (c. 1650–c. 1735), professor of anatomy and surgery at the University of Genoa.[106] The latter already used wax-injection techniques to display blood vessels, then, dismayed by the ruinous onset of decay, he sought to make full-body models that would allow human anatomy to be demonstrated 'without exciting the feeling of horror men usually have on seeing corpses'.[107] Thus he encouraged Zumbo to move away from crafting deceased bodies in the colours suggesting putrefaction which were so marked in his sculptural works such as the *Triumph of Time* (c. 1690). Desnoues continued to work wax with François de la Croix, previously an ivory carver, exhibiting models in 1711 at the Académie royale des sciences in Paris and setting up a cabinet there.[108] In the following decades Desnoues' models were exhibited in London for both lay and medical audiences, then in the 1740s by Benjamin Rackstrow, who set up a commercial museum showing 'anatomical figures' and 'curiosities' between c. 1765 and 1799 – a prominent business among a number of (sometimes temporary) exhibitions of this kind in the city.[109] His models were presented for learning and entertainment, for 'improvement and delight'; then in 1753 they were purchased for medical instruction at the University of Dublin.[110]

In Bologna the artist Ercole Lelli (1702–1766) made significant advances with widely admired anatomized bodies sculpted in living poses. His two male écorchés (flayed figures showing muscles), in the 1730s, were carved in wood to adorn the lector's seat at the University's Archiginnasio Anatomy Theatre, where public dissections were held.[111] Lelli's models, commissioned in 1742 for the Anatomy Museum of the Institute of Sciences (Istituto delle Scienze), included a male and a female nude – Adam and Eve – and four figures with wax muscles meticulously crafted onto human skeletons whose approved proportions were ensured by selecting bones from numerous bodies. Some with hair and glass eyes, these figures conveyed the impression of life, their gestures and emotional expressions evoking the biblical narrative of the Fall. Viewed as a series, the models revealed deepening layers of muscle ending with two memento mori skeletons (again male and female), one holding a scythe, like the figure of Death. Lelli's moralizing models, regarded by some as more suitable for artists' instruction than for medical students, were displayed to attract diverse viewers, just like the Anatomy Theatre's annual ritualized dissections.[112]

Life was suggested by different means in Anna Morandi Manzolini's (1716–1774) anatomical waxes, which represented body parts as though animate and sentient, but without dramatizing bodies in the ways that Lelli's works did.[113] In Bologna, from the 1740s Morandi worked with her husband, Giovanni Manzolini (1700–1755), who had been assistant to Lelli, and she gained international recognition as a leading modeller. After Manzolini's death she continued to make highly acclaimed models, receiving major commissions and a university position. Her methods involved taking casts from her dissections (of bodies from a hospital in the city) and sculpting wax, often onto bone, which she displayed at her household studio to medical students and visitors on the Grand Tour.[114] Important among Morandi's numerous productions of idealized body parts were the organs of sense – the eye, ear, nose, mouth and hand – which she modelled as though actively involved in sensing: wax eyes looked in different directions, for instance, while hands touched soft fabric or withdrew from thorns.[115] Morandi skilfully manipulated her working materials, which were pliable and durable, the properties of wax lending it particular suitability for fashioning anatomy. This malleable substance readily adopted bodily contours and it could be tinted with pigments in subtle tones to display skin, muscle and viscera.[116] Unlike ivory, which was carved to create anatomical models of the eye, the ear and miniature male and female bodies, wax, according to Lucia Dacome, 'seemed to bear itself the features and textures of life'. It was enlivened and especially powerful given its uses in magical and religious practices such as the making of spells (in the form of dolls) and figures of Catholic saints as well as ex-votos displayed in churches.[117]

In Florence anatomical ceroplasty flourished at the Royal Museum of Physics and Natural History (known later as 'La Specola').[118] Under the directorship of Felice Fontana (1730–1805), who was inspired by the Bolognese modellers, the museum workshop's anatomists and artisans produced hundreds of waxes for viewing by scholars and the wider public when it opened in 1775. These idealized models of the human male and female body, shown whole and in parts, allowed detailed exploration of bones, muscles, blood and lymph vessels, nerves and organs. The making process entailed the dissection of bodies (brought entire or in part from a local hospital and orphanage), guided by illustrations in established anatomical books. The resulting preparations, or wax copies of these, were cast in plaster to create moulds for the coloured wax components of each model, and thus a single ceroplastic body was composed from multiple flesh bodies. To form fine vessels and nerves, wax-covered wire and thread were applied before the entire model was varnished.[119]

Decaying flesh was replaced with wax, admired for its 'moist appearance which perfectly imitates the state of life', and from deceased bodies models were skilfully worked into forms that demonstrated functional relationships between anatomical parts in the living body.[120] Full-body figures with expressive faces reclined on luxurious drapery and silk cushions so that their insides could be viewed, and models of the head and torso whose eyes were closed might have appeared, with their unblemished complexions and robust, reddened organs, to be sleeping rather than dead. Contrasting with some models of heads and upper bodies which bore expressions suggesting they had died, seemingly animate, conscious waxes were staged as though yielding to their anatomical display, inviting visual inspection from the surface to deep within the body. The movement of viewers' eyes from the bodily exterior to the interior was encouraged by one female model, for instance, which holds a long plait of hair while pointing to her exposed abdominal viscera, her braided hair echoing the intricate interweavings of her lymph vessels.[121]

Models' postures were not only attuned to the requirements of anatomical exposition but were informed by classical sculpture. At La Specola's workshop Clemente Susini's (1754–1814) alert female figures were, for example, influenced by the *Venus de' Medici*, which was widely admired as an ideal of bodily beauty.[122] One such late eighteenth-century wax model lies awake in padded comfort (illus. 57); the removable skin of her trunk allows abdominal muscles and deeper internal organs – including lungs,

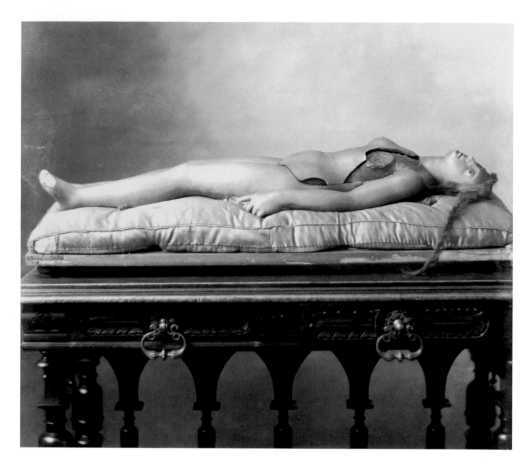

57
Wax anatomical
model, 1771–1800,
by Clemente Susini,
undated photograph,
probably early 20th
century.

liver, intestines, and uterus with foetus – to be studied (at a later date the model sustained damage to the trunk and left foot, as visible in illustration 57, which has now been repaired).[123]

'Living' models constructed to look partly intact and partly dissected allowed simultaneous outside and inside views of the body. This double view was presented by an 1818 life-size model produced by Francesco Calenzuoli (1796–1829), who had been assistant to Susini (illus. 58).[124] With hair, an open gazing eye and smooth skin, one half of the head is alert and the other half, like the torso, is anatomized to reveal the brain, lung, liver, intestine, uterus and blood vessels. A removable heart permits closer study from different angles and thread-like lymphatic vessels spread outwards from their nodes, lacing over organs in an intricate pattern. The model's split structure, part living surface and part bodily depth, echoes the divided structure of the living/dead memento mori but in wax form without any visual indicators or symbols of decay (see illus. 53). Exterior flesh tones and vibrant inner colouring in reds and pinks enliven this

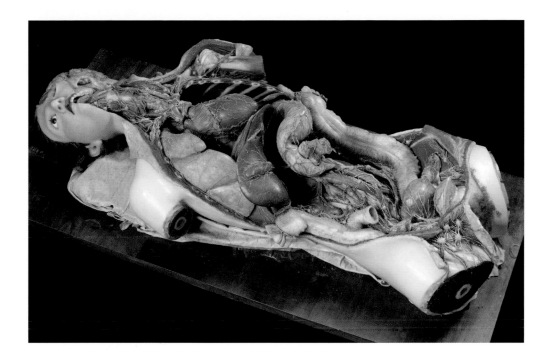

58
Wax anatomical
model, 1818, by
Francesco Calenzuoli.

anatomical body both inside and out. Yet surface signs of life, in the open-eyed facial expression, for instance, are restricted because most of this wax body's interior has been revealed – this interior is much more pronounced than that, for example, of the anatomical Venus (see illus. 57), whose openable torso could be re-covered to maintain its almost seamless pale wax skin (prior, that is, to the damage on the upper left torso). By contrast, the three-dimensional internal organs in Calenzuoli's model are made immediately manifest, the (implied) anatomist's act of cutting away to reveal deeper anatomical parts visibly staged by two severed ends of the large intestine, which are tied with ribbon. The convention of the living cadaver seems further subordinated to the demands of dissection with the deletion of limbs – rather than contributing to the appearance of an animate body, the limbs are reduced to an abbreviated frame for the model's viscera with their sectioned muscle and bone made visible. According to Martin Kemp and Marina Wallace, this treatment of limbs was common in models of the abdomen, providing a 'raw directness' that reinforced their 'real-ness'.[125]

However arresting and intricate, such models were critically evaluated by some. In London, during the late 1760s to the 1780s, William Hunter, Scottish-born anatomist, physician and man-midwife, found 'wax-work art' and 'wax-figures' wanting, especially those by 'masters . . . careless in their imitation'.[126] To Hunter these figures were so tawdry, with a shew of unnatural colours, and so very incorrect in the circumstances of figure, situation and the like, that, though they may strike a vulgar eye with admiration, they must appear ridiculous to an Anatomist.[127]

Hunter's view of such wax models was perhaps shared by other anatomists, many of whom by the 1770s no longer featured them in newspaper advertisements for their lectures.[128] At Hunter's private anatomy school – a commercial as well as educational enterprise like other such schools in London – he strongly advocated an anatomy learned through rigorous scrutiny of dead bodies, also teaching the subject with live human models at the Royal Academy of Arts, and his commitment to what Kemp refers to as an 'uncompromising empiricism' informed his approach to illustrations, models and preparations.[129] Although Hunter acknowledged that anatomical study yielded 'evident proofs of the astonishing art of the Creator', he advised that its 'more immediate purposes' were to 'lay a foundation' for the practice of medicine.[130] What, then, were the implications of Hunter's approach for his anatomical renderings of animated cadavers?

An indication is provided by Hunter's *The Anatomy of the Human Gravid Uterus Exhibited in Figures*, published in 1774 with life-size engravings.[131] Here he differentiated between the 'representation' of an object, on the one hand, 'exactly as it is seen' and, on the other, as it is 'not actually seen, but conceived in the imagination'.[132] Hunter aligned himself with the former approach to produce pictures, he claimed, bearing the 'mark of truth'.[133] Rather than idealizing the body or synthesizing multiple observations of dissected bodies into a single image, Hunter required faithful illustration of specific, singular dissections.[134] The brothers John and Charles Bell, anatomists, adopted a similar strategy in their early nineteenth-century illustrations: they rejected the 'vitious practice of drawing from the imagination'.[135] In seeking to 'copy accurately' their images featured anatomized bodies lying lifeless with closed eyes.[136] Hunter's productions, however, were still suggestive of life despite his insistence on scrupulous attention to deceased bodies. For instance, in the *Gravid Uterus*, with engravings of artist Jan van Rymsdyk's drawings, an umbilical cord is glossy as though still part of a living body.[137] The drawings were made from Hunter's preparations that had been injected with wax to preserve the shape of living blood vessels, and with other fluids that maintained the fresh appearance and position of organs.[138] Such operations were not considered deviations from the representation of bodies exactly as seen, and they were deemed necessary in making important aspects 'demonstrable'.[139]

59
Plaster cast of
a woman's torso,
opened uterus and
foetus, c. 1770,
made for William
Hunter, displayed
in the Museum of
Anatomy, University
of Glasgow, 2007.

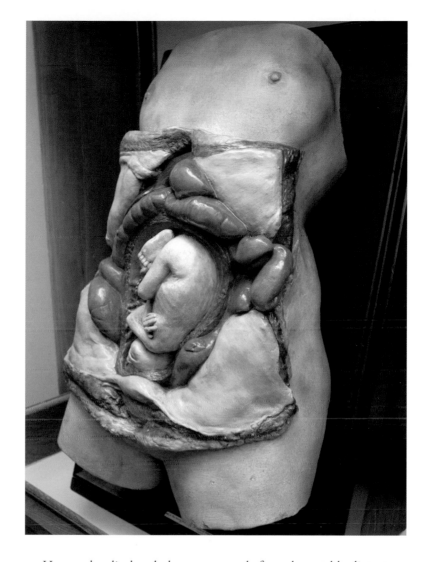

Hunter also displayed plaster casts made from deceased bodies, especially those bodies that were only occasionally available and difficult to
preserve in a 'natural state', such as pregnant women – and these casts were
similarly enlivened.[140] Unconvinced by wax models, Hunter nevertheless
considered figures cast in wax, plaster or lead directly 'from the real subject
[the dead body]' to be 'very correct in all the principal parts', and thus an
asset to 'modern Anatomy'.[141] Unlike composite models derived from
many anatomized bodies, Hunter regarded casting in plaster of Paris from
single dissections as a method that ensured that the size, shape and situation of parts were 'exactly as in nature herself' and therefore 'almost as
good as the fresh subject' – that is, a recently deceased body.[142] Thus

Hunter saw continuity between anatomized body parts in the flesh and in plaster, especially as the latter was derived from physical contact with the former.[143] In his view, the 'art' of casting allowed anatomists to 'preserve a very perfect likeness' of subjects, yet the creation of such a likeness would replace signs of death with those of life.[144] For example, pregnant women's torsos and abdomens, when dissected and cast, appeared not freshly deceased but fleshily alive (illus. 59).[145] Skin and muscle was moved aside to bring the deep interior, including the foetus, into view. But although adult head and limbs were omitted – a truncation which denied such casts the facial and gestural repertoire of anatomical waxes made to seem alive – life was still suggested.

This was done, firstly, with colour: plaster was painted in shades of red and pink to resemble living flesh. Colouring casts in this way was a response to Hunter's concern with deceased bodies:

> every hour that [the dead body] . . . is kept, it is losing something
> of its fitness for anatomical demonstrations; the blood is transuding,
> and bringing all the parts nearer to one colour, which takes off the
> natural and distinct appearance.[146]

Casts were painted, then, to avoid the disadvantage of chromatic depletion that reduced the utility of the decaying dead, and to grant casts, instead, the 'natural' look of the living body. Second, it was possible to imbue casts with 'life' by forging connections between these plaster renderings, fleshy preparations and engravings in teaching and museum display.[147] For instance, Hunter's descriptions of preparations, given in lectures, could inflect students' perceptions of related casts. A preserved opened uterus with foetus, for example, was narrated for students as though the baby was in a living slumber, shaping students' viewing of corresponding casts: 'As the child lies in this snug position there is a strong impression of a pleasant sleep, a seclusion or retirement from the World, it is very expressive.'[148] In Hunter's museum, anatomical preparations were displayed beside corresponding engravings in the *Gravid Uterus*, creating visual linkages between preserved body parts and printed versions.[149] And if in the plates of this atlas a sense of life was conveyed by the internal organs' appearance of 'fullness and texture',[150] this life was also suggested by the shapes and tangible textures of three-dimensional casts.

If colour supplied the appearance of life, it also accentuated depth when bodily layers of skin, muscle and tissue were differentiated (see illus. 59). But even subtly painted casts could only approximate the fine overlay of membranes which Hunter explored in dissections and preparations, such as the human foetus that currently still floats inside its gossamer amnion in a fluid-filled glass jar at the University of Glasgow's Museum of Anatomy.[151] While plaster bodies were formed from surface impressions, flesh could be probed more deeply to show, for example, how 'strata' are 'blended and entangled' with other parts.[152] Thus preparations were, Hunter asserted, of 'infinite use to Anatomy'.[153] Since the early decades of the eighteenth century anatomists and medical practitioners had increasingly made and collected these, preserving painstakingly dissected body parts – Hunter particularly valued preparations that would 'shew the very fine and delicate parts of the body', such as the ear and eye, and those that displayed anatomical 'structure distinctly' – as well as 'anatomical curiosities, or rarities of every kind'.[154] When Hunter referred to rarities he did so in a context where this category of material entity had shifted somewhat from its earlier formulation, which encompassed a profuse variety of eclectic and singular items, towards a focus on bodily parts defined as 'uncommonly formed', 'diseased' or difficult to obtain, such as the 'pregnant uterus and its contents'.[155] And in making preparations, Hunter sought to preserve the living appearance of tissues and vessels.

To display the routes taken by fluids through the living body Hunter injected blood vessels with mercury or wax coloured with pigments in either black, white, verdigris or yellow (from egg yolk).[156] As he explained, 'filling the vascular system with a bright coloured wax, enables us to trace the large vessels with great ease, renders the smaller much more conspicuous, and makes thousands of the very minute ones visible.'[157] He was especially interested in the uterus' 'net-work' of arteries which are partly seen on the outside, then 'disappear by plunging deeper and deeper into its substance'.[158] Maintaining the lifelike qualities of anatomized parts required dexterous manipulations. With regard to the placenta, Hunter

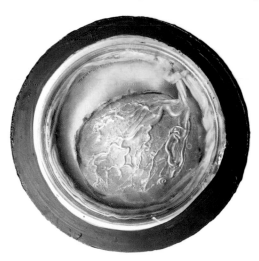

instructed, it should be acquired after childbirth in a manner which was 'slow, cautious, and gentle, leaving it principally to the gradual pressure from the mother, and very gently pulling by the naval string' so that it was not 'bruised or torn'.[159] Next it must be immersed in a basin of warm water to remove blood, before preserving it in spirits, almost as it was when still alive. The placenta's intricate blood vessels could then be revealed by injecting with mercury, as in one preparation where the vessels' 'serpentine' convolutions were made prominent and the umbilical cord kept attached and coiled around the inner edge of the glass jar (illus.

60).[160] Selected aspects of the living body – such as the flow of blood through vessels – were thus made visible via the dead. And they were viewed in a context where anatomists carefully arranged and posed preparations within their jars, suggesting movement, for instance, in order to enliven them.[161]

William Hunter's preparations and plaster casts were not, however, intended for the eyes of the merely curious. While, in London, the anatomy theatre of the Company of Surgeons (precursor to the Royal College of Surgeons of England), with its legal supply of publicly executed felons for dissection, was opened to people regardless of gender, class and age, Hunter's private anatomy school, at his Great Windmill Street residence from 1767 onwards, was not.[162] His anatomical preparations were displayed in the gallery of his museum in orderly rows, and other parts of his collection (such as animal horns, medals, minerals and articles from the Pacific) were grouped according to type (his shells, stuffed birds, quadrupeds, zoophytes and paintings occupied other spaces in the house).[163] Hunter would remove preparations from his museum for demonstration in his lecture theatre, passing smaller ones around so that each student could carefully look at (but not manipulate) them 'in his own hand'. However, Hunter insisted that 'strangers' or people with 'idle, or even malevolent curiosity' were not admitted and although students had permission to take a 'friend' to lectures this was not allowed when the 'organs of generation, and the gravid uterus' were being examined.[164] So unlike commercial anatomy exhibits – including, at Rackstrow's Museum from the 1770s, a figure of a pregnant woman with imitation blood 'flowing through glass vessels', the heart 'in action' and lungs 'mov[ing] as in breathing'[165] – which were open to any man or woman who was willing to pay the entrance fee, Hunter's preparations, described as 'perhaps the finest collection in Europe', were shown to a more restricted audience of medical students, doctors, surgeons, scholars and other eminent visitors.[166]

Still, the 'defect[s]' of preserved body parts, whether 'wet' (in spirits) or 'dry', were recognized, especially their loss of 'natural appearance', and Hunter cautioned that they were supplements to, rather than 'substitutes' for, a dead body. Yet they enabled demonstration of 'intricate, confused' or otherwise 'invisible' parts.[167] So when private anatomy schools in London offered students opportunities to learn anatomy by dissecting the dead, especially from the mid-eighteenth century onwards,[168] casts, preparations and illustrations, with their animate dimensions, were significant in that process. Such educational aids were generated through dissection and, in turn, they informed perceptions of it. Instruction in the 'essentials of solid anatomy', Hunter asserted, required both a 'plentiful supply of dead bodies' *and* a 'competent stock of preparations': the former was

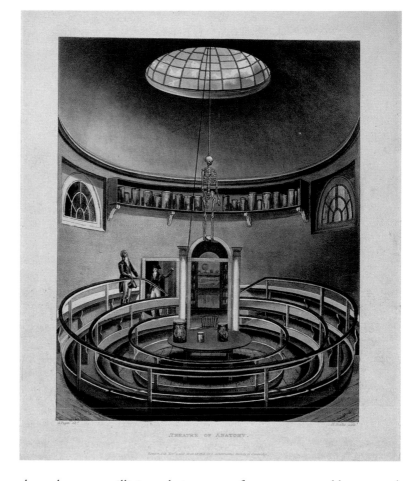

THEATRE OF ANATOMY.

dependent on an illicit trade in corpses from graves, workhouses and hospitals, the latter Hunter made and collected, as did his brother John Hunter, to the admiration of 'all men of science'.[169] Indeed, such was the perceived importance of large anatomical collections by the 1780s that 'modern Anatomists' were, William Hunter observed, 'striving, almost every where to procure' them.[170] How the twin concerns of obtaining bodies and making anatomical collections preoccupied anatomists during the nineteenth century is explored in the next two chapters, which analyse social and material processes of museum formation.

Bodies after death figured as animated entities in practices of display, from relics to rarities and preparations. They have been reconfigured over time in changing materials and have been caught up in shifting modes of viewing and engaging with them. Given the emergence of approaches that sought, by the late seventeenth century, to depict anatomy devoid of 'ornament and misleading representations', what was to become of animated anatomies? In an early nineteenth-century printed image of the anatomy theatre at the University of Cambridge a visitor is invited to view a human skeleton suspended from the domed skylight (illus. 61). Although articulated, the skeleton hangs from a rope without any suggestion of life. In the centre of the theatre the table is occupied not by a body in the process of dissection but instead by specimens preserved in three cylindrical glass jars: conjoined twins in one and a foetus or newborn in another. A display case of similarly preserved specimens is elevated above the entrance to the theatre. Through the door, two antechambers are just about visible – the first fitted with shelves holding further specimens and the second a display space showing what appears to be a wax model that is half intact and half 'dissected' to reveal the skeleton. Here there might be traces of memento mori but expressions of life on the part of the dead are not apparent. This was not, however, a visual indicator that animated anatomy had died – even though some anatomical atlases and wax models made during the nineteenth century highlighted the deathly condition of the dissected deceased.[171] Rather, anatomized bodies came to be visualized and materialized as very much alive through further anatomical practices involving, for instance, twentieth-century museum and photographic displays, as explored in later chapters.

Three
NERVE CENTRE: MUSEUM FORMATION I

William Hunter had observed, from his London-based school in the second half of the eighteenth century, that anatomists 'almost every where' were seeking to acquire large collections of preserved body parts.[1] Over the following century anatomical museums were created and expanded, not everywhere, but rather in particular places where multiple social, cultural and material factors gave rise to them. This chapter, and the next, trace the formation of the Anatomical Museum at Marischal College within the social relations and cultural practices that emerged throughout the nineteenth century in the city of Aberdeen, in Scotland and further afield. During the early decades of the 1800s diverse collections containing human remains co-existed in Aberdeen: body fragments defined as antiquities, curiosities and anatomical preparations were obtained by scholars, anatomists, doctors and surgeons for display in various settings, from the houses of wealthy collectors to public exhibitions, and from universities to learned societies. But by the late 1850s some parts of these collections began to gather at one particular site, the Anatomical Museum, thereby forming the beginnings of a centre for the display of anatomy in this region. Chapter Four goes on to analyse how this initial drawing together of material objects was consolidated, *c.* 1860–90, when the Anatomical Museum, dedicated to the collecting, display and study of human and comparative anatomy, was built and developed.

The wider pattern of museum formation in nineteenth-century Britain saw many substantial collections owned by individuals sold or given to public museums, while educational institutions expanded their museums on a grand scale for the purposes of science and medicine.[2] The teaching of anatomy shifted from private (or extramural) schools to university medical schools, royal colleges and teaching hospitals, and the Anatomy Act of 1832 brought in new regulations regarding the supply of bodies for dissection.[3]

Alongside the enormous growth in institutionally based museums of anatomy and of pathology, commercial exhibitions of anatomy flourished, especially mid-century, but subsequently declined – with the former gaining authority as sites of medical education and the latter largely defined as suspect, if not corrupting, entertainments.[4] Museum formation was also a process in which a complex of interrelated sites of collecting and display were informed by the social relations, cultural encounters and politics of imperialism and empire.[5] In particular, many graduates of Scotland's universities took up medical and military posts overseas, participating in extensive networks through which human and animal body parts were trafficked.[6]

Museums have formed through the strategic and the serendipitous accumulation of material objects, but they have also been constituted in metaphorical terms. This chapter describes an early manifestation of Marischal College's Anatomical Museum as a nerve centre, while Chapter Four traces its expansion as a growing organic entity – an arbour of interwoven trees. In the account below, then, a 'nerve centre' emerges among differently located and composed collections each with their own modes of categorizing and displaying human remains. These sites of material accumulation were socially connected through the contacts maintained by the scholars and medical men who acquired and exhibited dispersed parts of the dead.

MUSEUM METAPHORS

Anthropologists, anatomists and scientists have used multiple metaphors to grasp and articulate material objects and their complex groupings as collections. Current anthropological research highlights the social relationships that are created and informed by interactions with material objects. Chris Gosden and Chantal Knowles argue that objects are always in a 'state of becoming', building up social relations during the processes of their production and use through which they are reshaped both physically and conceptually. Consequently each museum containing such material objects is a 'node in a set of connections', a nexus of social relations formed via its material holdings.[7] Nicholas Thomas develops the metaphor of entanglement to convey the social dimensions of material objects. He suggests that objects are integral to people's entanglement in social relationships, such as relations between kin, just as objects become entangled in people's and communities' stories and histories – narratives which inform those objects' meanings and values.[8] People and material objects are thus mutually interdependent. And rather than being discrete or bounded items, material objects are also caught up with other items, such as those used in processes of making, repairing and adapting; so objects get entangled with other objects.[9] Furthermore, as assemblages or collections of things gather, through the interactions of multiple persons and materials, associations between objects arise, generating further connections within and between collections.

While such anthropological metaphors accentuate the social dimensions of objects, especially the interpenetration of the social and the material, anatomists and zoologists working closely with museums in the early twentieth century mobilized technological and organic metaphors. Arthur Keith, who studied anatomy at Marischal College during the 1880s, came to see the Hunterian Museum at the Royal College of Surgeons of England (RCS) as a 'great ship' when be became conservator in 1908. This museum, he wrote, although 'moored' at Lincoln's Inn Fields, 'was really sailing through time, laden heavily with a rather miscellaneous cargo', some having come 'on board' in the eighteenth century with John Hunter's preparations, and many specimens having since then 'added to her load'. Closely reading the RCS's archival records, Keith saw this ship's many switches in direction after the Government purchased Hunter's collection in 1799 and the Hunterian Museum opened fourteen years later: 'with each change of captain the "sailing orders" had been altered.'[10] Keith's metaphor alluded to the diversity of the collection and the mutability of its purposes but also emphasized the continuity of the institution over the previous century, with its hierarchically organized staff headed by a single figure – the conservator/captain. The metaphor described massive material accrual over time in a vessel associated with powerful capacity for movement, storage and transportation; from this point of view the museum was an inexhaustible technology of acquisition.

An organic metaphor, on the other hand, was advanced by John Arthur Thomson (1861–1933), when professor of natural history at Marischal College. He envisaged a museum as a 'ganglion in education' within its region, a ganglion being an anatomical term for a nerve centre that operates within the nervous system of an organism.[11] One such ganglion is shown prominently in a book of diagrams – with which Thomson may well have been familiar, as a copy was held in Marischal College's Anatomy Department from the 1870s onwards – based on dissections by William Henry Flower (1831–1899) and first published the year before Flower's 1861 appointment as the RCS's conservator (illus. 62, top left).[12] Situated within the cranial nerves, the gasserian ganglion branches out and divides, connecting with other anatomical parts, including other ganglia. So by likening a museum to a centre that radiates nerve fibres in the body, Thomson conveyed the notion of a concentrated focal point of activity

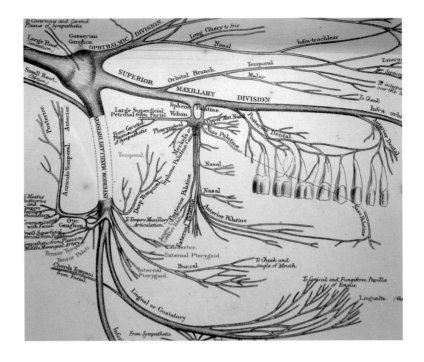

extending numerous lines of communication within a geographical region. Unlike the museum as self-contained vessel amassing its cargo in London, the Aberdeen-based gangliform museum was a growth receiving and transmitting messages (taking in objects and disseminating knowledge) as a centre in its northeast region, a centre connected with other centres.

Thomson – an associate of Robert Reid and Alexander Low as well as an influential teacher of Robert Lockhart at Marischal College, all of whom worked as professor of anatomy and curator of the Anatomical Museum – was convinced of the benefits that museums with vivid displays could bring to the education of both students and the public. His vision of the gangliform museum was fed by his theories about the 'inter-relatedness of things', as he explained: 'the world is a network of inter-relations. Nature is a vast system of linkages. There is a correlation of organisms in Nature comparable to the correlation of organs in our body. There is a web of life.'[13] The museum as ganglion was as inseparable from its material surroundings as the nervous system was from the human body. This metaphor was probably informed by Thomson's familiarity with anatomical work that would often construct likenesses between nerves and other material entities, as in nineteenth-century formulations of nerves as trees or as telegraph networks.[14] How something of a museum as 'nerve centre' came tentatively into being around 1860 in Aberdeen is described in what follows, focusing on the social and material aspects of this formation.

ANTIQUITIES AND CURIOSITIES

During the first half of the nineteenth century in Aberdeen, collections and displays of human remains featured in disparate settings, including the private collections of wealthy individuals and public exhibitions intended for the education of everyone. Prominent among the former was that owned by Alexander Thomson (1792–1868), gentleman and scholar. A graduate of Marischal College, where he studied law, zoology, botany, geology and literature, Thomson travelled in Europe and drew on his connections with doctors, military and naval officers and others to assemble his museum at his home, Banchory House, just outside Aberdeen.[15] As testimony to his learning and status, by the 1840s he had amassed over 300 eclectic items, many displayed on the walls and in the glass cases of his museum: an alligator skull, artefacts from Bali, China and New Guinea, toys, weapons, a unicorn horn, a model of an 'Indian boat' and metal votive offerings from Rome in the shape of arms, hands, eyes and a heart (votive offerings, or ex-votos, of this type were placed at Catholic shrines to promote and give thanks for healing in specific areas of the afflicted person's body). Among many antiquities – including fragments of glass, charred wood and ashes excavated at the ancient city of Pompeii, which was destroyed by volcanic eruption – were the hand of a female mummy with her 'coffin' and a 'figure of an Egyptian female in wood, containing the mummy of a foetus'.[16] Regarded as rare antiquities, mummies were eagerly sought by collectors. As bodies, or parts thereof, which had endured over lengthy spans of time, they were as fascinating as the embalming techniques used to preserve them, and this fascination was fuelled during the 1820s and '30s by mummy-unwrapping events held at private residences and in medical institutions. In London's Charing Cross Hospital lecture theatre and at the RCS, for instance, layers of coverings were removed from mummies to reveal their secreted ornaments, such as scarabs, as well as the human remains inside.[17]

Alexander Thomson was a committed collector, but he also distributed items, including preserved human remains, to worthy organizations and institutions. To the Aberdeen Medico-Chirurgical Society (AMCS) he donated some chemical apparatus in 1820, and to Marischal College three human skulls for anatomical study.[18] Thomson was also willing to lend objects to temporary public exhibitions such as one that opened in October 1840 on Union Street, in Aberdeen's central commercial area. At this four-month *Exhibition of Objects Illustrative of the Fine Arts, Natural History, Philosophy, Machinery, Manufactures, Antiquities, Curiosities, &c.*, visitors could view, from Thomson's own museum, an alligator, Egyptian papyri and a case of East Indian shells among over 1,000 other 'articles' from a number of lenders – including some preserved human remains.[19]

The exhibition was organized by the Aberdeen Mechanics' Institution to raise funds for this organization and in the spirit of opening museums to the wider public. As the exhibition catalogue announced via a quotation: 'every mind can learn to see, and to relish, the true and the beautiful: it is a common gift, which should be cultivated in all, from the Throne to the Cottage'.[20] Established in 1824 for working men and tradesmen, the Institution held lectures and aimed to provide access to educational materials such as books and three-dimensional models.[21] Their 1840 exhibition displayed items loaned from gentlemen, medical men, university professors, artists, ministers and several women mostly residing in the Aberdeen region but also in Birmingham and Sheffield. The Montrose Antiquarian Society made a contribution (a stuffed vampire bat) as did the Surgeons' Hall (a preserved serpent) at the Royal Society of Surgeons of Edinburgh (RCSEd). The intention was that visitors would see 'a collection of the works of nature and art, of greater extent and variety than has ever yet been brought together in the North of Scotland'.[22] And indeed, jostling for space in two rooms, a hall and staircase were paintings; preserved animals, birds and insects; clothing; fossils; items gathered in Scotland, Greenland, Brazil, China, Africa and many other places.

Within this admittedly crowded arrangement, human body parts appeared in a case of 'curiosities' – this term having long been used to refer to non-Western peoples' artefacts.[23] Among over 50 objects from North America, British Guiana (Guyana) and New Zealand (which became a British colony in the same year as the exhibition) was a 'tattooed head from the South Sea Islands' lent by Robert Dyce, a Marischal College lecturer in midwifery. This clustering was telling: the head was displayed with clubs, knives, poisoned arrows, 'beautifully carved' paddles and headdresses worn by 'natives'. Along with an 'Indian war club, neatly carved, and having one of the teeth of a chief, killed with it, inserted in it', and a 'necklace made of human bones', many of these articles were associated with war or with the beauty of fine workmanship. In this display context, the tattooed head – and a further 'preserved head', in the same case, provided by William Pirrie, professor of surgery at Marischal College – was positioned as an object both of violence and aesthetic interest.[24] As such, these body parts, defined as curiosities, were differentiated from those parts designated as antiquities: age and the modes of treatment they had undergone, as well as their geographical associations, were factors in such a differentiation.

Robert Dyce's tattooed head was just one of the treasures brought from his substantial personal collection into public view at this exhibition. Others included cases of butterflies, beetles, locusts and shells from Mauritius, Rio de Janeiro and the Cape of Good Hope. Dyce's collection may have been inherited from his father, the physician William Dyce

(1770–1835), who had also lectured on midwifery at Marischal College and was an active collector with extensive overseas contacts.[25] The collecting practices of both these men, like Alexander Thomson's, entailed active contributions to other collections amassing elsewhere in the city. Notably, the Dyces were involved in the Museum of the AMCS, discussed later – a society at meetings of which father and son displayed not their 'curiosities' but their medically related objects.

NATURAL AND ARTIFICIAL BODIES

Human remains, defined and treated as antiquities and curiosities in private collections and public exhibitions, were also gathering in university collections in Britain during the first half of the nineteenth century.[26] Here, bodies – either preserved or modelled – were produced and displayed as sources of knowledge for different subjects studied in increasingly distinct spaces. If in early modern cabinets of curiosities there were profuse category-defying objects and displays of striking eclecticism, in eighteenth-century collecting practices different principles of ordering had emerged, classifying items and narrowing the foci of collections to selected specialisms.[27] Early nineteenth-century curiosities were valued, as in Aberdeen, but they were subject to divisions which also mapped out different kinds of collectable human body parts.

In Aberdeen, prior to their fusion in 1860 which formed the University of Aberdeen, King's College and Marischal College were each acquiring collections, the latter perhaps more successfully.[28] At King's it had been proposed in the 1750s that students should have 'access to collections of natural and artificial bodies, digested in proper order', the 'natural' consisting of parts and preparations of fossils, minerals, vegetables and animals, and the 'artificial' encompassing models, prints and paintings of instruments and machines.[29] Although it was some time before a collection gathered momentum, by around 1800 a three-room museum was in operation but was suffering from lack of college investment. Plans for an anatomical collection had stalled.[30]

By this time at Marischal College, preserved human bodily parts and models thereof were being collected within two main assemblages. The first of these, kept in an 'apartment', was the apparatus used for explorations and teaching in natural philosophy (encompassing astronomy, hydrostatics, pneumatics, electricity, mechanics and optics).[31] This collection had grown during the eighteenth century, expanding especially with the activities of Patrick Copland (1748–1822), who constructed much of the equipment for his experiments and demonstrations with an assistant, John King.[32]

63
'Head of Despair',
late 18th century,
possibly by Patrick
Copland, in wood,
metal and hair.

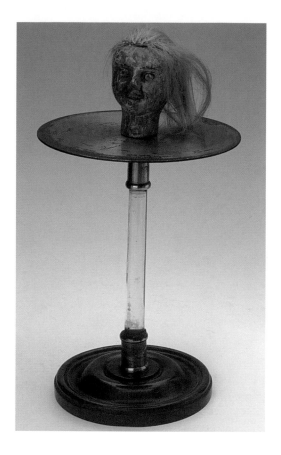

One such device, possibly made by Copland, was a model – the 'Head of Despair' – which he used in electrostatic demonstrations (illus. 63). Its hair would stand on end, during intentionally dramatic lessons for students, when the metal scalp and supporting stand were charged by an electro-static generator.[33] Purchases from instrument makers also expanded the collection, such as a brass model of an eye, by W. & S. Jones in London, used to teach optics (illus. 64). By looking through this, the workings of the eye and the effects of spectacles could be viewed.

A second assemblage, located in the museum set up during the mid-1780s to house the articles which had been accruing in the library over the previous century, consisted of a

> small but increasing collection of specimens in the various depart-ments of natural history, especially in mineralogy; also a good many serpents and other animal productions, preserved in spirits; together with a considerable number and variety of natural and artificial curiosities.[34]

64
Brass and glass
model of the eye with
spectacles, late 18th
century, by W. & S.
Jones, London.

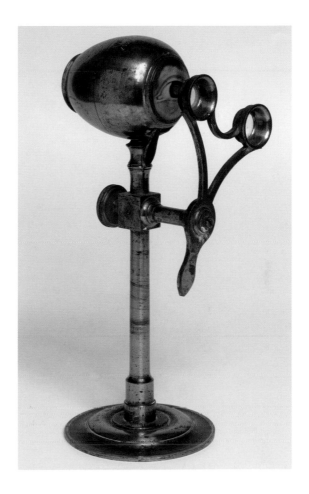

64
Brass and glass
model of the eye with
spectacles, late 18th
century, by W. & S.
Jones, London.

Further accruals were facilitated by William Knight (1786–1844), professor of natural philosophy. He encouraged Marischal College's numerous alumni, for instance, who sent articles from India and other parts of the world and was keen to receive more from the well connected and the well travelled.[35] The Museum was 'remodelled and extended' in 1823, and the collection continued to expand so that the many assorted items it boasted a decade later included, for instance, an 'umbrella . . . used by persons of distinction in Eastern countries', ostrich eggs, a crocodile and a 'piece of cheese petrified into a stone'.[36]

Into the Museum, under the rubric of the 'artificial curiosity', came human body parts in the flesh and bone, and in fabricated form.[37] Knight himself presented a 'model of a Chinese lady's foot, taken at Canton [Guangzhou]' (illus. 65).[38] The plaster-of-Paris foot, overlaid with silk bandages and embroidered layers of fabric, was fitted with a shoe as worn in life.[39] Five human heads also arrived in the 1820s, all obtained from

New Zealand. One, from a chief, 'finely preserved', was given by Lieutenant Reid of the Royal Navy, along with a 'large and heavy War Club'. Another head, tattooed and also recorded as that of a chief, was from King's College graduate and ship's captain Christopher Nockells, who travelled in the Pacific. The Marquis of Huntly, chancellor of the university, donated two heads of 'warriors', and one of a female was presented by Charles Forbes, baronet, MP and previously a successful merchant in Bombay (Mumbai). Forbes also gave to the Museum an Egyptian mummy, with two wooden cases covered in 'painted figures of animals and hieroglyphics on all sides both within and without', and considered to be 'in a state of perfect preservation' (illus. 66).[40]

While bodies were assembled as artificial curiosities, they were further categorized, and grouped with other items, according to their geographical origin. The mummy, for example, was additionally designated as an antiquity.[41] Thus human remains were incorporated into early nineteenth-century museum practices that deployed multiple, sometimes overlapping, categories in efforts to organize collections of body parts. Artificial curiosities were valued according to their state of preservation and the quality of work

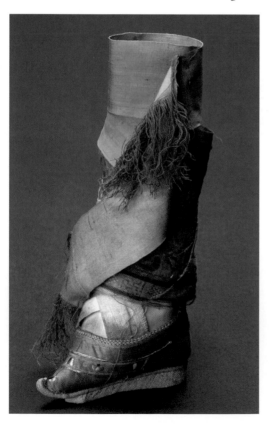

65 Model of a Chinese woman's compressed foot, 19th century, plaster of Paris and silk.

discernable upon them. Differentiated from these human remains, on the other hand, were those – without apparent embellishments or fabric wrappings – that were defined as 'natural curiosities'. For example, the 'skeleton of John Brockie hanged for murder in 1676, prepared and given by Dr M. Mackaile' was recorded in the Museum's inventory with, and possibly displayed beside, several pairs of deer horns and that of a 'sea unicorn'. Perhaps the bony nature of the human skeleton and that of these animals' preserved parts were seen to have instructive affinities among the Museum's other diverse natural curiosities – including a bird of paradise, 60 phials containing serpents, a scorpion, dried fishes, a very large Arctic bear and a white fox, 'some hairs from the point of the tail of an elephant' and 'the whiskers of a Tiger'. And again, the category of the natural curiosity was here undergoing further classificatory work as selected horns, skulls and skins of animals were also defined as objects of 'natural history'.[42]

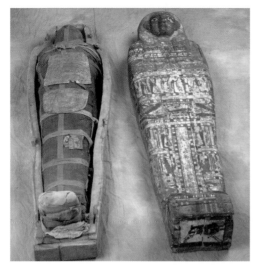

66
Mummy of a woman,
from Egypt, dating
to 300 BC–AD 150.

Body parts defined as curiosities, either artificial or natural, were valued in Marischal
College's museum – which, by 1845, was fitted
up as the Natural History Museum.[43] As
described above, this museum had been
attracting objects through social connections
between university teachers, students, doctors,
surgeons, missionaries, military officers and
others, and thereby gaining recognition as
potentially significant in generating knowledge.
But these body parts were largely differentiated
from collections that were gradually being
acquired, sometimes with difficulty, through
the anatomy teaching practices conducted elsewhere in the college.

ANATOMY IN EMBRYO

During the first half of the nineteenth century, when Aberdeen's medical
school was 'in embryo' – that is, not yet fully established – the facilities
and materials for the study of anatomy at Marischal College were initially
sparse but were beginning to grow, though not with ease.[44] For the first
two decades Charles Skene, professor of medicine, held an anatomy course
in a small classroom in a corner of the college's courtyard.[45] This accommodation had serious shortcomings: it was considered too cramped to
adequately accommodate dissecting, lecturing and the secure storage of
anatomical preparations in one space. In the late 1820s Alexander Ewing,
lecturer in anatomy and physiology, was also concerned that in the classroom 'the smell is very bad, and the air so tainted as to be unhealthy. It is
impossible to keep it clean, as there is no separate place for the dissections.'[46] These conditions were endured, however, for as Ewing reported,
it was here that the 'structure of the body [was] minutely described, and
illustrated by demonstrations from the *subject* [the dead body], preparations
and drawings, &c.'; students were also permitted to dissect for themselves
under Ewing's direction.[47]

As Marischal College owned no 'proper' anatomy collection, and provided no assistance for making preparations, Ewing purchased and made
his own, while also borrowing some belonging to Skene.[48] These Ewing
carefully carried to the classroom when required, given that there was no
place to keep them on site. He regarded his dry and wet preparations,
drawings, engravings, casts and books of plates as 'sufficient' for teaching

purposes, but saw the situation as far from ideal, especially as valuable preparations had been damaged for lack of appropriate accommodation for them.[49]

Teachers of anatomy at Marischal College would have been keenly aware that their collections, and the space available for display, paled in comparison with the museums developing elsewhere in Scotland and England. At the RCSEd there was notable expansion. Charles Bell's collection of around 3,000 items, admired as 'particularly rich in surgical pathology', was purchased in 1825; John Barclay bequeathed his substantial collection of human and comparative anatomy; and the new Surgeons' Hall that housed these acquisitions opened in 1832, including to the public.[50] At the University of Glasgow the newly built Hunterian Museum featured a Hall of Anatomy that displayed William Hunter's preparations and casts. Hunter had bequeathed his museum, at his London anatomy school in Great Windmill Street School, to his alma mater, and it was shipped to Glasgow in 1807.[51] Five years later visitors could view hundreds of preparations in wall-mounted presses (cupboards with shelves) and on tables, all 'arranged and displayed with a degree of science and taste'.[52] The Hunterian Museum was known to attract medical students to the city. However, although its holdings were used by professors to illustrate their lectures, students' entry was limited to one visit each year, as noted in 1830, and members of the public were charged for their admission. Medical students, who regarded the anatomical preparations as important in their learning, pressed for greater access to the collections.[53] In other cities collecting also continued apace.[54] In London the Anatomical Museum of Guy's Hospital, for example, boasted thousands of preparations in its 1829 catalogue – these having been obtained on site from deceased patients who underwent dissection and from doctors who gave preparations to the institution. Despite its considerable size, this collection was still regarded as an 'infant', indicating the extent of further growth to mature adulthood that was clearly anticipated.[55]

This was museum-building for the study of anatomy on a different scale to that taking place at Marischal College. There anatomists, largely relying on their own stocks of preparations for their classes, lacked both a major bequest of a sizable collection and the institutional finances to purchase one. With sufficient funds, anatomical preparations could be bought at auction – as, for example, when Joshua Brookes's museum at his private anatomy school in London was auctioned in 1828 with sale catalogues distributed to Edinburgh, Glasgow, Paris and other urban centres.[56] But this was not an acquisition route available to Marischal College's anatomists. In any case, forming and maintaining a substantial collection depended to a large extent on anatomists' access to human and animal remains, especially on their access to human bodies obtained for dissection.

Before the 1832 Anatomy Act the bodies of executed criminals (felons) had been legally assigned for dissection in Britain.[57] Two centuries prior to this act, anatomists in Aberdeen had been granted two bodies per year, those of executed men 'being notable malefactors', especially 'rebells and outlawis'. If these were unavailable anatomists were allowed 'bodies of the poorer sort' who died in hospitals, 'abortive bairns, foundlings; or those of no qualitie, who [. . . had] few friends or acquaintance that [. . . could] tak exception'.[58] But by the end of the eighteenth century, demand for corpses required to teach and learn anatomy far outweighed this allocation and students in the Aberdeen Medical Society (renamed the Aberdeen Medico-Chirurgical Society from 1811 onwards) were involved in resurrectionist activity: taking recently buried bodies from their graves so that they could be dissected – a practice that was rife in many regions.[59] Senior members of the AMCS, by 1818, tried to combat the problem, impressing on students 'the pernicious effects of raising bodies from the Church yards'.[60] Throughout Scotland families and communities protected the recently buried with devices such as iron mortsafes, which locked over each grave to prevent access to the coffin (see illus. 34, centre top), and by building watch houses in graveyards from which resurrectionists could be detected and deterred.[61]

Widespread fears of losing loved ones to anatomists' dissecting tables were fuelled by the scandal surrounding the activities of William Burke and William Hare in Edinburgh. During the late 1820s the two men were involved in killing people and selling their bodies to anatomist Robert Knox for dissection at his private school; Burke was hanged for his crimes and dissected at the University of Edinburgh's medical school.[62] In Aberdeen there were strong local concerns about anatomists' treatment of the dead. Reported in the press in December 1831 were angry reactions among the 'lower classes' to Andrew Moir's recently built private anatomy theatre and especially to the presence of decomposing body parts in ground at the back of this establishment; a 20,000-strong crowd gathered and destroyed the theatre by fire.[63] This was not an isolated event. Forceful public opposition to the practice of anatomy – when it was associated with grave-robbing or even murder and when inappropriate methods for disposing of the dead were seen to be used – was demonstrated, especially among the poor, whose bodies were most vulnerable to acquisition for dissection. There were protests in, for example, Sheffield, Liverpool and Cambridge.[64] Anxiety about, and resistance to, the prospect of dissection after death for a person's own body or for their relatives were strong and underpinned by complex factors including feelings of repugnance in response to this invasive treatment of the body, its association with the punishment of murderers, and Christian beliefs that the deceased body must remain intact at burial so that in the afterlife the soul would be secure and physical resurrection on the Day of Judgment prepared for.[65]

Despite criticism, the Anatomy Act of 1832 made it lawful for anatomists (who were now required to obtain a licence from central government, and were overseen on their premises by HM Inspector of Anatomy) to receive the bodies of those who died in poorhouses/workhouses, hospitals, asylums and prisons if they were unclaimed by relatives or friends for burial.[66] In Aberdeen a funeratory was established, as in Edinburgh and Glasgow, which took in the bodies of 'paupers' from institutions (including Aberdeen Royal Infirmary, the Royal Lunatic Asylum, the House of Refuge for the destitute, Old Machar Poor House and the St Machar Poor House), as well as from private residences throughout the nineteenth century and beyond.[67] Many bodies were claimed by relatives who could afford the cost of a burial, but those remaining, if not overly decomposed, were allocated to teachers of anatomy and of surgery at Marischal College (and at King's College, where there was also some medical teaching until the institutional fusion of 1860, when this was located solely at Marischal College).[68]

Thus it was the bodies of the destitute, abandoned or socially isolated that anatomists obtained. For each body they paid an agreed set sum to the funeratory using funds from the fees paid by medical students. After a maximum of six weeks undergoing dissection, the bodies were buried at Footdee Cemetery near the city's harbour.[69] The Anatomy Act required all anatomized bodies to be 'decently interred'.[70] However, it imposed no requirements regarding the retaining of human skeletons and tissue which were preserved for the long term as anatomical preparations for medical education. Such practices that stocked museum shelves, although not authorized, were therefore not ruled out by law.[71]

In the three decades following the Anatomy Act anatomists in Aberdeen remained anxious that the number of bodies available to them was 'insufficient' even to illustrate lectures, and that teachers were frequently without any for several weeks at a time. With the body supply regularly swinging from inadequate to 'barely sufficient', they were keen to make and acquire preparations for their collections.[72] It was in this context, at Marischal College – which was rebuilt during 1836 to 1844 according to designs by architect Archibald Simpson – that Allen Thomson, professor of anatomy from 1839, conducted his teaching. Around this time, a collection, belonging to Marischal College rather than to individual anatomists, was gradually beginning to gather. Human skulls included those of two men hanged for murder in Inverness and Aberdeenshire, probably preserved after they were dissected at the college.[73] The importance of the skull in the examination of anatomy and the classification of humankind into 'varieties' had been emphasized since the late eighteenth century, and anatomists in Aberdeen welcomed donations of preserved skulls from private collectors, such as that of a 'European' and two from Java given by Alexander Thomson.[74] Three skulls from North America came from John James Audubon, ornithologist, probably through his connection with William MacGillivray, museum conservator at the RCSEd during the 1830s, then professor of natural history at Marischal College in the 1840s.[75] A human skull from MacGillivray's own natural history collection, which was kept in Marischal College's Natural History Museum until his death in 1852, also joined the anatomy acquisitions.[76]

Anatomical preparations would have been accumulating too. Allen Thomson's emphasis on topographic anatomy required students to dissect in order to accurately learn and remember the 'position, form, appearance & texture of the parts', but this 'analysis of the structure of the dead body' was also conducted with the use of preparations.[77] During the early 1830s Thomson had visited museums – in London (at the RCS and Guy's Hospital) and further afield in the Netherlands, Germany, Italy and France – taking notes on human skulls, foetuses and preserved organs, making drawings and compiling a list of those preparations, human and comparative, that he intended to make for his own teaching purposes.[78] Thomson most probably made and displayed such preparations at Marischal College (although none are now extant). His lectures were also illustrated with many 'beautiful diagrams', which he drew on paper for hanging on walls and sketched in coloured chalk on blackboards.[79] Works on paper obtained for Marischal College's anatomy collection allowed enlarged versions of small bodily parts to be viewed more easily, for example the bones of the human skull, including the ear (illus. 67).

Thomson's successor, Alexander Jardine Lizars (from 1841 to 1863), also saw educational value in illustrations and atlases, adding to Marischal College's collection of anatomical plates and volumes. A. J. Lizars had taught at his brother John Lizars's private anatomy school in Edinburgh and also acquired his brother's anatomical preparations, which John Lizars 'had collected from the field presented by his practical rooms'.[80] So A. J. Lizars was equipped with his own collection for teaching when in Aberdeen. Accommodation for teaching at Marischal College, by 1845, included an anatomical theatre with an adjoining dissecting room, and an anatomical museum fitted with glass cases and a gallery, in addition to rooms for anatomical preparations. Along with this spatial provision, expansion of the resources for teaching anatomy continued in the area of paper-based illustrations for temporary display on walls.[81] The anatomist and surgeon Richard Quain's *Anatomy of the Arteries of the Human Body* of 1844 was acquired, for instance. This comprised 87 lithographic drawings

67
Edward Mitchell,
illustration of bones
in the cranium,
engraving from John
Barclay, *The Anatomy
of the Bones of the
Human Body*, new
edition by Robert
Knox (Edinburgh,
1829), Plate 8.

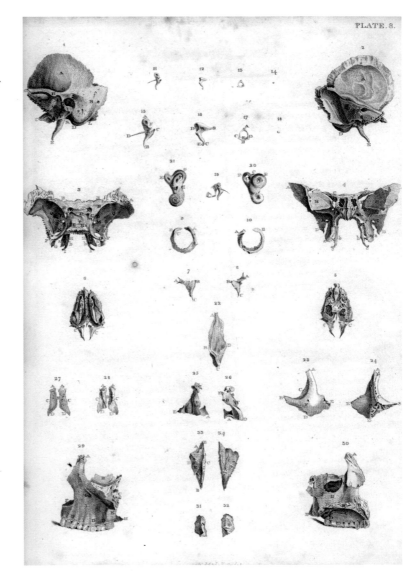

PLATE. 8.

of figures at life size by surgeon Joseph Maclise, with an accompanying descriptive volume (illus. 68, see illus. 139). Such images were often displayed for study in dissecting rooms, where they could be compared with bodies being anatomized.[82] A. J. Lizars's own volume, an anatomy textbook for students (1844), added to teaching resources at Marischal College and generated prestige. The work was especially praised in the medical press for its 'novel and interesting' sketches – depicting the nerves and ganglia, for instance – which provided 'correct and judicious views', some derived from examination with a microscope.[83]

68
Joseph Maclise,
illustration of blood
vessels and muscles in
the arm, lithographic
drawing from Richard
Quain, *The Anatomy
of the Arteries of the
Human Body* (London,
1844), Plate 26.

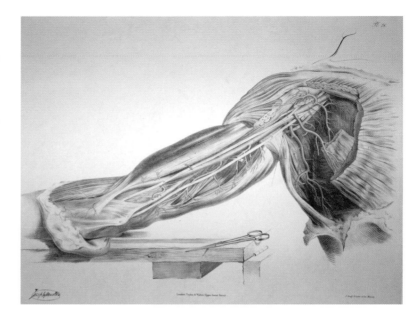

Further anatomical images enhancing Marischal College's collection were supplied in John Lizars's *A System of Anatomical Plates of the Human Body* (1822–6), with 101 plates engraved by another brother, William Home Lizars, in Edinburgh. These images were 'faithfully drawn' by the author/anatomist and the engraver, from dissections conducted by the former and his skilled assistant, all with the aim of 'scrupulous correctness' and with reference to previous influential anatomical works.[84] Plate XCVIII shows, for example, the lymphatic vessels of the heart, liver and intestines (illus. 69). The aim was to provide 'some substitute for the [dissecting room] subject' when bodies were difficult to procure and there was, therefore, 'scarcity of *material*'.[85] Medical opinion on the plates confirmed that with them John Lizars had 'displayed, with great felicity, the anatomy of the human body'.[86]

Producing and collecting such images of anatomy for display in teaching situations prompted students to make and compile their own paper versions. One such student at Marischal College in 1856, Angus Fraser, made notes on lectures given by Alexander Lizars, working into his notebook numerous sketches of anatomical parts in pencil, ink and watercolour.[87] For example, Fraser illustrated the pancreas, within an outline of a truncated body (illus. 70). He labelled eight anatomical parts (a to h) with a key in the manner of an anatomical atlas, thus appropriating established visual and textual conventions in this mode of learning through interrelated drawing and note-taking.[88] By so doing the student composed and collected his own anatomical figures, as many of his fellow students would

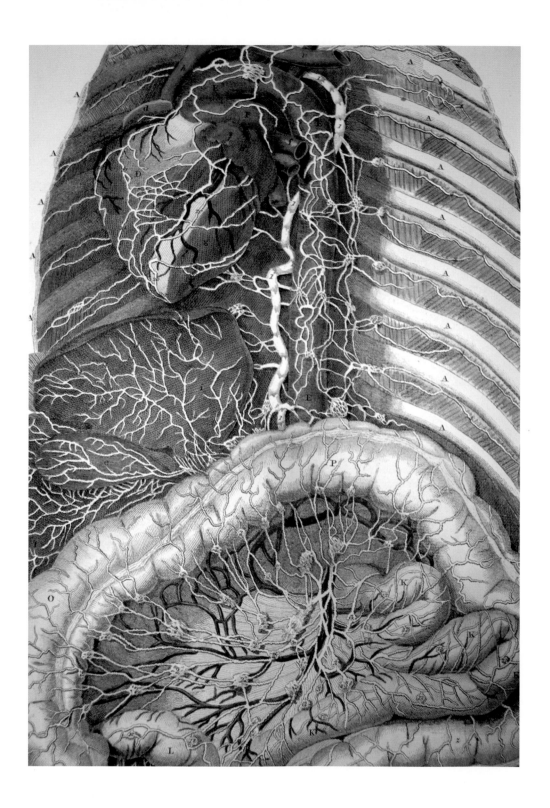

70
Angus Fraser,
drawing, in a
notebook, of the
pancreas within the
human body, 1856,
ink and watercolour
on paper.

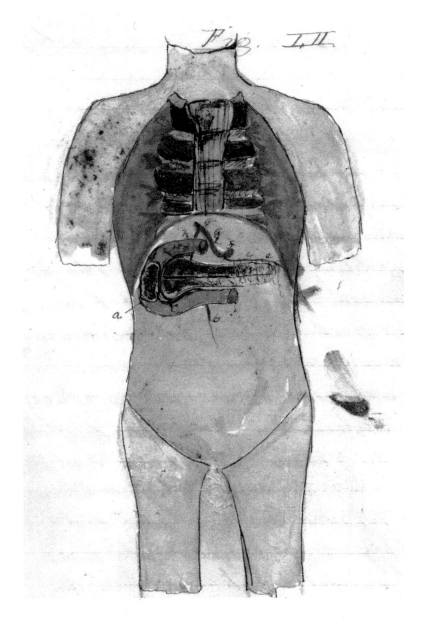

70
Angus Fraser,
drawing, in a
notebook, of the
pancreas within the
human body, 1856,
ink and watercolour
on paper.

69
William Home Lizars,
illustration showing
lymphatic vessels and
organs, engraving
from John Lizars, *A
System of Anatomical
Plates of the Human
Body* (Edinburgh,
1822–6), Plate XCVIII.

have done, to aid his immediate learning and for future reference. Within the material and visual culture of anatomy by the 1850s, then, students as well as teachers were generating anatomical collections in paper formats.

INTRACTABLE OBJECTS

While anatomists at Marischal College were using their own private collections in their teaching, overseeing donations to the college's anatomy collection, such as skulls, and acquiring portfolios of anatomy on paper, further collections of preserved human remains were being gathered by learned societies based in Aberdeen. The AMCS's Museum was perhaps the most ambitious of these.[89] This society provided an educational forum for medical students and senior practitioners, including local anatomists, doctors and surgeons, to discuss matters of interest and concern – and here there was momentum for its museum's collection to expand. Yet the process by which this museum came to embrace comparative and human anatomy as well as natural history and botany became more difficult than anticipated, and part of the collection was eventually transferred to Marischal College in the late 1850s.

In the 1820s, however, members of the AMCS had high hopes for the as yet limited Museum at the society's building in the city centre. Concerned that it was in a 'state of absolute starvation', one of the AMCS's main priorities was to obtain a 'proper collection of anatomical preparations', notwithstanding the low funds available for this. In particular, it was agreed that two skeletons (one male, one female), as well as preparations of the blood vessels, the lymphatic vessels and the nerves, should be 'procured as speedily as possible'.[90] Contributions to this museum were sought and the AMCS's members responded swiftly. An Aberdeen doctor presented a blood-vessel preparation, for example, and an adult male skeleton was received from Alexander Ewing following his election as keeper of the Museum in 1822. Joshua Brookes, from his private anatomy school in London, also presented an adult skeleton and an injected preparation of an arm.[91]

What the AMCS was able to draw in from its members was, however, dependent on what those members chose to keep for their own private collections. While they retained many of their most prized medical items, though, they were prepared to offer them for temporary display at the AMCS's meetings. When medical 'cases' were discussed with reference to living patients, post-mortem examinations and dissections, members demonstrated and exhibited relevant preparations and instruments. William Dyce, for instance, read a paper on equipment used in midwifery and displayed to the meeting a 'lever of his own invention' from his private collection and laboratory.[92] Doctors and surgeons who preserved body parts from patients during the course of their work would show and debate these preparations at the AMCS. They reported on physical afflictions and deaths – some involving extreme suffering, suicide, poverty and addiction – in order to cultivate and disseminate medical knowledge. In one case, for example, that of a servant girl, her feet had separated at the ankle due to 'gangrene produced by exposure to cold', the girl having slept at night in a wood; one of her feet, preserved by the medical practitioner involved, was observed at the meeting.[93] Selections from medical practitioners' own collections, kept in their homes and/or places of work, were thus temporarily circulated as exhibits. These exhibits were clearly derived from the bodies of local people. And so it was these bodies that also yielded material for the Museum of the AMCS when members chose to permanently pass on their preparations.

In addition to its members' gifts, the AMCS also aimed to boost its holdings by cultivating wider, geographically distant, social connections (especially with their medically trained acquaintances who were based overseas) through which they could expand their collection. In this process of contact-building, certain members of the AMCS became key intermediaries. William Dyce was particularly well connected. For instance, he communicated with William Chalmers, surgeon in the East India Company's service, when the latter sent an elephant skull and bones.[94] Further contributions to the Museum were forthcoming: birds were sent by a surgeon in Sydney, and medicinal plants arrived from India, Ceylon (Sri Lanka) and Mauritius.[95]

Two major donations received in 1822 marked a degree of success in acquiring items, but also highlighted difficulties in transporting, preserving and incorporating them into the AMCS's Museum. When Dr James Strachan – Deputy Inspector of Hospitals in Halifax, Nova Scotia – sent some 'indigenous' bulbs, seeds and plants, they made a 'tedious passage across the Atlantic', so much so that they became difficult to identify. In particular, their labels had 'separated during the voyage from the rotting of the cords with which they were attached'.[96] The problem of decay during transit also arose with Dr George Alexander's shipment of 29 'specimens of comparative anatomy and natural history' from Prince of Wales Island (Penang). The 'Head of a Native of New Zealand' was 'much injured by insects' and – again – labels were missing from the cargo that included bottles of snakes; parcels of shells; scorpions; roots; coral; and skeletons of two tigers, a flying fox and a crocodile (illus. 71).[97]

This latter reptile incurred expenses to prepare it for display, prompting discussion at the AMCS regarding the item's purpose at a time of low funds. The skeletal 'present' was evaluated as 'highly ornamental to the Museum',

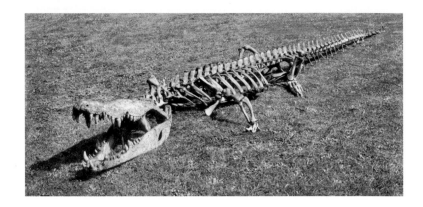

but unfortunately 'of a nature that scarcely admits of being made sub-
servient to the purposes of the Society'. The AMCS recorded the request that
members wanting to give 'rarities' should bear in mind the 'low state' of
the finances available for dealing with such museum gifts.[98] The rarity in
this context was, then, defined as a somewhat unnecessary, costly ornament.

From the early years of its museum-expansion campaign, then, the
AMCS became overburdened with specimens perceived as too demanding
in relation to available resources: they were vulnerable to decay, difficult
to identify, costly to maintain and awkward to assimilate into the Museum
as sources of appropriate knowledge. By the 1830s there were moves to refocus the collection, to establish 'the most advisable mode of rendering it
useful to science', and it was proposed that specimens unconnected with
anatomy should be sold or exchanged for others. Although the specimens
of natural history were not removed at this stage, the Museum was 'put in
proper order' and the value of pathological anatomy was highlighted
along with renewed requests to medical members in private practice and
public institutions to help increase holdings in this area. Following this,
acquisitions continued to be received in 'healthy anatomy' – such as a
uterus and foetuses 'at different stages of gestation' – and preparations of
pathological body parts also arrived. One surgeon, for example, presented
23 such preserved parts including an ulceration of the stomach and a
piece of diseased kidney.[99]

Alexander Lizars became a member of the AMCS when he joined
Marischal College as professor of anatomy and in the early 1840s he
contributed to the Museum a preparation of breast tissue after exhibiting
it at a meeting. Efforts to maintain the Museum were made over the next
few years, as when Robert Dyce presented, for members of the AMCS,
demonstrations on 'different modes of making preparations' and how best
to preserve their colour.[100] Offering assistance with the restoration of
preparations – such as refilling their glass jars with preserving fluid,

replacing their degraded lids and revising labels – Dyce also helped to rearrange the Museum with its curator, surgeon Robert Smith.[101] But, despite these efforts, by the mid-nineteenth century the Museum had become too costly and time-consuming to maintain, and its material holdings were disintegrating. Many preparations in methylated spirits required further preservation and some were 'putrid': in February 1859 the curator reported that of the Museum's 162 preparations, 118 were 'good', 22 'doubtful' and 22 'worthless'.[102] The same year, the AMCS calculated that the continued costs of maintaining 'perishable article[s]', including those in spirits and the dried botanical specimens, could no longer be met. These objects were simply too intractable, too demanding in resources and attention to properly maintain over time. The stuffed birds in the collection had already been given away; they were transferred to the Natural History Museum at Marischal College in 1856, 'with expression of the grateful remembrance of past kindness received' from that institution.[103]

So it was decided that the best way to preserve the preparations in the AMCS's Museum was to dispose of them in order to offer them a potential future – that is, to hand them over to Marischal College, where the professors were trustees of the AMCS and where it was (thought to be) likely that permanent and paid curators would be appointed.[104] A senior representative of the college had already 'pledged' that any preparations presented – which were deemed 'valuable' – would be treated with all due care. Clearly this transacting of preparations involved judgements of value on the part of recipient as well as giver. With the movement of the AMCS's preparations to an institution regarded as a safer repository, collections of human remains in the city were gathering at what was coming to form a centre at Marischal College. How this composite collection – of preserved human bones and preparations as well as anatomies on paper – was shaped into the Anatomical Museum during the second half of the nineteenth century is explored in the next chapter.

From the late eighteenth to the mid-nineteenth century human remains were acquired, preserved and exhibited in various contexts in Aberdeen and its region: private collections, temporary public exhibitions, university collections and a medical society's museum. Preserved bodies and body parts were assimilated into the categories of antiquity, curiosity and healthy and pathological anatomy. They were dispersed across various sites – with their different strategies of display – which were connected through the involvement of anatomists, surgeons, private collectors and medical practitioners in the city and beyond. Collections of human remains were made, sustained and circulated through social relations established predominantly among men of wealth, learning and professional standing within the locality who were also able to draw upon a wide network of medical, military and other contacts overseas. Preserved body parts were inherited and gifted within familial relationships between fathers and sons, and between brothers. They were also donated as a means to express connection with, and continued loyalty towards, educational institutions. Furthermore they were mobilized in interactions between teachers and students to disseminate anatomical knowledge. If collections of bodies and body parts registered these social relations, they were also made possible through patterns of social disconnection, as when preparations were made from the bodies of the destitute who were unclaimed after death. These socially disconnected or isolated bodies came to be a significant source for anatomical collections, and preparations made from them were most often associated with those who had dissected and preserved them, rather than the persons whose bodies they had once been part of.

Unlike the Hunterian Museum at the RCS, which Arthur Keith imagined as a ship, museums in Aberdeen did not go 'sailing through time' accumulating an extensive 'cargo'. In the winter of 1859–60 the Museum of the AMCS was divided and distributed: the anatomical, botanical and natural history collections were transferred to appropriate rooms at Marischal College, pathological preparations were offered to Aberdeen Royal Infirmary, and a small selection of human bones was retained in the much reduced Museum of the AMCS for medical students' use.[105] This donation to Marischal College, in addition to the anatomy collection already building up at this location, formed something of a 'ganglion in education', to use John Thomson's metaphor – that is, the beginnings of a nerve centre for anatomical display that was both a material and a social formation. Here there was a convergence of collections, but there was also divergence: while preserved body parts defined as anatomical preparations were assembled together, others designated as 'antiquities' and 'curiosities' were located and displayed elsewhere in Marischal College. And human remains continued to feature in further settings in the city, where preserved body parts, such as skulls, were persistent components of private collections (see illus. 16). No single metaphor can fully capture the shifting complexities of museum formation and, as the next chapter shows, nineteenth-century perspectives on the Anatomical Museum offered up yet another organic analogy through which the collection and display of bodies was described and imagined.

Four
SKELETAL GROWTH: MUSEUM
FORMATION II

The small museum, off the old dissecting-room, was a pleasant arbour
of white bones, and old flesh, and models: man and his correlates met
here to exhibit their comparable features. The union of the dead
taught us the unity of the living. The series of seven skeletons was
alone a fine lesson in how the human 'moves upward, working out the
beast'. There were greater places; but none more lovingly tended . . .
It grew, here a little and there a little, out of reverence for the great
scientific traditions and for the great pioneers of modern science.[1]

The Anatomical Museum at Marischal College, Aberdeen, was thus
described, in the late nineteenth century, as a growing formation – an
arbour, or latticework of intertwined plants – where tree like skeletons
offered an education in evolution. Unlike the sixteenth-century imagery
of the arborescent skeleton with its memento mori messages (see illus.
52), this later display of bones, many articulated into living postures, was cultivated as part of 'modern science'.[2] For the anatomist John Struthers the
tree was a resonant image: when lecturing on evolution to medical students
in Aberdeen he declared that 'life doesn't rise, dyentlemen [sic], like the
steps of a ladder. It is a tree.'[3] Here aspects of the anatomist's teaching and
research, from the 1860s onwards, drew on Charles Darwin's work
regarding 'variation, natural selection, adaptation, [and] survival'.[4] As
Darwin wrote in *On the Origin of Species* (1859):

the green and budding twigs may represent existing species; and
those produced each former year may represent the long succession
of extinct species. At each period of growth all the growing twigs
have tried to branch out on all sides, and to overtop and kill the
surrounding twigs and branches, in the same manner as species

and groups of species have tried to overmaster other species in the great battle for life . . . so by generation I believe it has been with the great Tree of Life, which fills with its dead and broken branches the crust of the earth, and covers the surface with its ever branching and beautiful ramifications.[5]

It is, then, perhaps no surprise that one of Struthers's former medical students, William Mackenzie, should adapt the metaphor of the tree to describe the Anatomical Museum, which his teacher had 'lovingly tended', skilfully and untiringly converting 'fine monster[s]', such as whales, into 'fine museum specimen[s]'.[6] The Anatomical Museum's growth had gained momentum from 1863 onwards when Struthers, appointed as professor of anatomy, a position he held for 26 years, was keen to fully establish Aberdeen's medical school. Defining anatomy as the most 'fundamental' subject in medical education (pathology being second and physiology taught separately from anatomy but with some cross-referencing), he regarded a new anatomical department as essential.[7] This would provide facilities for rapidly increasing numbers of students at a time when 'modern progress in practical anatomy' required particular methods of learning – and to achieve this Struthers placed what he termed 'museum-making' at the forefront of his strategy.[8] For Struthers recognized that anatomical museums in medical schools were widely regarded as central to students' education as well as sources of status and prestige for institutions.[9]

During the period *c.* 1860 to 1890, at Marischal College, the Anatomical Museum expanded through intensive gathering of deceased human and animal body parts, and the on-site 'converting' of these into legitimate specimens (the latter term by now regularly used to refer to dissected and preserved body parts as well as the term 'preparation'). In addition there was strategic purchasing of commercially available anatomical models. The Anatomical Museum's growth, though often at the time attributed to Struthers's own dedication and industry, was facilitated by his interactions within a wide field of social relationships in which anatomical collecting took place. Donors, especially medical men whom Struthers had taught, obtained human bones overseas for the collection, and those who were instrumental in obtaining animal remains included naturalists, a taxidermist, museum conservators, the proprietor of a menagerie, merchants and ships' captains. Museum-making was an unavoidably collective endeavour and Struthers's work relied on collaboration, particularly with his assistants in the Anatomical Department, even if it was not necessarily represented as such. So while parallels were drawn between museum development and organic growth, the Anatomical Museum's material accretion was also a social and cultural process.

The Anatomical Museum flourished at a time of unprecedented museum expansion in Britain and elsewhere, which produced staggeringly large collections for scientific study and public viewing.[10] Such expansion, as Susan Sheets-Pyenson notes, was characterized by 'constant international imitation and cross-fertilization' so that 'concepts and innovations freely travelled the museum circuit'.[11] When architectural styles, classification systems, display strategies and other techniques were observed in one site to be used as models for another, intermuseal influences reverberated between museums. Thus anatomical museums grew in relation to other museums and cultural displays, yet they were necessarily located in particular places – this interplay of local and distant sites crucially inflecting their development.

From the Anatomical Museum's architectural 'shell' to the composition of its exhibits and the practices that sustained it, the following sections explore the exhaustive work at Marischal College and the wide-ranging relations that enabled a flourishing of displays comprising remains of the dead. Material, embodied and performative aspects of museum-making and anatomical display were significant in establishing the Anatomical Museum as an authoritative site for medical teaching and learning, as was the careful management of relations between this museum and popular or commercial exhibitions.

SHELL AND CAST

In 1869, six years after John Struthers's arrival in Aberdeen, Marischal College's new Anatomical Museum's 'shell' or architectural structure was built (employing local masons and carpenters), although the 'museum proper, or collection . . . was still to form'.[12] Under a glazed roof, there were 350 ft (106 lineal metres) of glass-fronted wall cases on the ground floor and the gallery (which was also fitted with rail cases), as well as floor space for large skeletons.[13] Just as Struthers measured bodies in his anatomical research, so he attended to the museum's dimensions, as he explained in his *Osteological Memoirs*:

> the habit of making careful measurements is a valuable one to the anatomist; it gives an exactness and finish to our knowledge, whether of large things or small, and enables us to use proportion in the recollection of facts.[14]

With such an approach to knowledge, Struthers was particularly adept at using measurement to marshal an argument, an advantageous skill when campaigning for more university space and resources.

Following Struthers's move from Edinburgh, he had not hidden his disappointment at the facilities available for teaching anatomy at Marischal College: the modest anatomical collection around 1863 comprised a few human skulls and anatomical books, together with some preparations donated by the Aberdeen Medico-Chirurgical Society. If Struthers's predecessors, Allen Thomson and Alexander Jardine Lizars, used their own private collections for teaching purposes, these were most probably taken with their respective owners when they left employment at Marischal College. What Struthers found in their wake was decidedly lacking – a motley assemblage whose validity and suitability was not readily apparent. As Struthers reflected: 'I can never forget the depression I felt when . . . I was shown all that was for an Anatomical Museum.' The rooms were inadequate given the growing medical-student body; the dissecting room, in particular, was in urgent need of 'enlargement' for 'working space, and on the score of health'.[15] Expanded space here, as in other universities, was seen as essential if students were to acquire the requisite knowledge. Thus Struthers set about transforming what he saw as a 'thing of shreds and patches' into what he would later describe as a 'commodious, convenient and handsome suite of anatomical rooms . . . not equalled by any in the United Kingdom, though those of Edinburgh University were larger'.[16] Sizable buildings indicated the perceived importance of anatomical knowledge, and museums, with prestigious architectures and authoritative displays, were important in the development of university disciplines.[17]

By 1881 Marischal College's new Anatomical Department was built, at the back of the building and without impressive 'ornamental exteriors', but with prestige and authority amplified by its internal constitution.[18] The old lecture room and dissecting room were replaced with more spacious ones. There was a larger laboratory for microscopic anatomy and separate work rooms for the professor and the attendant. An 'injecting room' (for injecting bodies with solutions to help preserve them and for filling blood vessels with coloured fluids to make them easier to see) communicated, via a mechanical lift, with the 'dead room' or mortuary in the newly excavated basement, where there were also rooms for preparing specimens.[19] The interconnecting rooms, 'opening into each other', were considered especially conductive to anatomical work. In particular, the Anatomical Museum was well placed for study: one door opened into the lobby of the lecture room and another (in the corner of the museum) from the dissecting room 'by which the students enter when they wish to study specimens'. Dissecting room and museum, both about 55 x 30 ft (17 x 9 m) and lit from the roof, were also routed together with a doorway from the one-wall gallery of the former to the gallery of the latter.[20]

Establishing space for anatomical study involved situating that space in time, linking the present with a meaningful past. 'Modern' facilities were custom-built for then current purposes but they were also deliberately associated with selected historical figures and styles through sculptural display. Neoclassical portrait busts, in plaster-cast copies, were installed of John Barclay (1758–1826) with the year 1863 embedded in its base (the year of John Struthers's professorial appointment), John Hunter, dated 1873 (when the new lecture theatre was authorized) and William Harvey (1578–1657) and Georges Cuvier (1769–1832), both dated 1881 (when the new anatomical buildings opened; see illus. 29). Displaying plaster likenesses of elevated individuals, dated in this way (rather than with their own birth/death years), created an authoritative lineage for the Anatomical Department, and consequently for its museum, associating it with the 'great scientific traditions'.[21]

Plaster casts of classical sculpture were also obtained for the 1881 opening, made by Domenico Brucciani's pre-eminent London firm that supplied many museums collecting casts around this time. Three blocks of the Parthenon frieze with figures on horseback graced the Anatomical Department (see illus. 89, far left), as did the distinguished statue the *Germanicus* and the Berlin Adorante (see illus. 29).[22] Struthers also acquired casts of *L'Écorché* (*Figure of a Flayed Man*), originally sculpted with classical proportions by Jean-Antoine Houdon in 1767, and *Smugglerius* (*Écorché of Man in the Pose of the 'Dying Gaul'*), the original having been cast by Agostino Carlini in 1775 from an executed smuggler's body dissected by William Hunter for the Royal Academy of Arts in London.[23] While the *Germanicus* displayed the muscular male body with a smooth surface of skin, the muscles of *L'Écorché* and *Smugglerius* were exposed with skin removed. Such figures were exhibited in dissecting rooms during the late nineteenth and early twentieth century, as at London's St Thomas's Hospital (see illus. 95, far right), where their musculature (with or without 'skin') could be studied. By placing casts in Marischal College's Anatomical Department, John Struthers created continuity with predecessors who had explored anatomy through the classical form since the sixteenth century.

Antique sculptures from Italy and Greece had been eagerly sought by early modern aristocratic and wealthy collectors, either original or in marble, bronze and plaster copies.[24] During the eighteenth century, portrait busts and figures assumed prominent places in the libraries and museums of individuals and institutions.[25] Struthers's display of plaster copies in a site dedicated to anatomical learning echoed these conventions. It also mobilized a 'classicizing aesthetics', with plaster écorchés highlighting the 'normative male body' and providing, as Martin Kemp and Marina Wallace note, an 'exemplar of heroic perfection'.[26] In addition, plaster-cast horse and bear heads, which Struthers again obtained from Brucciani, highlighted the current interest in comparative anatomy, and skeletons of these along with many other creatures could be viewed at the Anatomical Museum to enable comparison of their bony structure.[27] Building a 'shell' for anatomical study within a suite of new rooms and establishing this as an institutional asset with an assemblage of casts thus asserted authority by alluding to the past while also signalling the current agendas of anatomy as a 'modern science'.

ANATOMICAL ACTUALITIES

The idealized, 'living' classical body, with smooth plaster skin or surface musculature, was displayed in a context where anatomical knowledge was gained through observation of deceased bodies whose skin was cut away to allow deeper exploration. As John Struthers wrote with regard to the medical student:

> The new world of science is dawning upon him, especially the revelation of the interior of the human body. His work is largely objective . . . all he requires is at first to be shown the method, to be helped out of the habit of trusting to word-knowledge. What I mean here is that the individual has to be trained, shown how to use his observing powers, to get his knowledge at first hand from nature, in the laboratory, not to trust to the word-knowledge obtained from lectures or books.[28]

An overly 'bookish' approach to anatomy, where undue reliance on unquestioning reading allowed students to passively 'rest in words', was rejected.[29] Moving away from word-knowledge towards 'modern methods' for learning anatomy, Struthers stressed the necessity of study in museums, and in laboratories where dissection and microscope work was conducted.[30] Here students were advised to 'investigate for yourself, dissect, analyze, observe, verify, systematize from the actualities'.[31]

This 'practical' learning was widely recognized as necessary if students were to access 'exact information' and develop their 'mental discipline'; by dissecting and studying specimens themselves, students would obtain a 'fullness of knowledge', a 'reality' that could not be gained from words heard in lectures or read in books.[32] From this perspective, knowledge that was valuable was 'well-assimilated' and comprehended, not simply 'mechanically-gathered' for later repetition.[33] Thus anatomists expected every student to be 'handling and seeing, and really knowing all that can be shown to his eyes and felt by his hands'.[34] This was work for body and mind, as Struthers explained: 'new facts and principles . . . gradually unfold themselves under the patient exercise of observation and thought, the combined use of the bodily and mental eye.'[35] Onus was placed on each individual to 'look at nature with your own eyes, to observe and think for yourselves', to 'walk on your own feet', so that students' eyes, ears and hands were their key 'instruments' for effective learning.[36] When Struthers asserted that anatomy was of 'fundamental professional importance', he did so at a time when medical students were increasingly expected to be industrious and orderly.[37] While some dissecting-room activity, especially in the 1830s and '40s, was reported as rowdy and coarse, during the second half of the nineteenth century anatomists stressed the necessity of disciplined practical study in the adoption of approved professional conduct.[38]

Learning to observe anatomical actualities, then, required particular bodily actions and mental work in designated spaces where 'nature' – that is, human and animal bodies – was made to seem directly apprehensible. Enabling students to gain knowledge in approved ways, Struthers 'set his face against words', which was not to reject lectures (indeed he remarked on the 'stimulus' of the 'living voice' when heard in lectures) but rather to ensure that his teaching was, above all, 'demonstrative' – an approach favoured in other medical schools, such as at University College London, where teachers 'endeavour[ed] to impart a knowledge of things, in opposition to a knowledge of words'.[39] Declaring that the most 'vicious' lecturing consisted of 'cramming or grinding', which overloaded the student's memory (especially in preparation for exams), Struthers instead combined the 'exhibition of objects and phenomena with the enunciation of ideas and principles', displaying bodily interiors so that 'concrete images of things' not 'verbal descriptions' were retained in students' minds.[40] Words were necessary but they were subordinated to things made to appear more actual than words (even though words – in the form of labels, narratives and anatomical descriptions as indicated below – were significant in constituting that actuality). To gain anatomical knowledge at 'first hand' was to observe in what was regarded as an unmediated way, free from interference – such a pursuit of objectivity having emerged forcefully in mid-nineteenth-century scientific practices.[41] And for the 'objective method' to be performed and learned, anatomists taught with bodies in the flesh, on paper and in the form of three-dimensional models.[42]

Deceased bodies were considered absolutely essential for anatomical learning: freshly dissected parts were to be shown in lectures, anatomists insisted, and each student was to dissect for themselves. But supplies of bodies were often unreliable, varying according to geographical location, with significant repercussions for teaching practices.[43] In Scotland, Glasgow reportedly had ample 'material' in the 1870s due to the larger 'pauper population', and one suggestion (though not implemented) was to transport bodies by railway, at night, to other medical schools in need of them, for example at Edinburgh University.[44] In mid-nineteenth-century Aberdeen, numbers of unclaimed bodies obtained from the funeratory were considered 'very scanty', and available only 'irregularly'. These 'uncertain and fluctuating circumstances' continued into the 1880s.[45] John Struthers's first year at Marischal College coincided with a decline in numbers and, although these sometimes increased, he monitored them closely, remaining sensitized to periodic downturns and deficiencies measured in relation to rising student numbers.[46] In years when fewer bodies were procured, therefore, students' opportunities to dissect were correspondingly reduced. Thus, while bodies were usually divided into parts, with each student paying a 'small sum' for each one they dissected, the total proportion of the whole body that a student might dissect was heavily dependent on the extent and regularity of their medical school's supply.[47] An amendment to the Anatomy Act in 1871 eased problems of shortages slightly by extending the period that bodies could be kept for dissection (before burial) to eight weeks.

Alongside dead bodies, a range of resources for practical study was produced and utilized, with carefully preserved anatomical collections assigned high pedagogical value, especially given the instabilities of corpse acquisition. Displays highlighted salient anatomical aspects: bones, joints, muscles, organs of sense and viscera. The human body was studied both 'topographically' (in terms of the arrangement and relations of structures within regions) and as 'systems of organs which fulfil definite functions', such as the vascular and the nervous systems.[48] Struthers offered visual instruction with blackboard sketches and diagrams which he drew during his teaching sessions, 'filling in the outlines as he proceeded'. His drawings on paper, made by his 'own hand, and many of them direct from nature', provided longer-lasting visual investigations and records of his dissections.[49] Large-scale anatomical wall charts and atlases were also purchased for teaching. Students at Marischal College could view, for instance, Francis Sibson's *Medical Anatomy* (1869), which claimed advantage over decaying bodies on dissecting tables with its colour illustrations (illus. 72).[50]

The validity of these images was reinforced by Sibson's description of the meticulous procedures adhered to in their making and the 'mechanical aids' that ensured their 'precision': from his dissections he traced 'outlines' of organs to provide 'groundwork' for the coloured drawings and lithographs that William Fairland 'executed with untiring care'. Sibson consequently referred to the illustrations as 'literal transcripts' of bodies. Although he stressed that these transcripts represented organs 'exactly as

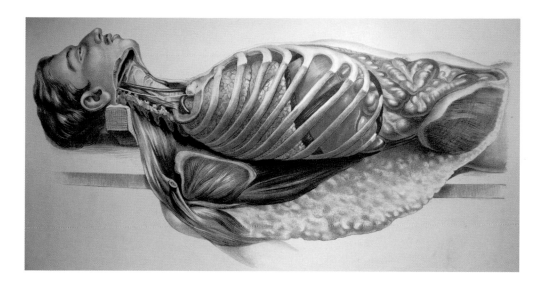

William Fairland,
illustration showing
ribs, organs and
blood vessels,
coloured lithograph
from Francis Sibson,
Medical Anatomy
(London, 1869),
Plato X.

they were found after death', they were not so literal as to prevent the suggestion of life beneath the body's deceased surface: the vibrant anatomical interior, with bright red blood vessels, was made to contrast with grey, deathly skin. Indeed, Sibson acknowledged that 'accurate representations' of the dead were deficient in conveying knowledge of the body as it was before the 'departure of life'. So his atlas also included pairs of illustrations, one body depicted dead beside the same body with internal organs (their size and position) shown as though alive. This visual doubling furthered Sibson's aim to communicate living 'physiological truths', especially of respiration and circulation; it illuminated descriptions of the lungs' movements when breathing, the heart's motions and sounds when beating.[51]

Further volumes available to students in the second half of the nineteenth century sought, in smaller, more affordable formats, to provide 'good practical illustrations' with an emphasis on 'correctness, clearness and simplicity'. According to one publication of 1880, again used in Marischal College's Anatomical Department, overly embellished illustrations with illegible labels were a source of 'erroneous ideas', leading students into a 'maze of wonder and uncertainty'.[52] To guard against this, images were visually pared down, rendered as uncomplicated lines that students' eyes and fingers could follow without getting lost (illus. 73). Plainness was linked with practicality, and, like the hugely successful *Anatomy, Descriptive and Surgical* (known as *Gray's Anatomy*), first published in 1858, this book was designed for convenient use while dissecting and its illustrations were akin to Henry Vandyke Carter's simplified compositions with integrated labelling as published in *Gray's*.[53] The 1880 atlas urged students to verify all textual descriptions in the dissecting room, reinforcing the importance

73
Illustration of the
'topography of
the abdomen' from
J. Osborne-Walker,
*The Descriptive Atlas
of Anatomy* (London,
1880).

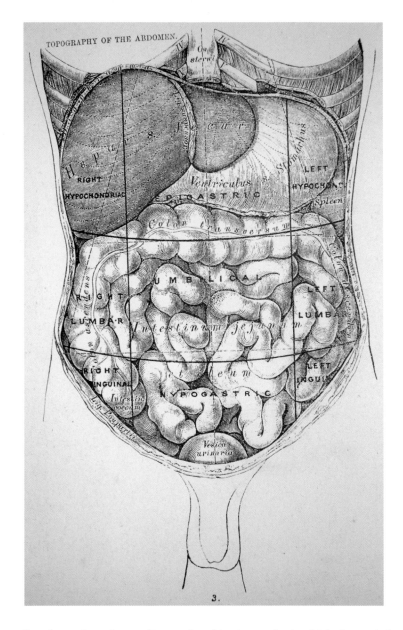

of work conducted according to the objective method, which demanded far more than studying printed illustrations. As Struthers insisted, the properly rigorous use of books was necessarily in conjunction with the study of recently deceased bodies and preserved specimens. Furthermore, while mechanical means of producing precise anatomical images, of seemingly minimizing or at least regulating human intervention, were valued positively,[54] as in Sibson's atlas, attempts to learn in ways deemed mechanical – that is, perfunctory or uninvolved – were viewed negatively. Students were not expected to be passive 'onlookers', but to become demonstrably involved in learning, especially in active observation.[55]

Facilitating this in practice required close work with bodies, human and animal; it necessitated sustained museum-making. Students' skills, both visual and manual, were gained by dissecting, but learning to observe also took place in museums where a wider range of specimens could be proximately and unhurriedly examined on shelves even if glass cases prevented tactile contact with them (while protecting them from 'the ever-recurring cost and trouble of dusting').[56] So, although anatomists would not generally allow bulky, delicate or especially valuable museum specimens to be moved, they also sought to provide specimens that students could 'handle', while endeavouring to protect these from 'injury' due to carelessness or simply to their carriage backwards and forwards.[57]

PROTOTYPE

Forming a museum took time. As Struthers pointed out in 1876, after thirteen years in Aberdeen, the Anatomical Museum was 'as yet only growing'.[58] Some of this growth was achieved through comprehensive collecting practices, described later, but it was also stimulated by observation of museums regarded as exemplary models for designing further ones. Struthers was well acquainted with museums in Edinburgh, Glasgow, St Andrews, London, Dublin, Paris, Berlin and Vienna. At Marischal College he was very familiar with the museums of natural history (encompassing geology and zoology), of botany and of pathology. What he envisaged for the Anatomical Museum was based on three 'models' in particular, museums that (around 1863) he regarded as especially relevant, authoritative and inspiring: the Anatomical Museum of Edinburgh University, that of John Barclay at the RCSEd and the Hunterian Museum at the RCS in London.[59]

Barclay's collection, displayed at the RCSEd from 1832, was particularly rich in comparative anatomy and Struthers had used this for teaching in Edinburgh from the mid-1840s.[60] Here Struthers regarded the skeletons of larger animals, including an elephant and ostrich, a horse and dolphin, as the most compelling part of the collection, making drawings for his classes on comparative osteology (the study of bones) and teaching in the museum space among Barclay's collection if relevant specimens were too large for moving to the lecture theatre.[61] Edinburgh University's Anatomical Museum also featured comparative anatomy in addition to 'normal and pathological' human anatomy. However, in the 1870s, according to William Turner, professor of anatomy and this museum's curator, it was in 'miserable condition' regarding space. It was 'blocked up' with many thousands of specimens, so much so that many animal skeletons were stowed in boxes and there was hardly a 'gangway for students to move about in'. Specimens needed to be 'properly arranged' and the manuscript catalogue made available in print.[62] Progress was made by 1884: the expanded Anatomical Museum in Edinburgh's newly built medical school boasted spacious glass cases, two galleries, spiral staircases, an Italian mosaic floor and furniture monogrammed with *AM* (illus. 74).[63]

John Struthers also 'took some hints' from the Hunterian Museum at the RCS.[64] Hunter had amassed in excess of 13,000 human, animal and plant specimens, healthy and pathological, for studying and teaching anatomy and surgery during the second half of the eighteenth century.[65] Rehoused in the RCS, the collection continued to expand. In the 1850s the gallery shelves held a comparative series of specimens in glass jars showing organs in different animals categorized according to function. On the ground floor, skulls and bones of vertebrates were displayed in wall cabinets, with the larger articulated skeletons on platforms in the centre.[66] An

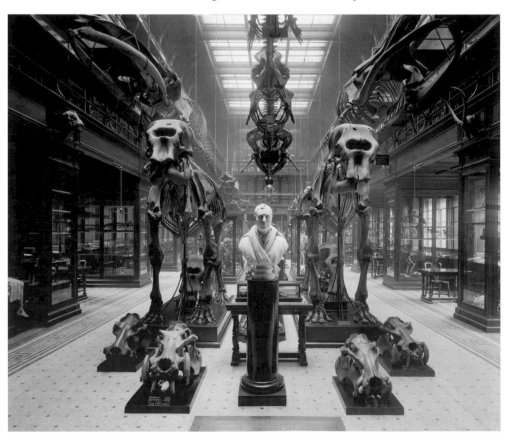

74
Anatomical Museum at the University of Edinburgh Medical School, 1895, photograph by Harry Bedford Lemere.

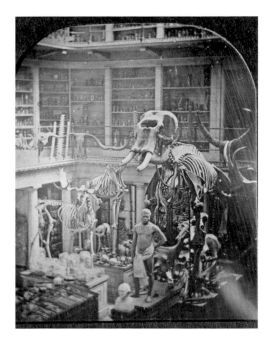

75
One of a pair
of stereoscopic
photographs of the
Hunterian Museum,
Royal College of
Surgeons of England,
London, 1852.

1852 stereoscopic daguerreotype offered a three-dimensional view of the museum showing a bust of John Hunter before a plaster cast of an African man, and the skeletons of an elephant, Irish elk and a giraffe minus its skull (illus. 75). The following three decades, during William Flower's conservatorship, saw growth in the collection of comparative osteology, with skeletons of vertebrates, including whales, camels and crocodiles, exhibited prominently.[67]

By using the Hunterian Museum as a source of inspiration, Struthers drew from what was widely regarded as a centre of science. Within Aberdeen's medical community this view was expressed in 1868, for instance, by a pathologist at the Royal Infirmary who, when applying for a position as museum assistant to William Flower, explained that Aberdeen was 'too far removed from the centres of scientific activity so placing me at a considerable disadvantage'.[68] Flower underlined the Hunterian Museum's authority and influence when he described it, in 1881, as the 'predecessor and prototype' of anatomical museums in Britain, America and many in Continental Europe. Nevertheless he recognized the Hunterian's 'faults of construction and arrangement' – especially the separation of bottled from dried specimens, casts and models, which could not be accommodated on the same narrow gallery shelves.[69] Flower preferred the possibility of arranging displays in which specimens could be positioned alongside and therefore in connection with relevant objects in different media.

When museum-making in Aberdeen, Struthers aimed for a 'smaller scale' anatomical museum with a 'select collection' suitable for a provincial university rather than one on the 'metropolitan scale' aspiring to 'universality'. Within the architectural context and spatial constraints of Marischal College, Struthers abandoned his initial plan for a 'large general anatomical and pathological museum' combining 'normal' anatomy with specimens of diseases and malformations, and concentrated instead on the Anatomical Museum as 'separate' from the college's Pathological Museum. While some malformations were displayed in the former, the latter was the main site where the pathology collection developed. A further distinction was maintained between the Anatomical Museum – this, primarily of human anatomy with a comparative collection comprising parts of 'the

76
Articulated
skeletons from the
Anatomical Museum,
c. 1860–1900, in the
Anatomy Department,
Marischal College,
University of
Aberdeen, c. 1900,
photograph.

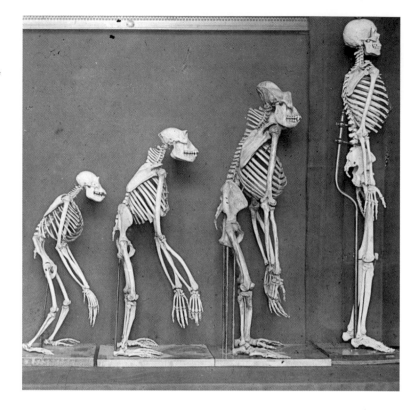

76
Articulated
skeletons from the
Anatomical Museum,
c. 1860–1900, in the
Anatomy Department,
Marischal College,
University of
Aberdeen, c. 1900,
photograph.

higher animals, constructed like the human body on the vertebrate type, as serve to illustrate human structure' – and the zoology collection in Marischal College's Natural History Museum (which opened to the public from the 1860s onwards; see illus. 157).[70]

In the Anatomical Department Struthers instructed medical students to keep 'their eye on the object', to learn from careful observation, whether of an enormous elephant skeleton or tiny human foetal bones (see illus. 90).[71] Displays of skeletons demonstrated relations between humans and apes, and students admired how Struthers made the 'evolutionary idea run in the valley of dry bones, so making the bones live' (illus. 76).[72] In addition to enhancing students' learning, Struthers saw potential in the Anatomical Museum for 'promoting an interest in biological science in the city and district'.[73] How this museum was formed mainly for anatomical learning but also for the wider dissemination of science is explored next with attention to the social relations of collecting and the practices that constituted the collection as a valuable source of anatomical knowledge.

Conducting lessons in anatomy required numerous museum specimens produced from deceased human and animal bodies, which anatomists obtained via their social networks. Struthers mobilized extensive social connections with wide geographical reach, and drew substantially on the local region, to yield a profusion of bodily parts to the extent that he became well known in Aberdeen as an avid and determined collector. He received regular praise in local newspapers for his educational work: an 1886 edition of the *Aberdeen Weekly Journal*, for instance, published a sympathetic description of him as an 'enthusiastic scientist' who was 'honourable' and authoritative (though with minor 'blemishes' of 'fussiness' and 'personal vanity'), accompanying this text with a portrait sketch of Struthers in full academic dress. Following this he was humorously caricatured in the *Bon-Accord* as a rag-and-bone man (illus. 77) – a gatherer and recycler who would collect unwanted items from house to house with a horse-drawn cart.[74]

In this image the Anatomical Museum was a wooden barrow, trundled around by Struthers busily acquiring skulls and calling out, according to the caption, 'The highest prices given for OLD BONES'. A package, labelled 'Bones with Care', and a travel tag addressed to Marischal College perhaps

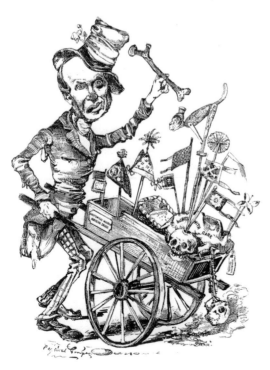

77
Caricature of John Struthers in an 1886 issue of the Aberdeen newspaper *Bon-Accord*. The label on the barrow reads 'ANATOMICAL MUSEUM, MARISCHAL COLLEGE'.

referred to human remains sent to the museum from many distant places. The toy monkey wearing a hat had a dual function. First, it represented an organ-grinder's monkey, which would often accompany this familiar street performer, and by implication the anatomist was such a performer (a mechanical grinder of human organs?) with a museum-cum-barrel-organ on wheels.[75] Second, the monkey alluded to Struthers's commitment to Darwin's theories.[76] This interrelation of the learned and the popular is an apt theme with regard to anatomical collecting and display to which this chapter later returns. But here, with regard to the anatomist as collector, a further aspect of the image is especially pertinent: although in the caricature Struthers publicly gathers human bones (whereas rag-and-bone men dealt with animal bones), in practice the process of acquiring human remains was much more discreet than Struthers's more publicly visible quest for animal remains – especially in the case of bodies obtained for dissection, which remained a matter of considerable discretion.

Struthers's own private collection provided a foundation for the Anatomical Museum in which it was displayed, although it was kept in its own cases and therefore clearly demarcated as his property.[77] He was deeply attached to this collection, declaring, after his retirement in 1889: 'these specimens follow me everywhere; they went with me to Aberdeen; they sojourned there; and now they have followed me back here' – Struthers was speaking in the Museum of the RCSEd, where he was president and to which he presented this private collection in 1896.[78] By then his collection numbered over 1,600 specimens, including human bones, hearts, lungs, blood vessels, nerves and tendons, having grown in the Anatomical Museum at Marischal College alongside the collection belonging to the institution, the two collections differentiated yet informing one another.[79] This was not unusual: from the early nineteenth century, private collections in Britain had often formed 'a seed for an institutional museum', as in Glasgow and Edinburgh.[80]

Many of Struthers's own specimens were prepared from human bodies brought to dissecting rooms for teaching and research. Anatomists expected to keep such specimens as records of their findings to be deployed in various ways: as museum displays, exhibits at scholarly meetings and (when drawn) as illustrations in scientific publications. Their positions of power in relation to the dead obtained for dissection enabled the appropriation of body parts which in many cases were largely disassociated from specific deceased persons through the execution of anatomical work. During the 1850s in Edinburgh Struthers preserved malformations of the intestines and an instance of a double uterus.[81] Dissections at Marischal College produced a 'series of specimens illustrating variation of the vertebrae and ribs' as well as others relating to the supra-condyloid process of the humerus (a bony growth near the elbow on the upper arm bone), one of Struthers's research interests – and probably the bone held up by the anatomist in the caricature (see illus. 77).[82] While these specimens accrued to his own collection, the dissecting room was also a site of collecting for the Anatomical Museum, as in the case of an interesting 'variation' in a man's wrists discovered in 1869 – the bones as well as the ligaments were cleaned and preserved.[83]

This route from dissecting room to museum was routinely traversed so that body parts could be preserved for further observation and teaching. The dissecting room itself was dependent on supplies of bodies obtained from the funeratory, which received deceased paupers from Aberdeen's poor houses and infirmary. From there carefully managed acquisitions were

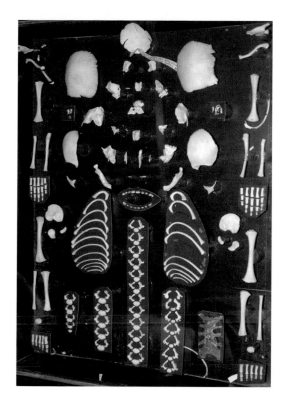

78 Case displaying disarticulated bones of a foetus at the stage of development shortly before birth, late 19th–early 20th century.

made. Each unclaimed body was discreetly transported to Struthers's department – in a shell (coffin) and in a 'decent and orderly manner' – by the funeratory's superintendent and porters, who also took the dissected 'remains' of each person back to that institution before interment. This transit of bodies was mostly conducted after dark.[84]

Two notable aspects of Struthers's private collection were foetal and comparative anatomy and these, especially the latter, were also comprehensively developed in the Anatomical Museum from the 1860s onwards, so that private collection and institutional museum developed in tandem.[85] For example, from human foetuses Struthers prepared blood vessels, such as those of the liver, and a malformed heart for his own collection in the 1840s and '50s. Similarly, for the Anatomical Museum, he purchased a series of nine articulated foetal skeletons mounted in standing position and arranged in ascending order to show growth during nine months of gestation.[86] Obtained in 1873, along with a further 'young' skull (see illus. 103), they were most probably bought from Maison Tramond, the Paris-based supplier of osteological specimens that also devised boxed displays of symmetrically arranged disarticulated foetal skeletons, including ossicles of the ear and tiny teeth (illus. 78).

Comparative anatomy – which became central to the Anatomical Museum – also figured in Struthers's private collection. The latter incorporated, for instance, a large part of the 'considerable museum' formed by Robert Knox (1791–1862), whose forte, according to Struthers, had been 'bringing comparative anatomy to the explanation of human anatomy'.[87] Knox's collection had passed to Struthers via two previous owners, both of whom taught anatomy in Edinburgh: Henry Lonsdale purchased most of it in 1842, then gave it to Peter Handyside in 1845, and Struthers bought it about two years later, along with Handyside's preparations.[88] Knox's specimens were dissected and preserved with assistance from his brother Frederick Knox, who was in no doubt about the importance of collecting for the practice of anatomy: without museums, he declared, 'the profession would be in the state of man without a language.'[89] In compiling his collection, Robert Knox was influenced by Georges Cuvier, with whom he studied in Paris (1821–2), and whose collection of comparative anatomy at the Muséum d'histoire naturelle (formerly the Jardin des plantes) he much admired.[90] Motivated by these interests during the 1820s and '30s, Knox acquired specimens of human anatomy, especially bones, but also, for instance, skeletons of fish, birds and snakes, and crania of larger mammals.[91]

At Marischal College, Struthers moved outwards from his private collection to expand the Anatomical Museum, drawing on his social and material environment to assemble numerous vertebrate animals for comparison with 'human structure'.[92] He lost no time in persuading the Aberdeen Medico-Chirurgical Society to release its crocodile skeleton, which it had retained when it transferred its anatomical preparations to Marischal College in 1859. Struthers hoped to keep it for the Anatomical Museum but reluctantly returned it after a decade on loan (see illus. 71).[93] With a small annual university fund Struthers purchased further specimens from commercial dealers. Horse and sheep skulls already cleaned, labelled and mounted on stands, for example, were obtained from Moore Brothers, a firm of osteology dealers in Liverpool. But the raw material of dead animals and their parts, obtained at a lesser cost in the local region and prepared in-house for the Anatomical Museum, was considered a richer source of skeletal specimens. When out walking in the country Struthers would search for suitable animal remains, for example the bones of sheep that he 'picked up on the hills'.[94] The carcases of a horse, cow, dog and boar were acquired locally and that of a red deer was secured from Queen Victoria's nearby estate at Balmoral. This bone gathering led the anatomist (and/or his assistants), aided by workers such as butchers and gamekeepers, from the city's slaughterhouses to royal grounds.

Beaches and harbours provided access to animal parts that were particularly valued by Struthers for research and for display in the Anatomical Museum. Arrangements made with ships' captains sailing from Scotland's northeast coast to the Arctic proved particularly productive. Struthers acquired, for instance, the bones of a Greenland bear and a seal from whaling ships. He was keen to explore cetacean anatomy, particularly in terms of anatomical variation and adaptation, and whalers again helped the anatomist obtain remains of these mammals. Parts of ten Greenland right whales from Davis Strait (between Baffin Island and Greenland), for example, were acquired in this way during the 1870s.[95] After dissecting and examining pelvic bones and rudimentary hind limbs, making life-size drawings from dissections, writing descriptions and recording tables of measurements, he retained some of the specimens for his own collection and for the Anatomical Museum, then donated others to museums at the universities of Edinburgh and Glasgow, and the British Museum.[96] For the anatomist, specimens could thus either be conserved or distributed to further museums, thereby consolidating the collections in Aberdeen, enhancing his status as a museum donor and presenting gifts that might be later reciprocated.

When whales washed up or became stranded along the coast, from Dundee to Peterhead and Wick, Struthers would either visit the site in person or secure parts of these creatures with the aid of his contacts. Either way Struthers was dependent on local cooperation for the success of his collecting endeavours.[97] During the 1880s Struthers continued to anatomize whales, accumulating numerous osteological specimens, some arranged in series, to enable comparison, some forming 'striking preparations' in the Anatomical Department's lobby.[98] In 1884 a beluga whale, previously trapped in salmon fishing nets at Caithness and obtained by Adam Mackay, one of Struthers's students, was brought to the anatomy rooms at Marischal College, where it was photographed and rapidly dissected. The viscera, including sections of the 91-ft (27.8-m) intestine, were transferred temporarily to the Anatomical Museum for further examination.[99] The same year, Struthers relocated his anatomy class to Aberdeen's Recreation Grounds, a setting regularly used for sports and by touring menageries and circuses, where a 50-ft (15-m) great fin whale was exhibited.[100] Having been stranded at Nairn (near Inverness), the whale was purchased by an Aberdeen whale-oil merchant and transported to the city as a popular attraction.[101] Here Struthers was allowed to temporarily work on the whale, giving a 'demonstration of the characters of this species' for his students, and measuring it with Robert Gibb, his assistant and attendant of the Anatomical Museum from 1872.[102] He then purchased its skeleton, which Gibb helped to clean, articulate and suspend from the ceiling of the Anatomical Department's corridor (see illus. 89).[103]

The collection and anatomical examination of whales intersected with a range of industrial, commercial and exhibition practices. This was particularly apparent when Struthers had tried to purchase a 40-ft (12-m) humpback whale in January 1884. The mammal had initially appeared in the Firth of Tay near Dundee, where it was wounded by whalers in pursuit. Fishermen then towed it, dead, into Stonehaven harbour, near Aberdeen. There Struthers made measurements, and photographs were taken by Aberdeen photographer George Washington Wilson (1823–1893). At auction Struthers was outbid by John Woods, a Dundee whale-oil merchant, who exhibited the 16-ton mammal at his yard.[104] It became a major attraction for thousands of people curious to see a 'giant of the deep' and willing to pay the admission fee.[105] Struthers was invited to dissect the whale at the exhibition site, with assistants including Gibb and several whalers. When they arrived to 'perform' the strenuous task they were undeterred by the difficulties noted by Struthers, namely a crowd of spectators admitted by Wood and a military band also arranged by this 'astute proprietor', not to mention a snowstorm which periodically drove them from their task.[106]

That the whale's viscera was decomposing did not help the procedure – as Struthers later wrote, 'we tried to preserve the heart, but our hands went through it.'[107] Bowels, flesh and blubber were moved to barrels for conversion into manure and oil.[108] Pelvic bones, rudimentary hind limbs and vertebrae were packed off for study in Struthers's Anatomical Department. The whale was then embalmed, and a wooden backbone and rib-cage inserted so that this 'wonderfully-restored' (and lighter) creature could be toured to Aberdeen (where it was shown in a marquee at the Recreation Grounds), and then to Glasgow, Liverpool, Manchester and Edinburgh.[109] Scientists, naturalists, professors and students flocked to see the whale, as did children from charitable institutions who were invited to view it without charge.[110] At the end of its eight-month tour, John Woods permitted Struthers to retrieve the rest of its bones and to prepare the skeleton in Aberdeen, so that Woods could then donate it for exhibition at the Dundee Museum. The significance of these remains was inflected by the extensive reporting the whale received during its journey from capture to exhibition: numerous telegrams and newspaper articles produced narratives of the hunt with harpoons and explosive bombs, of its transportation in wagons and train trucks which formed a peculiar funereal procession.[111] Struthers's own anatomical account, recognizing the cruelty of the kill, praised the whale's 'great strength' when fighting furiously for life in waters coloured red by so much blood.[112]

Struthers's access to the whale's anatomy was enabled by the work of whalers, fishermen and a merchant, and had to be negotiated in the context of various commercial uses of the carcase. But this navigation through the industrial processing of the whale, including phases of exhibiting, was of benefit to the anatomist, who gleaned from it valuable material for display in a range of venues. During the Aberdeen leg of the whale tour, Struthers gave a public lecture on parts of its skeleton, explaining the existence of rudimentary structures in terms of the 'doctrine of evolution', and exhibiting enlarged drawings of the whale based on photographs by George Washington Wilson.[113] At the 1884 meeting of the British Association for the Advancement of Science in Montreal, Canada, he delivered a paper on this whale (*Megaptera longimana*), concluding that the thigh bone is 'a vestige of a more complete limb possessed by some ancestral form from which the Megaptera is descended'.[114]

At Marischal College, Struthers attended to the whale's skeleton, as one student recalled, tirelessly 'gathering facts':

> day after day, for hours on hours, those observations went forward
> . . . until one imagined some great Cetacean tailor dictating
> measurements for winter furs in the Kara Sea [of the Arctic Ocean].
> But the anatomist revelled in the details, which were to determine
> the species.[115]

Preparing the skeleton for display was a lengthy procedure – it had to be cleaned, drained of oil and bleached in the sun – and Struthers was reluctant to return it more speedily to its owner. He explained to Woods that until oil had stopped oozing from the bones it would smell too much to be placed in a museum – Dundee Museum would have the skeleton, he promised, 'as soon as it is in a fit state to be put in the museum without offence to the nostrils of the visitors'.[116] In the meantime, students remarked that the odour in the anatomy rooms of Marischal College was 'like the deck of a Greenland whaler'.[117] At the end of 1889, the year that Struthers retired, the Tay Whale, as it became known, was sent in railway wagons to its Dundee destination.[118] Two years later Struthers visited the skeleton, which he considered his 'old friend', and which was by then on public show; he gave a lecture and provoked great laughter by presenting the Dundee Museum with a hair of the whale's beard in a small phial – and he was rewarded with a 'valuable walking-stick, made of a unicorn's horn and gold mounted', sent by Woods as a 'token of respect' for the anatomist's 'great interest' in the whale.[119]

NATURALIST AND TAXIDERMIST

The interrelated processes of collecting, dissection and display were sustained through Struthers's social relationships with relatives and friends, (former) students, medical associates, local doctors and workers in various industries.[120] There were, however, particular persons, whom Struthers acknowledged in publications, who were especially helpful in their contributions to the Anatomical Museum. Many whalers participated in Struthers's collecting practices, but the efforts of one particular ship's captain, David Gray (1828–1896), of an established whaling family at Peterhead, were made prominent. Gray was known, as Struthers noted, for his 'very large experience in the Greenland whale fishing', and he was also a keen naturalist, making detailed studies of the habits of whales and seals, and collecting animals as well as artefacts when sailing in the Arctic.[121] In the 1880s Gray answered Struthers's anatomical queries, supplying whale measurements and a drawing of a Greenland right whale. The captain's son, Dr Robert Gray, had studied with Struthers and he also gave the anatomist accounts of whales and a drawing 'made from nature' while employed on his father's ship, the *Eclipse*.[122] On one of David Gray's voyages he had a wooden model of a captured right whale made (at one inch to the foot): this he exhibited at the Aberdeen meeting of the British Association for the Advancement of Science in 1885 and William Flower obtained it for the British Museum (Natural History), where he was director (1884 to 1898).[123] A copy of the model also went to the Anatomical Museum at Marischal College (see illus. 87, centre).[124]

Another of Struthers's local collaborators in collecting, George Sim (1835–1908), based in Aberdeen, also examined and sketched stranded whales during his frequent excursions to beaches in the area.[125] Sim became an esteemed naturalist to whom Struthers acknowledged 'frequent obligation' for often providing 'viscera of various animals' to the Anatomical Museum.[126] By giving, and having these animal parts accepted, from the late 1860s onwards, Sim gained status as well as privileged access to anatomical activities: in 1884–5, for instance, he assisted Struthers in measuring a great fin-whale, and in dissecting the Tay Whale at Dundee.[127] Indeed, the naturalist's practices of collecting and display overlapped, in some ways, with the anatomist's. Like Struthers, Sim scoured the local terrain for potential specimens. He regularly explored rock pools, coastal areas and woods, travelling by foot, train and tricycle. Just as the anatomist sought fish and birds for the Anatomical Museum, so Sim would collect for his own purposes. However, unlike Struthers, Sim also acquired insects and crustacea, finding these already dead or catching them in traps.[128] He recorded the appearances, habits and sounds of creatures in notebooks – in which he also described his thoughts, feelings and dreams – along with observations of the weather and the coastal conditions most conducive to collecting.[129] In April 1867, for instance, in the early hours of one morning he went to the beach to see what might have been 'cast up' by the unusually rough sea. He found a 'beautiful confusion', among which were 'onions, carrots, greens, turnips, rhubarb, berry-bushes, ivy, holly, and lilies', and he picked up some salmon, trout, haddock and eels killed by this vegetable wreck.[130]

Combining activities as a naturalist with business, Sim opened his Aberdeen taxidermy shop in 1862, following an apprenticeship with a tailor and subsequent training with an Edinburgh-based taxidermist (illus. 79).[131] He purchased skins, such as wild cat, badger, polecat and goat, so that they could be 'stuffed' or 'dressed'. He made rugs from deerskins and fashionable jackets from fur, according to clients' specifications, and mounted deers' heads and horns for clients including Captain Alexander Gray of Peterhead, David Gray's brother.[132] Sim also skinned animals himself, and in the process he would discover innards of possible interest

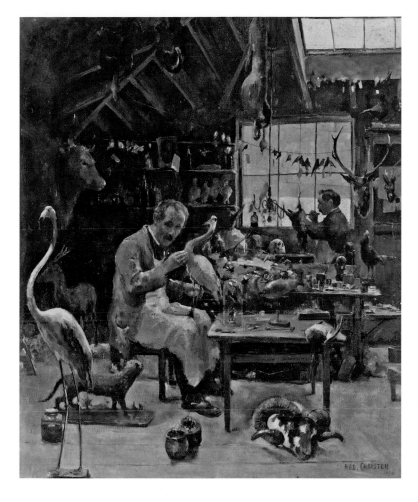

to Struthers: he noticed a 'strange anatomical peculiarity' in a squirrel skeleton in 1868, for example, which he gave to the anatomist.[133] There were frequent transfers of viscera, in particular, from Sim's workshop to the Anatomical Museum at Marischal College.[134] For the taxidermist was primarily concerned not with internal organs but with the preservation of skin with scales, fur or feathers (and selected bones), from which he created specimens, sculpted with lifelike 'form, proportions and attitude', so that they resembled their living versions.[135] A flamingo, for instance, was made to retain its proper shape and plumage (illus. 80). In this way the taxidermist fashioned animals for public exhibitions, shop windows, domestic interiors and for sartorial show, unlike the anatomist, whose main concern was to display 'internal structure' to advance anatomical understanding.[136]

The collecting practices of Sim and Struthers were thus complementary when they sought to preserve different parts of animal bodies, just as their

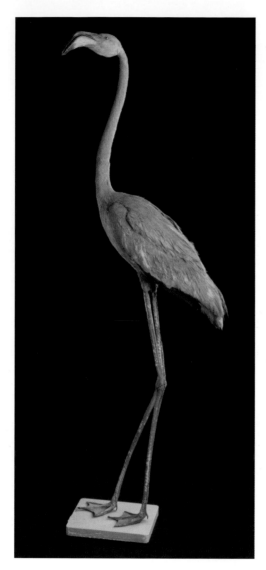

80
Flamingo, prepared by George Sim (of Aberdeen), late 19th century.

interests, social relationships and museum activities intersected. Both Sim and Struthers visited institutions such as the Muséum national d'histoire naturelle, presented specimens to the British Museum (Sim donated crustacea in 1868 and 1878) and purchased specimens from the same commercial model maker and osteological supplier, Maison Tramond.[137] They both operated within a culture of collecting, which was both local and international, where natural history was a burgeoning field of popular as well as learned enquiry.[138] Both were active members of the Aberdeen Natural History Society, begun in 1863, which held regular evening meetings at Marischal College, sometimes in the Anatomical Department.[139] Its members were men from the university and town who conducted fieldwork and collected botanical, geological and zoological specimens, exhibiting and discussing these at their gatherings. In 1885 women were encouraged to join the society and to take part in local excursions to the coast and woods where they would search for seaweeds, shells, flowers, grasses and mosses.[140]

Another regular participant in the Aberdeen Natural History Society was Robert Gibb, Struthers's assistant and the Anatomical Museum attendant. He and George Sim went on many local excursions together over many years, collecting birds' eggs, investigating a small beached whale in 1877 and hunting for bats in the cathedral of Old Aberdeen in 1891. They visited public museums in nearby towns where birds, fish and insects were displayed and also scrutinized private collections, including that of another George Sim (of Gourdas) in Aberdeenshire (illus. 81).[141] While Gibb formed his own collection of natural history, he also spent much time gathering material for Struthers to use as specimens when teaching comparative anatomy.[142] Sim joined Gibb on these searches, going 'in quest' for creatures such as mussels required for microscopic study: at the pier, Sim recorded in June 1877, 'we had to take off shoes and stockings to reach them, water bitterly cold'.[143]

During these trips the taxidermist made observations and conversed with his friend about shared natural-historical interests. Thus Sim became familiar with the Anatomical Museum, not only gifting to it but communicating with others about its holdings. Sim's 1879 correspondence with Charles Darwin on issues relating to heredity, for example, referred to the museum's preserved legs of a cow, and her young, which both showed the same 'peculiarity' of three toes on her fore feet.[144] Here the taxidermist disseminated information regarding the museum's specimens, citing them to bolster his scientific communications. This was not unlike Struthers's approach to specimen circulation: in 1864 he had written to Darwin regarding his anatomical research interests on the 'supra-condyloid process

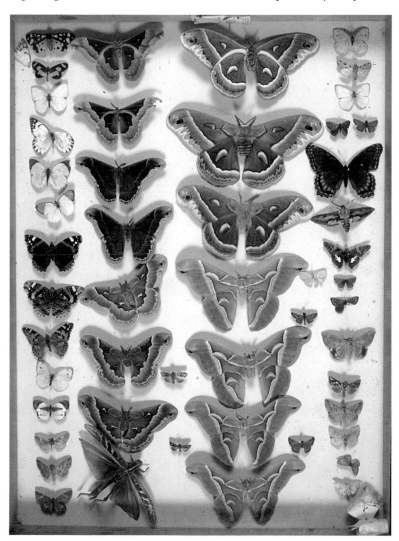

81
Case displaying butterflies, moths and a locust, collected by George Sim (of Gourdas, Aberdeenshire), late 19th century.

in the human arm . . . in relation to the subject of variation' – offering to send some of his many specimens for Darwin to 'inspect'.[145] Thus it was in this context of social connection, collaboration and communication that the Anatomical Museum's displays were expanded, viewed and discussed.

EXTENDED CONNECTIONS

So the Anatomical Museum grew within its locality but also within a nexus of social connections extending through Britain and overseas. To obtain animal skeletons, Struthers utilized Aberdeen-based industries involved in international trade, such as the meat-preserving works where meat and fish were packed in tins for export. Through one such firm, with connections in Australia, Struthers acquired the bones of an emu, apteryx and large turtle.[146] While these were probably purchased, Struthers also drew animal remains to the Anatomical Museum through exchanges with other organizations and museums. When elected as a member of the London-based Anthropological Institute of Great Britain and Ireland in 1873, Struthers gave two human skulls to its museum and, in return, he could anticipate assistance with further acquisitions.[147] Indeed, through the institute, he obtained the bones of several apes (see illus. 76).[148]

Reciprocity, to facilitate museum-making, also characterized Struthers's interactions with the RCS in London. When, in 1868, Struthers sent a tiger's clavicle to William Flower, the latter responded by offering to help procure bones for the Anatomical Museum. Three years later Struthers enlisted his help in evaluating a gorilla skin and skeleton offered for sale by a dealer in London. Unable to view these in person and with 'little faith in the completeness of skeletons not prepared by an Anatomist', Struthers sought Flowers's opinion. A report on the gorilla was swiftly returned and, although this animal was too young for Struthers's purposes and therefore not purchased, he thanked Flower for his efforts with the promise of a 15-ft (4.6-m) whale skeleton. This had been recently delivered to Marischal College from a nearby beach and, as the Anatomical Museum already held a similar skeleton, Struthers had intended to prepare and save it 'for some chance exchange'. Now Struthers explained to Flower, 'it would give me much pleasure to present it to your Museum' – but, Struthers insisted, Flower must not hesitate to decline if the whale was 'not worth Museum space'.[149] Such exchanges, with their expected etiquette, were an important aspect of relationships through which collections accrued. Thus anatomical specimens were simultaneously sources of knowledge and resources for establishing and strengthening social and learned connections.

Former students fuelled the Anatomical Museum's expansion when they sent animal and human remains from overseas as gifts in return for their education at Marischal College, their alma mater. For instance, George King, superintendent of the Calcutta Botanic Garden in the Indian Medical Service (1871–98), gave the bones of a camel, a young elephant and a crocodile.[150] Between 1860 and 1900 over one-third of medical graduates from the University of Aberdeen went overseas to work in imperial service and the military, independent practice and private companies.[151] From their destinations these men, often in senior positions, sent bones to Struthers for the museum. In accompanying letters they expressed thanks to an admired teacher, and explained where and how they originally secured their contributions.[152]

Since the early 1850s Struthers (then in Edinburgh) had encouraged students, when travelling or working abroad in future, to send him human skulls and pelves, which would aid in studying the 'different races of man' and 'different individuals' in terms of their various anatomical 'forms and dimensions'.[153] Many bones were forthcoming, especially skulls, the collection of which (whether from the recently deceased or from ancient burial sites) was gaining momentum at university, college and medical-school museums in Europe, North America and Australia.[154] One 'old student' of Marischal College, when working at the General Hospital in Calcutta (Kolkata) in 1867, sent a human skull he had obtained in the Andaman Islands ten years previously, and also promised further skulls of the 'natives of India'.[155] Another 'old pupil', in London in 1870, sent two skulls from Australia, explaining that 'they were brought to a friend of mine by some of the natives, who got them from the burying place, and as you see have no hesitation in selling for a few pence.'[156] Whether or not indigenous people participated in such acquisitions – and contemporary accounts would suggest not, given their aversion to the disturbance of graves and their attempts to protect their dead – the meanings they attributed to the skulls were largely displaced by the collector's narrative, and then again overlaid when they came into use as anatomical specimens.[157] Fuelling Struthers's skeletal collecting was the conviction that any conclusions regarding 'differences of race', in order to be 'reliable', had to be founded on the 'examination of a series of specimens'. So ever-growing numbers of bones were required, as were systematic methods using instruments such as the glass-box craniometer that Struthers designed for measuring the cranium (or a plaster bust or a living head) with 'perfect accuracy'.[158]

Human skulls were sent as single contributions to the Anatomical Museum, such as that of a 'North Chinaman' sent from Chefoo (Yantai) in 1873 by a surgeon, or they arrived in batches, especially during the 1880s, such as a box of eight conveyed from Ceylon (Sri Lanka).[159] Six skulls from Borneo were also delivered. According to the doctor who sent them, four were 'taken from the houses [of] native interior tribes . . . during recent expeditions made [by colonial authorities] for the suppression of head-hunting'; taking heads for scientific purposes was, on the other hand, regarded by those same authorities as legitimate.[160] A 'consignment of skulls' was dispatched from Calcutta by William Simpson, an 1876 graduate appointed as Health Officer in that city (1886–97), and a previous acquaintance of Struthers's daughter, Mary Masson, who lived in Melbourne. Simpson offered to send skulls as 'specimens of Burmese, Chinese, Indian and nearly all of the gradations between' if Struthers was interested in 'skeletons of different nations'.[161]

The relocations involved in a medical career could give rise to an extended sequence of presentations, as did John Robb's movements. From Zanzibar he dispatched the bones of a hippopotamus (prior to 1882). Then, as a surgeon in charge of the Civil Hospital's Medical School and the Lunatic Asylum at Ahmadabad, in Gujarat, India, he sent four male 'Hindu' skulls – these having been obtained from the dissecting room – and the skin and bones of a crocodile shot by an Aberdeen friend of Robb's in the Bombay Civil Service. The package was shipped from Bombay (Mumbai) to Liverpool and onwards to Struthers in Aberdeen.[162] Skeletal remains, whether animal or human, travelled these routes to the Anatomical Museum mostly from colonial contexts, especially in Asia, where medical men in positions of authority could exert their power to acquire them directly or through intermediaries. Whether body parts were drawn to the Anatomical Museum through extended connections or through local relations, once they arrived work was required to convert bones into recognizable museum specimens. Aspects of this work, and those who performed it, are discussed next.

ORGANISM AND ARTEFACT

The difference between 'natural objects' and 'art' was outlined by William Flower in the late nineteenth century by focusing on the role of the museum curator in relation to these two categories. 'Specimens' of art, which the curator must 'preserve and exhibit', Flower suggested, 'come into his hands very nearly in the condition in which they will have to remain', for example a picture or a statue which, he argued, only call for 'mechanical' tasks such as cleaning and repairing before they are ready to exhibit. By contrast, natural objects 'require special methods of preservation' and, in many instances, their value as museum specimens depends entirely upon the skill, labour, patience, and knowledge extended upon them. In specimens illustrating biological subjects the highest powers of the museum curator are called forth.[163]

Thus art was assumed to have already been made or completed when it entered a museum, whereas natural objects called for work to fashion them into museum exhibits. Specialists in this kind of work could clearly discern it when inspecting specimens, so that preserved body parts were not simply regarded as instances of anatomy but as demonstrations of the methods used to prepare and display them. So one commentator explained in the 1880s: 'the anatomist comes to the museum quite as much to see methods of mounting and preservation as to see the specimens.'[164]

Whether defined as art or derived from nature, once incorporated into a museum an object became part of an institution that Flower described metaphorically as a living entity: 'A museum is like a living organism – it requires constant and tender care. It must grow or it will perish.'[165] Quoting another senior museum director, Flower emphasized the necessity of never-ending acquisition: 'when the collections cease to grow they begin to decay. A finished museum is a dead museum, and a dead museum is a useless museum.'[166] In Flower's view, a museum also required maintenance by a curator who, with 'his staff', would keep it in a 'state of vitality', for specimens required appropriate arrangement, labels and protection from dirt, devouring insects, damp and bleaching light.[167] As Flower advocated, a curator was needed in a museum like a minister in a church, a school-master in a school and a gardener in a garden; he would ideally be a man of education and 'natural ability' with manual dexterity and good taste as well as 'moral qualifications', especially 'indomitable and conscientious industry'.[168] Thus Flower identified the skills and moral qualities of the central figure considered essential in the growth of any museum. As an 'organism' the museum required not only a constant influx of material objects that were appropriately treated, but personnel with particular dispositions.

MASTER OF DETAIL

The elevation of the curator as the key figure in the life of a museum tended, however, to obscure others involved in museum-making. Just as an anatomist's collecting practices depended on his multiple social relationships extending beyond the medical school, so his display practices – fundamental to his curatorial role – were reliant on his working relationships within it. Dominant views of Marischal College's Anatomical Museum associated it predominantly with Struthers's work as professor, yet this work was enabled in important ways by assistants. When senior university officials, according to newspaper reports of Struthers's retirement in 1889, referred to the museum as his 'creation' and an 'enduring monument to his name', they identified it so closely with the anatomist that the involvement of others was occluded.[169] This identification was made in a context where the Anatomical Museum's growth was sustained by the activities of many persons organized such that the outcomes of those activities accrued mainly (though not exclusively) to Struthers's profile. The structure of authority manifest in the division of anatomical labour, and the different values assigned to work within this, were to the anatomist's benefit. In his professorial role, performing and gaining recognition as an authoritative figure, Struthers was seen as a reliable guarantor of the Anatomical Museum's scientific and pedagogical importance, just as the expanding collection amplified his status – and, indeed, helped form him as a successful anatomist.

Struthers was himself unreserved when emphasizing 'the amount of time, consideration, and personal labour' expended in forming an anatomical museum 'worthy of a University'. Teaching was his daytime priority, so museum-making, especially preserving specimens, filled evenings and holidays. He regarded this as 'extremely interesting work, both in the doing and in the result', and others appreciated it as an indicator of his dedication – one medical visitor described the Anatomical Museum as a 'labour of love'.[170] Discipline and control were especially important, as one student observed of Struthers: 'in the dissecting room he moved like a master of detail', with an approach that required every anatomical structure to be laid out 'in perfect order'. Such 'exacting' requirements produced valuable museum specimens, which were authenticated and therefore legitimized for display by the procedures they were (seen to be) subject to.[171]

Most of the Anatomical Museum's animal skeletons Struthers initially obtained 'as carcasses, to be dissected first, or as bones in the rough state, requiring to be macerated [cleaned] and otherwise prepared before being mounted'.[172] He described this requisite specimen-making as mainly 'the work of my own hands', carried out mostly at his own expense with only modest university funds. Although carcasses were not expensive – that of a horse in 1864 'did not cost a shilling', Struthers recalled – they did, however, cost him 'a good deal of time and trouble to clean and put up'.[173] Fluids for preserving, glass and other materials needed to mount specimens were costly, but it was their shaping in the hands of the anatomist that really defined their worth. Many admiring viewers flocked to see the shilling horse once it was presented by Struthers as a striking articulated skeleton – a 'new' specimen, the 'first thing of the kind that Aberdeen University ever saw', he claimed.[174]

Struthers's experiments with methods of preservation also enabled tactile as well as visual exploration of specimens, which enhanced their educational utility. For example, series of brains, human and comparative, originally prepared by the 'old spirit process', were removed from their spirit-filled jars and specially preserved in a 'moist state', the lobes stained with pigments in different colours. Lying under a simple, removable glass shade (to keep off dust) in the dissecting room and museum, these were easily available for demonstration and could be 'handled freely'. Using particular concoctions of fluids to stabilize them, Struthers had found that museum specimens from human bodies – such as the bladder, prostate, uterus, heart, joints and dissections of the hand and foot – no longer needed to remain immersed in spirits. Suspended in dry glass jars, thus avoiding the 'optical distortion' caused by looking through liquid, they could be conveniently removed for 'closer examination'. He also preserved larger dissections – of ligaments, muscles, blood vessels, nerves and viscera – by his moist method, and displayed them without containers, thereby exposing 'a great many more views' than was possible when sunk in open basins filled with spirits.[175]

Anatomical work was recognized as physically demanding, requiring 'bodily strength and activity'. Allen Thomson, when professor of anatomy at the University of Glasgow, emphasized that a man in his position performed 'a great deal of manual and bodily work', drawing on all his 'senses and muscular powers'.[176] This labour was integral to the senior anatomist's knowledge-making practices – just as practical study was to students' learning – and here proficiency was represented in terms of masculine bodily alertness and stamina. But this was not solitary work – preparing specimens could involve painstaking, delicate action with the scalpel or heavy sawing, and such tasks enlisted the labour of others.[177] At the University of Edinburgh's Anatomical Museum, William Turner praised the 'eminently skilled man' who assisted him, and there was also a 'charwoman' for the very necessary cleaning.[178]

Struthers was certain that professors of anatomy, pathology, natural history and botany were 'naturally the curators' of the university museums associated with those subjects, as in Aberdeen, but he also emphasized how useful a skilful attendant – an 'intelligent, neat-handed servant' – could be, when 'working under the directing head'.[179] Within the Anatomical Department's hierarchy at Marischal College the museum attendant's role was to preserve and mount specimens and assist throughout the department as appropriate. His position was subordinate to the professor's chief demonstrator and assistant demonstrator, who prepared dissections and illustrations for teaching and helped to instruct students in practical classes.[180] But it was not as lowly as that of the dissecting-room servant or porter, a job that men were reluctant to take and quick to leave, especially, as Struthers pointed out, as this employment was 'neither attractive nor healthy'; a man taking on the so-called 'menial' duties of this post would sweep rooms, tend fires, wash dead bodies prior to taking them into the dissecting room, scrub the tables therein and help students by, for example, getting their dissecting clothes washed.[181]

Museum attendant Robert Gibb was certainly appreciated by Struthers as 'faithful' and dedicated – the professor credited his help in forming the Anatomical Museum, commended his 'intelligent interest in the work' and was grateful for the extra hours of assistance Gibb willingly gave.[182] As a 'genuine working-man naturalist' Gibb was keen to help in collecting animal parts, dissecting whales and measuring and articulating skeletons – which included sculpting small wooden 'bones' to replace missing ones.[183] In one dissecting-room photograph (or informal group portrait) he perhaps indicated his strong investment in this work producing anatomical specimens: with telling gestures, he held and pointed to the carefully preserved human bones (see illus. 91).

Museum specimens in the making thus passed through many hands, from the acquisition of deceased bodies and body parts to dissection, preservation, mounting and display. Multiple contributors and practitioners included, for instance, those at an Edinburgh glassworks who supplied specimen jars according to Struthers's specifications with diameters of 6 and 12 in. (15.25 and 30.5 cm), and a philosophical instrument maker in the same city who constructed metal rings for the all-important sealing of jars.[184] Museum specimens thus had many producers but they were attributed mainly to Struthers, whether personally crafted by him or made under his direction. This was partly due to his position within the university's medical school, where his demonstrations of anatomical knowledge were afforded respect and his command of specialist techniques was acknowledged. His private collection – exhibited in the Anatomical Museum – was seen as testimony to his abilities in preserving specimens, both wet (immersed in spirits) and dry. The latter included dried and varnished bones and organs, some with intricate wax-injected blood vessels and painted parts.[185] Two preparations from the 1870s, for example, displayed the position of muscles, arteries (in red) and nerves (in white) at the base of the skull and top of the spine (illus. 82). Struthers's signature on labels explicitly linked specimen with anatomist, so that viewers derived anatomical knowledge while also appreciating the maker's skill. As William Flower asserted, 'a properly-mounted animal or a carefully-displayed anatomical preparation is in itself a work of art, based upon a natural substratum.'[186]

The 'art' of cutting, manipulating, painting and framing therefore enhanced the appeal and status of natural objects, without detracting from their perceived inherent naturalness.

Struthers performed these techniques according to particular codes of conduct, thereby guaranteeing the legitimacy of specimens as seen within his scientific networks. His own comportment and that which he expected of staff was significant: rendering anatomical actualities visible through the methods advocated by Struthers and his contemporaries required disciplined, earnest industry, diligence and exactitude.[187] The relentless labour and patience of individuals, as Lorraine Daston and Peter Galison argue, were considered 'dutiful virtues' of the scientific personnel of the time, and their work was regarded as 'constitutive of the careful, empirical methods of science'.[188] Large-scale exhibits such as massive mammal skeletons were seen as impressive manifestations of such scientific work – the bones and cartilages of an Indian elephant, obtained in Multan and presented by Dr John Gunn in 1873, took two years to clean and prepare, and then an entire autumn to articulate with metal rods and wire.[189] From such a process, specimens emerged as multifaceted: they could be observed as tangible anatomical parts, appreciated as evidence of skilled techniques, and recognized as special gifts from respected persons connected with Marischal College.

Different viewers might interpret specimens in different ways but those specimens' meanings were guided, though not determined, by Struthers, who exerted considerable influence over their display and uses by medical students within the Anatomical Museum. And although the collection was

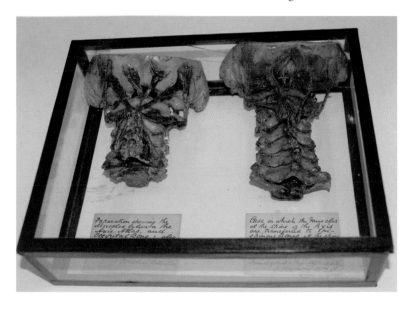

82
Dried preparations of the human skull, spine and muscles, prepared by John Struthers, 1870s.

not catalogued, handwritten labels, signed and/or dated by Struthers, supplied descriptions and probably named significant donors, especially those who gave large animal skeletons (see illus. 90). Struthers also circulated specimens beyond the museum through descriptions and drawings in scientific publications. Notably Struthers's articles in the *Journal of Anatomy and Physiology* explicated the museum's specimens within established anatomical discourse, discussing them in relation to specimens exhibited in colleges and universities internationally – for example in Edinburgh, London, Göttingen, Jena, Vienna, Leuven and Copenhagen.[190] This dissemination and networking of specimens via print had significant effects: while reinforcing the validity of Struthers's statements, scholarly references to specimens augmented their value while also strengthening their connection with his work.

The Anatomical Museum also benefited, however, from the acquisition of exhibits produced by prominent specialist manufacturers, though, again, Struthers's selection and assemblage of these left his own mark on them. Here there was considerable investment in anatomical models purchased from leading commercial firms through the second half of the nineteenth century, so that anatomy in wax, plaster and other materials featured strongly in displays. Students had to learn by dissecting, but supplies of human bodies for anatomical purposes fluctuated and, even when considered (temporarily) improved, as in 1868–9 and 1871–2, models displayed details that were difficult to observe through dissection.[191] Furthermore, like specimens, models were both educationally and socially meaningful: they were labelled with names of anatomical parts but they also carried the inscription, or trade label, of the well-known firms that made them. The recognizability of models' manufacturers, who developed signature house styles, acted as a reassurance of quality, thereby boosting the prestige of institutions that could afford their products. And models given to Struthers by distinguished anatomists – and labelled as such – were indicators of his, and by extension the museum's, learned connections.[192]

During visits to museums in Continental European cities Struthers selected particular models and osteological preparations from highly reputable firms which sold to anatomical museums in Europe, North America and

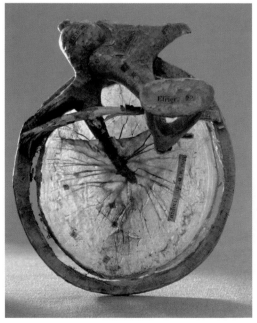

83
Model of the eardrum, an inner component from an enlarged model of the ear, 1879, by Auzoux, Paris.

Australia.[193] His trip to Paris in 1869 yielded an enlarged model of an ear made in robust paper paste by Louis Auzoux and, ten years later, another featuring an eardrum the size of a saucer (illus. 83) along with a horse hoof, a series of brains (for example, of the elephant, cat, rat and goose) and hearts (including of the tortoise and snake). Also arriving in 1879, a wax dissected hand by Maison Tramond was one in a sequence of purchases from that maker over the next few years: an exploded human skull (resembling illus. 2), part of a skull with modelled blood vessels and nerves, and wax models of the lymphatic vessels of the torso (see illus. 33) and of an anatomized foetus with umbilical cord and placenta. Following Struthers's visit to Leipzig around 1877, an intricate wax model by Dr Rudolf Weisker arrived at the Anatomical Museum (illus. 84).[194] Models of human anatomy were added to the museum almost every year during the 1880s, many displaying the head, brain and neck – such as Franz Josef Steger's painted plaster casts, again made in Leipzig (see illus. 38).[195] This influx built on a key acquisition: an exceptionally detailed life-size male human figure, one of the most expensive items in Auzoux's catalogue, which was displayed (probably with heart, lungs and other organs exposed) at the 1881 opening of the new Anatomical Department (see illus. 141). Struthers inscribed this figure with the year of its acquisition, the characteristic mark which he applied to many purchased models, sometimes accompanied by his own initials, to personally authorize their incorporation into the institution.

84
Wax anatomical model, c. 1877, by Rudolf Weisker, Leipzig.

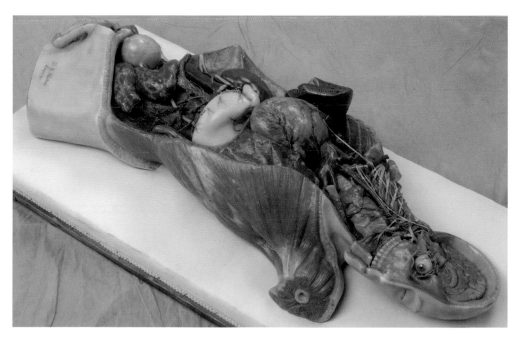

The Anatomical Museum's growth, in both the acquisition of specimens and the expansion of audiences to appreciate them, was also fuelled through the (managed) interaction of professional anatomy and popular or commercial displays. The latter were open to people across the social spectrum, including those without specialist anatomical knowledge.[196] As noted above, John Struthers used public exhibitions of whales to instruct medical students as well as to gain access to specimens, and one of his whale dissections was staged (by the mammal's entrepreneurial owner) as an attraction with musical accompaniment. In addition, the anatomist regarded shows featuring living people and animals as yet further productive sites for collecting. Although Marischal College's Anatomical Museum was primarily used in research and medical teaching, Struthers also invited a 'general audience' to it via his 'popular lectures'.[197] This opening up to a wider audience was described by Struthers in terms of his 'duty' to 'spread . . . knowledge among the people' which would be both intellectually rewarding for them and 'useful in its application to the preservation of [their] health'.[198] But this opening up also strengthened the anatomist's educational claim on specimens, as suggested below, thereby bolstering his local collecting practices while publicizing the Anatomical Museum's importance for scientific learning.

Live displays of animals were sites where anatomists sought rare acquisitions.[199] From the Berlin Aquarium, where many creatures were exhibited in ponds, cages and a grotto, Struthers secured, in the late 1870s, a life-size model and photographs of a young gorilla.[200] Menageries, displaying collections of beasts, birds and reptiles from around the world, were also sources for the Anatomical Museum. The well-known travelling menagerie established by George Wombwell supplied Struthers with deceased animals, including a giraffe, kangaroo, tigress and tapir which died during visits to Aberdeen, or soon after leaving.[201] Sent to Marischal College for dissection, their skeletons were carefully preserved. The route from menagerie to museum was also notable elsewhere. For instance, an Indian elephant, Chunee, having been transported from Bengal to London, was moved through a succession of display contexts: he featured in a pantomime and a menagerie, and after being shot he was dissected and his skeleton toured as a commercial exhibit prior to its display at the RCS's Hunterian Museum by the 1850s (see illus. 75).[202] The appropriation of animals for both entertainment and education is evident in the publicity for Wombwell's menagerie, which, during the second half of the nineteenth century, regularly brought to northeast Scotland hundreds of living 'specimens' and 'zoological curiosities', including elephants, leopards, polar bears, spotted and striped hyenas, zebras, llamas, serpents, monkeys, emus and kangaroos, all accompanied by a brass band.[203] Human performers were very much part of the menagerie's shows: its visits to Aberdeen brought a circus with a 'daring' lion tamer and tightrope walker, and a 'boneless wonder' was presented as a 'grotesque feature particularly interesting to students of human anatomy'.[204]

Displays of living people, regular occurrences in European cities during the nineteenth century, were of interest to anatomists seeking to observe and document physical differences and to delineate particular racial 'types'.[205] Living human displays, especially of peoples from colonial territories, could be seen in circuses, entertainment halls, zoological gardens, theatres and large-scale international fairs where villages were reconstructed and so called 'savages' performed.[206] Such displays were embedded in complex cultural politics that often tended to reinforce hierarchies of power; anatomists engaged with such displays as a means to further their expertise and expand institutional collections. Having seen two 'Bush-people' or 'Bushmen' (San) from South Africa exhibited in Edinburgh, around 1880 Struthers commissioned a London firm to make life casts of these people – probably Brucciani, who also supplied classical, écorché and bust casts to the anatomist (illus. 85).[207] The painted plaster figures, labelled 'Bush-woman' and 'Bushman', along with skulls in the Anatomical Museum, were designated as specimens for identifying 'anatomical characters' that might distinguish 'races'.[208] Both 'external form' and 'internal structure' were of import: the former described through observations and measurements of living people or casts thereof, and the latter discerned in studies of bones.[209] When William Flower had reported from the RCS on his dissection of a 'Bushwoman' – a woman who, as a girl of about twelve, had been exhibited in London and 'the provinces' – he had emphasized the urgency of this anatomical work, stressing that numerous races 'are passing away from the face of the earth', an argument that worked to strengthen the rationale for preserving her skeleton in his institution's museum.[210] In Scotland the large majority of recently deceased bodies in dissecting rooms were those of 'Europeans', and this heightened interest in full-body plaster casts of people deemed of different race.[211] Struthers commissioned a second pair of the 'Bushmen' (San) casts, and presented them to the Museum of the RCSEd.

Plaster casts of this kind were not only displayed in the anatomical museums of universities and colleges; they could also be seen in exhibitions operating as commercial enterprises in which combinations of 'ethnological' and anatomical specimens attracted attention.[212] Images of the Liverpool Museum of Anatomy in circulation c. 1877 appear to show two such casts in the foreground along with models and diagrams of

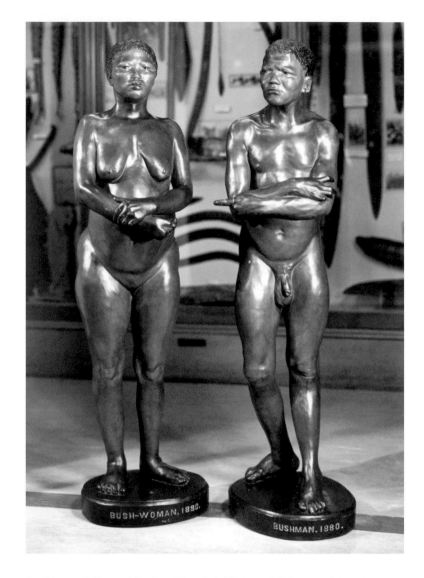

healthy and diseased bodies (illus. 86). This establishment claimed to provoke visitors' interest while serving as a 'public advantage' by promoting
health; it admitted men and women at different times, and the 'working
classes' at a reduced charge.[213] Commercial anatomical museums based at
dedicated premises or touring to temporary venues, and often displaying
more pathological than healthy specimens, offered visitors potential
improvement (in knowledge and health) as well as amusement. Proliferating
from the 1830s, especially during the 1850s,[214] attitudes to these exhibitions varied within and between locales. For example, Reimer's Anatomical
Museum was reportedly approved by Hull's town magistrates and other

gentlemen, but at Leeds's Music Hall in 1852 it was declared 'grossly indecent' and 'immoral', with specimens 'of inferior grade . . . suited only to a low and vitiated taste'.[215] Undeterred, the exhibition opened in London in the same year and subsequently at other venues in northern England.[216]

Commercial exhibitions of anatomy were regularly advertised for public viewing in Scotland's cities. In Edinburgh exhibition visitors viewed Signor Sarti's shows in the 1840s, which toured from London with collections including models of diseases, a life-size female figure 'of the Moorish Race' and a wax 'Florentine Venus' (see illus. 57 for an example). Dundee saw a return of Sarti's Venus and Anatomical Adonis in 1883, this time organized by a different proprietor.[217] Glasgow was treated to a temporary exhibition of Dr Joseph Kahn's Anatomical Museum in the year following its 1851 London opening.[218] In Aberdeen Sarti had opened his display in 1847, issuing local press adverts promising that it would impart 'useful knowledge' to everyone regarding common physical ailments and diseases.[219] Further temporary anatomical shows in the 'Granite City' included Herr Reimers's in 1857.[220] A decade later Dr Frederick Adair's Anatomical Museum opened only a few streets from Marischal College, exhibiting until 1876 and subsequently under another owner until at least 1885.[221] Adair's self-proclaimed 'costly and magnificent' collection – of almost 1,000 models of human anatomy, including those of the 'grand caesarean operation' and the 'effects of tight lacing' corsets, as well as many 'skulls of various nations' – was 'for gentlemen only' who were over eighteen and paid a shilling admission. Within this constituency, as large an audience as possible was sought through advertising in local newspapers as far as the islands of Orkney.[222]

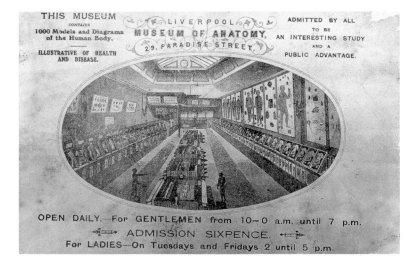

86
The Liverpool Museum of Anatomy, back cover of *A Descriptive Catalogue of the Liverpool Museum of Anatomy* (Liverpool, 1877).

Medical men became highly critical of commercial anatomical museums – especially when used to promote sales of suspect treatments, many for sexual diseases – and then encouraged prosecutions and closures (under the Obscene Publications Act) during the second half of the nineteenth century. In doing so they reinforced their own professional and moral standing.[223] As an anatomist in a senior position, Struthers would have been keen to distinguish his medical school's Anatomical Museum from those establishments losing educational credibility, even as his collecting and display practices traversed the professional/popular distinctions that were increasingly marked at the time.[224]

Although Struthers seems not to have openly opposed commercial anatomical museums, in strategic ways he expanded the audience for Marischal College's Anatomical Museum, claiming for it a weighty authority as a site of scientific display and thereby elevating it, like similar institutionally based museums, above those operating commercially. In addition to the Anatomical Museum's main purposes in university research and teaching, Struthers saw its potential to inspire interest in science within the local region, probably sensing that this interest might increase cooperation in his collecting pursuits. From the late 1860s onwards Struthers's public (often Saturday-evening) lectures, which were open to all – including working men and women – featured the museum's specimens and there were invitations to visit the displays in situ. The lectures proved 'exceedingly popular', with audiences appreciating Struthers's efforts to 'disseminate scientific knowledge', especially among those with few 'opportunities for instruction in scientific subjects'.[225] He publicly asserted that women should 'no longer be shut out' from 'literary, scientific and other intellectual culture', engaging them in learning with anatomical exhibits – unlike Adair's commercial museum – and supporting their claims to higher education at a time when they were not yet admitted as students of the university.[226] While a debated issue, there was public opinion in Aberdeen forcefully in favour of women's university instruction and examination, which was eventually allowed in the 1890s.[227]

Lectures given by Struthers to a 'general audience' on anatomical subjects, such as the 'organs of nutrition', were object-based, as for medical students.[228] Explaining that he would not 'give book knowledge', he instead took 'objects in his hands' and discussed them so that people could 'see and judge for themselves'. It was the Anatomical Museum, he pointed out, that enabled this way of learning.[229] When lecturing on evolution, for example, Struthers displayed various of the museum's animal skeletons with which, a local newspaper reported, he 'succeeded in popularizing the subject to outsiders [those external to the University]'.[230] Allowing controlled public access to the museum, either through its doors or by showing selected specimens as part of a programme of local educational initiatives, increased its visibility and reinforced its value. In turn this enhanced the anatomist's reputation as a collector determined not only to accumulate but to successfully use and disseminate knowledge through those objects.

The 1880s local newspaper caricature of Struthers as simultaneously collector and popular performer (see illus. 77) tapped into his dual strategy of acquiring specimens for medical education and disseminating science more widely.[231] Indeed, the caricature may well have even drawn upon, and playfully subverted, metaphors in Struthers's own public lectures in Aberdeen when he expounded that 'a true scientific lecture, no matter who should form the audience is . . . not [the "routine" and repetitive "perform-ance"] of a man turning the handle of the barrel "organ", but that of a musician playing an instrument.'[232]

Saturday, 19 October 1889, twelve noon until 4 o'clock: eminent members of Aberdeen's medical profession, many of whom Struthers had taught, along with some of the highest dignitaries and officials in the city, were invited to examine the Anatomical Museum. This was a publicized wit-nessing of the museum's growth to maturity, just prior to Struthers's retirement as professor. The assembly of at least twenty men was one in a sequence of occasions over the previous few years when distinguished per-sons, including scientific 'big-wigs' visiting for the 1885 Aberdeen meeting of the British Association for the Advancement of Science, had admired the anatomical collection and its arrangement.[233] Upon entry through the main door, viewers saw all four walls fitted with glass cases: on the ground floor to their right these were filled with osteological specimens, and to their left with soft preparations in jars of spirits; the wall behind them held blood-vessel preparations and that in front specimens of topographical anatomy. In the centre of the floor stood the larger skeletons and figures of the human form, including the 'extraordinary' 'Bushman and Bush-woman'. Enclosing this grouping were tables displaying specimens and models under removable glass shades. Of particular interest were the 'series of skeletons and brains of the higher apes ranged as in a procession . . . ending with the human skeleton and brain in their young and old state'.[234] Above the ground-floor exhibits, the gallery featured specimens of com-parative anatomy, models of the human embryo (those of the face and neck, which Struthers obtained in Germany, attracting particular attention) and 'bones of prehistoric man', while the collection of 'national skulls' was noted as 'considerable'. The event was reported as a great success.[235]

If museums were living organisms, as Flower had suggested, growing through the sustained accrual of specimens, Struthers as anatomist-curator became a cultivator, a gardener in an arbour. Through his museum-making the anatomist was also seen as a tailor, a rag-and-bone man, a master of detail. These multiple guises were enacted and ascribed within the network of social relationships that crucially gave shape to the Anatomical Museum. From local beaches to overseas hospitals, from learned societies to popular shows and from amateur collectors to commercial dealers, the diversity of this museum's sources was directly related to the range of the anatomist's social connections. Skeletal growth on a sustained and substantial scale was central to the Anatomical Museum's formation, and this process was both organic and social, personal and political, material and metaphorical.

Five
VISUALIZING THE INTERIOR

Following the nineteenth-century growth of museums of anatomy in teaching institutions, the rapid influx of human and animal remains was to continue alongside developments in techniques for making visible the interior of the human body and for analysing its exterior. If knowledge of the human body was gained, as anatomists agreed, by 'teasing' it 'to pieces' to reveal it from the inside, many bodies after death were utilized for this purpose alongside bodies of the living, which were becoming increasingly subject to anatomical exploration from the surface of the skin.[1] This chapter examines displays of bodies, alive and deceased, from the 1890s to the 1930s, when anatomy museums (as anatomical museums became commonly termed during this period) were, for the most part, firmly established within university medical education.[2] Summarizing the status of these museums in 1899, one anatomy professor explained that they had 'ceased to be a storehouse for a heterogeneous association of curios' and had assumed their 'proper place as an important factor in scientific education'.[3] Coincident with this recognition, indeed partly constitutive of it, were restrictions in public access to anatomy exhibits, which were coming to be firmly defined as the territory of professionals and their students.

Although conservators had begun to detect a problematic fixity in museums – their sturdy structures, both material and social, were seemingly resistant to change – anatomy museums were far from static during this period. Their growing collections, pulling in specimens from across the world, were displayed in new ways, especially with the use of photography and the making of images in a range of interconnected media. At Marischal College's Anatomy Museum investments in collecting and preserving specimens persisted, feeding expansion, while modifications in displays were facilitated by changing anatomical techniques and image-making practices. Continuities in exhibits were certainly maintained, but the Anatomy Museum also underwent a degree of strategic alteration; this twin approach ensured the enduring importance of this museum in the generation and communication of anatomical knowledge.

The following account examines how bodies were visualized, from the inside and outside, through the making and display of the Anatomy Museum's ever-enlarging collection of specimens and images thereof. The relevance and value of museum specimens was amplified by their movement between the Anatomy (previously Anatomical) Department's various spaces for teaching, research and exhibiting, movements through which key observational skills were cultivated. Of import then, was the development and utilization of the Anatomy Museum alongside, and in relation to, practices in the dissecting room, lecture theatre, anthropometric laboratory and Anthropological Museum.[4] The effects of the latter's removal from within the Anatomy Department to form a public gallery at Marischal College are addressed later in this chapter, which begins with an overview of stabilities and changes in the Anatomy Museum during the first few decades of the twentieth century. The material, visual and spatial processes of display during this period – which entailed particular kinds of embodied practices as well as intermedial connections, especially between museum specimens and visual images – were embedded in social and power relations, just as the practices associated with the Anatomy Museum were enmeshed in its local and wider colonial context.

DARK ROOM

In 1899 the Anatomy Museum's interior seemed to closely resemble its incarnation ten years earlier, when John Struthers retired from the professorship of anatomy. Within the familiar structure of wall cases, ground-floor exhibits and gallery above, there were striking displays of skeletons, including those of whales suspended from the gallery and of apes, now articulated into 'lifelike positions'.[5] As one local newspaper reported:

> the Darwinian theory of evolution at once forces itself upon the
> mind of the visitor on entering the hall, for the glass case in front
> contains a series of skeletons of anthropoid apes, including the gib-
> bon, chimpanzee, male and female gorilla, etc., their hands clasping
> the branches of trees, and by way of comparison the skeleton of a
> man stands erect at the head of the line. A series of skulls illustrates
> the types of races, among the more noteworthy being those of Maori,
> Chinese, and various tribes of Indians.[6]

87
Anatomy Museum,
Marischal College,
University of
Aberdeen, 1906,
photograph.

88
Anatomy Museum,
Marischal College,
University of
Aberdeen, 1929,
photograph.

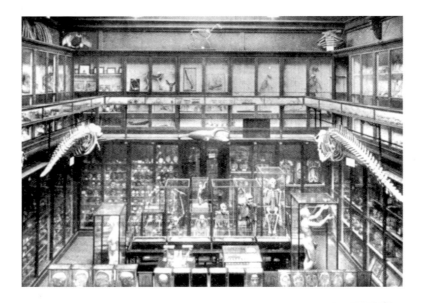

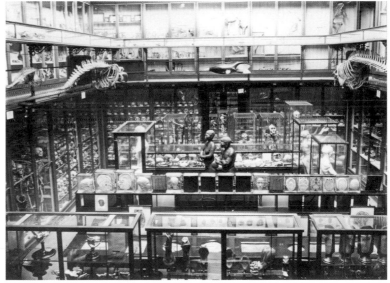

Such displays could still be observed in 1906, as shown in one of the
earliest photographs of the Anatomy Museum (illus. 87), and by 1929 they
had largely remained in place, as is apparent in a photograph published
in a specialist medical education journal (illus. 88).[7] So too had skeletons
of vertebrates for the study of comparative anatomy, some accommodated
in the Anatomy Museum and larger specimens arranged in the department's entrance corridor (illus. 89) and vestibule (illus. 90). The tendency
of collections to settle and sediment was an issue to which museum

89
Entrance corridor,
Anatomy Department,
Marischal College,
University of Aberdeen,
c. 1906, photograph.

90
Articulated skeletons
of animals including an
elephant and giraffe,
c. 1860–1900, in the
Anatomy Department,
Marischal College,
University of Aberdeen,
c. 1906, photograph.

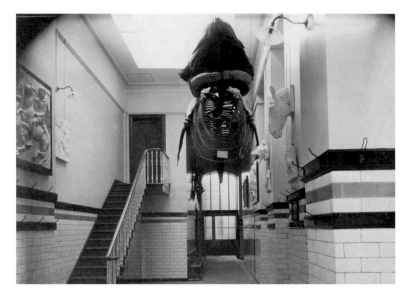

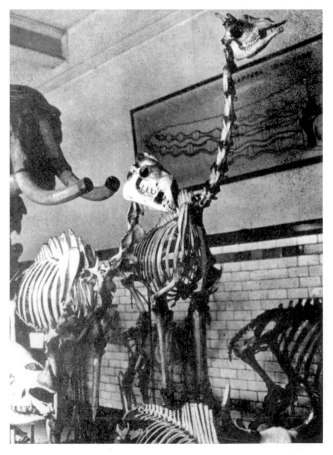

conservators had become alert. William Flower, for example, had noted 'difficulties of readjustment' caused by 'obstacles', such as the size and layout of museum buildings, and also by staff whose 'personal interests . . . grow up and wind their meshes around such institutions'. These, Flower warned, could cause 'passing phases of scientific knowledge' to become 'crystallised and fossilised' in museums.[8]

But at the Anatomy Museum certain continuities were actively sought and valued in a department also implementing changes – especially in staff, working spaces and exhibits – so that, around 1930, it was considered very much 'up-to-date'.[9] The collection of skeletal specimens, human and animal, was maintained and enlarged, as discussed later, especially through anatomists' contacts and former students in posts across the empire. Skeletons of a man and a woman were obtained, for example, from hospitals in the Andaman Islands in 1895 and Calcutta (Kolkata) in 1929.[10] Plaster casts purchased in the 1880s from Brucciani's firm, including a classical figure (see illus. 29), and those labelled 'Bush-woman' and 'Bushman' which were displayed in the Anatomy Museum after 1907 (see illus. 85), were joined in 1919 by more from the same firm; this time two plaster-of-Paris 'reproductions' of a cast originally taken in the Anatomy Department from a 'living muscular male' to show on its surface the points where nerves enter the muscles.[11] Late nineteenth-century models were kept in use, while new ones were bought around 1921 from the same suppliers in Paris: from the Auzoux firm a giant kidney (see illus. 40) and from N. Rouppert (successor to Maison Tramond) waxes including a model of the portal venous system (comprising veins, the liver, stomach and intestines; see illus. 146).[12] A series of wax models showing the development of animal and human embryos, obtained for the Anatomy Museum by Struthers on visits to Continental Europe, probably from Adolph Ziegler's studio in Freiburg, was augmented by further purchases from Ziegler's son Friedrich (see illus. 88, bottom).[13] All of these models bore their reputable manufacturers' distinctive styles, developed over the previous century. Complementing these commercial products were models made in the Anatomy Department during the early decades of the 1900s, such as those of the human embryonic nervous system and heart with blood vessels.[14]

Changing displays were perhaps most evident when the Anatomy Museum's fleshy specimens were involved – these prepared from bodies in the dissecting room. Certain shifts in techniques for producing specimens, and in strategies for displaying them, were preferred, as one scientific journal reported in 1888:

> The kind of specimens most valued for illustrating anatomy in a
> museum is now very different from what was sought for in the first

half of this century. Dried and varnished dissections showing blood-vessels, etc., are now looked on as nearly useless, and are kept only as historical relics. Elaborate dissections under alcohol . . . and sections of frozen bodies similarly mounted, are what the student and the practitioner most desire to see.[15]

At Marischal College, from the 1890s, specimens of the human head, neck, trunk and limbs were prepared according to these favoured methods. Bodies were frozen to retain their shape and sawn into several sections, either vertically or horizontally, to expose their anatomical composition. They were then suspended in glass jars filled with preservative: formalin, a solution of formaldehyde with its improved preserving properties, was now employed (as well as methylated spirits), and square museum jars (in addition to cylindrical) were used and praised for 'neither magnify[ing] nor distort[ing] the specimen in fluid'.[16] From around 1904, the heads of two females, aged 63 and 33, were exhibited as a series of sections extending the width of the Anatomy Museum (see illus. 87, bottom; 88, centre).[17] Time and resources were thus invested in museum specimens of this sort, for their pedagogical value was high, especially given the frequent shortages in the Anatomy Department's supply of bodies from the Aberdeen funeratory.[18] So specimens were preserved whenever possible, necessitating the purchase of museum containers to display them; in the first three decades of the 1900s six large glass-covered troughs and at least 240 glass jars were obtained for this purpose.[19]

Overseeing and conducting some of this museum work was Robert Reid, professor of anatomy (a post that carried with it the curatorship of the Anatomy Museum), and his successor Alexander Low (1868–1950). Reid had been a medical student at Marischal College, graduating in 1872, and after acting as John Struthers's assistant for a year he was appointed as an anatomy demonstrator in the medical school at St Thomas's Hospital, London. From 1877, Reid was lecturer in anatomy, credited with reorganizing his department at St Thomas's, before returning to Aberdeen as professor in 1889.[20] Low, also a Marischal College medical graduate, became Reid's assistant in 1894, and thereafter a lecturer. He was promoted to professor when Reid retired from this post in 1925, just as Low's successor, Robert Lockhart, would study in the same place and subsequently take up the professorship from Low in 1939. Here there were continuities in education that cut across changes in staff with relationships between anatomy teacher and student creating bonds that connected four generations of professors. By 1930 the Anatomy Department was staffed by a professor, two lecturers (in anatomy, and in embryology) and two assistants, all involved in teaching and 'scientific research'. Two 'technical assistants'

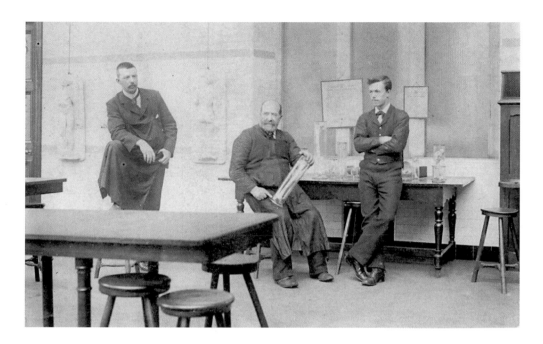

and two departmental attendants were also employed – one of these positions having been previously occupied by Robert Gibb from the 1870s for four decades, overlapping with his nephew, James Moir, who joined the department in 1895 and worked there for around 50 years (illus. 91).[21] Ties of kinship, then, whether familial or formed through learning, spanned a century from the 1860s to the 1960s, and this continuity in social connection was matched by the material stability – though with significant renewal and modification – in the Anatomy Museum.

Displays within the Anatomy Museum were conserved, created and utilized in the context of the Anatomy Department's wider complex of rooms, which were reconfigured over time. Part of Marischal College's 1895 extension involved rebuilding the anatomy rooms on a larger scale 'to meet the requirements of ever advancing science' and to accommodate more students (illus. 92).[22] Reid directed the replanning of rooms, expanding spaces for research and practical work but retaining the previous positioning of the dissecting room and lecture theatre on either side of the Anatomy Museum (illus. 93).[23] The latter was 're-furnished', as noted above, along lines already established, but with wall cases combined with newer elements, such as linoleum on the floor and glass cases arranged in the centre.[24] Electric lighting, providing 'brilliant' illumination, was installed throughout, and the walls were decorated with off-white enamelled tiles for sanitary purposes but also to maximize light, especially important in the dissecting room, where there were around 30 dissecting

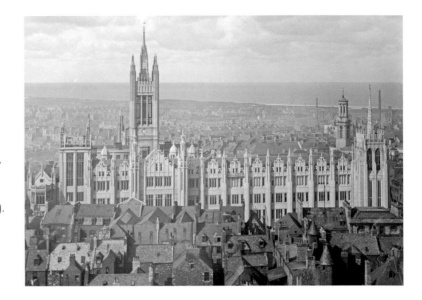

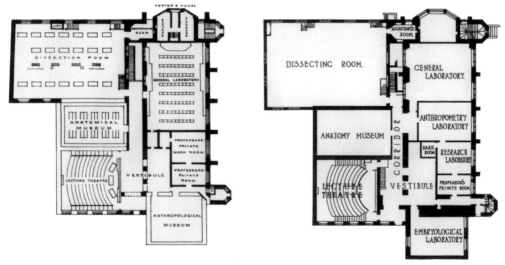

tables.[25] Here ventilators were fitted (students' habit of smoking in dissecting rooms was also discouraged) and there was a lift to the mortuary in the basement.[26] Leading from the dissecting room was the demonstration room, and the department's facilities now included the general laboratory and the anthropometric laboratory, which was also used as the Anthropological Museum. The professor's 'private room' adjoined his work room at the front of the department. The porter's house, located at the rear entrance, where the dead were delivered for dissection, had a parlour and a bedroom, and was probably the residence of Robert Gibb until his death in 1911.[27]

Between 1906 and 1929 the floor plans of the Anatomy Department indicate further changes: the porter's house ceased to be occupied as domestic space, the anatomy assistants were allocated a work area off the dissecting room (the latter had staircases to the attendants' work room and students' cloakroom on the floor below), and the professor's private work room became a research laboratory (see illus. 93). The Anthropological Museum was relocated and the embryological laboratory installed, with the anthropometric laboratory now assigned floor space taken from the general laboratory. The latter was equipped for students with tables for practical work in microscopic anatomy and neurology, radiographs (X-rays) for study, displays of bones, and frequently changed exhibits of specimens in glass cases.[28] A dark room had also been set up for photographic work in the department, where the use of photographs in anatomical research and teaching had been growing since the 1890s and was to further develop in relation to a variety of other media deployed in this context. The following sections of this chapter explore, then, the articulation of the Anatomy Museum with the aforementioned rooms through working practices in the department, and the implications of this articulation for displays of bodies. These displays were produced through interrelated media in order to constitute and disseminate anatomical knowledge.

DRAWING FROM DISSECTION

Methods of anatomical observation learned in dissecting rooms were trusted for their precision and veracity: dissecting was perceived as directly revelatory, as a practice that provided crucial access to the interior of the human body. For genuine knowledge to be gained, many hours of careful and patient work were required. The anatomy teacher Thomas Cooke (1841–1899), a surgeon at London's Westminster Hospital, for instance, emphasized the importance of practical work – entailing active visual and manual involvement – if students were to gain a 'sharp eye', 'trained hand' and 'educated finger'. Advocating the cultivation of this multi-sensory, tactile knowledge, Cooke's 1898 illustrated anatomy textbook, co-authored with his son Francis Garrard Hamilton Cooke, explained that in anatomy 'seeing and doing are understanding and nothing else is'. 'Doing' in dissecting rooms involved precise cutting, cleaning away fat and connective tissue, exposing and feeling anatomical structures. With practice the hands and eyes of the emerging expert would become so closely aligned that, according to Cooke, he would acquire an 'eye at the tip of his finger' – a 'digital eye' that could see the deeper parts of the body by means of 'tactile sensations'.[29] Furthermore, it was through practical work, as the Cambridge professor of anatomy Alexander Macalister explained, that a student of anatomy was

> educated to translate the impressions made by the objects of his study on his senses into words, this enabling him to check the descriptions in his books, or those taught in the lecture room, by comparing the realities under his hands with the verbal accounts of them given by his teachers.[30]

Checking or 'critically examining' in this way, Cooke advised, provided the 'foundation . . . which lies at the base of all true knowledge'.[31] Each student had, therefore, to translate their own disciplined sense impressions into anatomical description – and significant in this process was drawing.[32]

At Marischal College students' practical study in the dissecting room (illus. 94) involved learning to observe and describe the 'exact topography' of the human body's organs and structures, and to aid understanding of human anatomical parts they were compared with 'corresponding ones in other animals'.[33] Some animal dissection was conducted, such as that of a male chimpanzee in 1912, but it was human bodies that were prioritized. The dissecting room was furnished to accommodate around 300 students working in groups of about ten, with each group at a table.[34] Upon every table would not, however, have always been a whole body, as supplies of the dead from the Aberdeen funeratory regularly fell short. Few years saw 30 bodies available for dissection. There were critically low numbers from 1908 to 1920 – causing acute 'anxiety' among anatomists in Scotland, England and Ireland, Reid noted in January 1914 – and concerns about

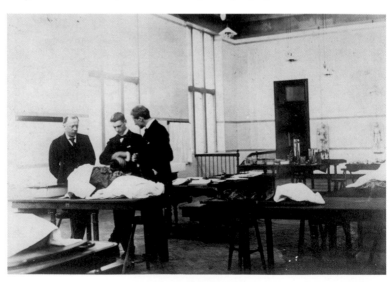

94
Robert Reid (far left) and Arthur Keith (far right) assessing a medical student in the dissecting room, Anatomy Department, Marischal College, University of Aberdeen, 1898–1901, photograph.

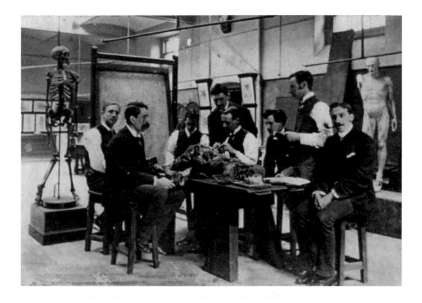

insufficiencies were expressed in Aberdeen during the next two decades, and beyond.[35] Times of scarcity necessitated prudent and careful distribution of dissecting tasks among students, crucially supplemented by the use of museum specimens and anatomical images. Bodies treated with preserving fluids and kept for several months before burial were dissected in regions – beginning with the 'extremities', then proceeding to thorax, abdomen, and head and neck – by students assigned specific 'parts'.[36]

Students were especially encouraged to make drawings of 'variations' and 'abnormalities' found during dissections.[37] Variations in the size, form and position of anatomical parts were considered 'normal' within a given range, but beyond this they were potentially identified as 'anomalies' – they could enter the category of the pathological.[38] On discovering interesting or extreme variations, students drew them, enhancing their understanding and providing a visual record for further study. Robert Reid's anatomy students at St Thomas's had made drawings from dissections (illus. 95), which he assembled along with his own rough pencil-and-ink sketches of variations – drawing was a way of collecting human anatomy as well as a means of learning from it (illus. 96).[39] At Marischal College, between the 1890s and the 1940s, standardized forms were issued to students for noting the age and sex of the numbered (not named) deceased person/body or 'subject' in which a variation was identified in the dissecting room, then sketched and briefly described.[40] One drawing, for example, by John Wilson was concerned with the sternalis muscle in an 80-year-old man's chest, and showed muscles outlined in pencil and ink, their fibres suggested in red (illus. 97). Other students used watercolours and crayons, some

96
Robert Reid's book
of assembled sketches
and notes made from
dissections conducted
at St Thomas's
Hospital, 1874–8.

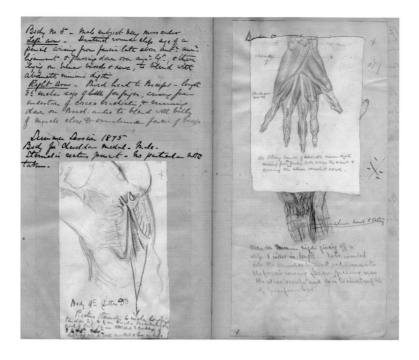

97
John Wilson,
annotated and
labelled drawing
from observations
of a dissecting room
subject, 1928.

aiming to capture the three-dimensional appearance of anatomical parts, such as those in the heart or foot, others opting for a diagrammatic approach. Women students, admitted to study medicine from 1895 onwards with practical anatomy classes sometimes held separately from men, also produced drawings.[41] All of these images utilized conventions, such as labelling, adopted from illustrated anatomical textbooks. Students' drawings were thus informed by authoritative images but they were also intended to relate exactly to what was observed so that, according to Reid's instructions, students would then be able to correct 'errors which have been handed down from book to book'.[42]

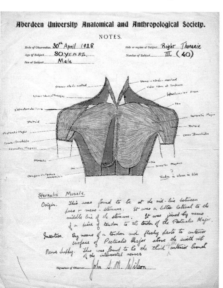

Drawing anatomical parts required close and sustained attention to dissections; learning to draw in this context was a matter of concentrated focus and the management of attention.[43] Manuals explaining how to dissect advised students to make sketches of parts because 'in no other way are the details impressed on the memory so accurately or is the eye attracted to points which would otherwise escape notice.'[44] Just as dissecting instruments were used to expose the part, so it was rendered again with marks on paper. To draw in this way was to gain knowledge.[45] Drawing refined observation and aided the translation of visual and tactile explorations into descriptions. Observations became drawings that were then linked to textual accounts via labelling techniques: the movement from tactile sensation to visual image on paper to inscribed word was eased by lines connecting each drawing with relevant anatomical terms. The act of drawing mediated fleshy specimen, visual image and text.

Such images produced by students were temporarily displayed in so far as they were submitted to anatomy demonstrators – who assisted Reid in teaching – and circulated in group discussions among fellow students.[46] But these novice images were not for museum display, unlike drawings created specifically for this purpose with close expert guidance, such as one key series that took central position in the Anatomy Museum (see illus. 88, centre row). These images depicted and named the components of over 30 anatomical specimens made under Reid's supervision around 1892.[47] Each specimen – an anatomical section cut either vertically or horizontally – was matched with a corresponding labelled image, the presentation of sectional views being a familiar mode of display used in anatomical atlases

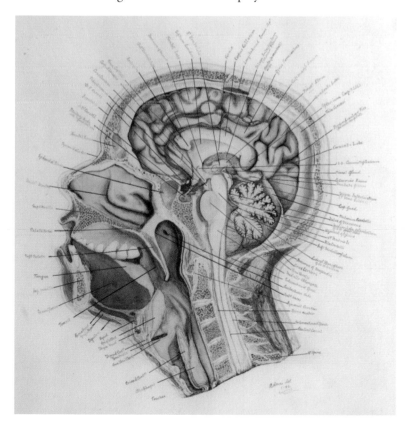

98
Alexander Don, pencil drawing and watercolour of the head and neck, 1892, based on a section prepared by Robert Reid and preserved as a museum specimen for the Anatomy Museum, University of Aberdeen.

and by three-dimensional models. For example, the 1877 English translation of Wilhelm Braune's atlas of topographic anatomy, in which Braune utilized the technique of sectioning bodies to great visual effect, was in the department's collection, as were plaster models of the thorax cast in a series of horizontal slices.[48]

The Anatomy Museum's images of sectioned specimens were drawn, and watercolour applied, by Alexander Don and Arthur Hugh Lister, both medical students already in possession of university degrees, the latter a science graduate from the University of Cambridge and nephew of the surgeon Joseph Lister.[49] Don and Lister produced images that bore close visual resemblance to the dissected specimens upon which they were based, while also clearly distinguishing labelled anatomical parts (illus. 98). When such images and specimens were displayed together – as one anatomist emphasized with regard to the pairing of preserved body part and drawing – the two were to be shown in proximity so that students could directly compare them: 'in this way salient points can be accentuated and the attention properly and immediately directed to the important facts which the [specimen] is designed to illustrate.'[50] So with the use of colour and label, such images supplied definition, selecting and augmenting the shape of relevant parts, and thereby helping to consolidate the very visibility of the specimen in particular ways.[51] The precise arrangement of images in the Anatomy Museum was thus significant in making visible the bodily interior as composed of specimens crafted in the dissecting room.

The spatial and conceptual drawing together of specimen and image was a display strategy favoured among museum conservators. William Flower, whom Reid respected as a great authority on museums, was critical of arrangements that separated specimens from drawings and casts, advising that related items should be located together 'in one spot' to provide a 'connected view' of them and to allow direct comparison of 'objects which must necessarily throw light upon each other'.[52] Charles Walker Cathcart, at the RCSEd, promoted similar intermedial displays during the 1890s.[53]

Further visual iterations of museum specimens were created at Marischal College when drawings of anatomical sections were photographed, as in the case of those made from one woman's body in 1906.[54] Reid reported on this process in the department's regularly published journal – the *University of Aberdeen Proceedings of the Anatomical and Anthropological Society* (*PAAS*) – the Aberdeen University Anatomical and Anthropological Society (AUAAS) having been founded in 1899 by and for medical students, and actively supported by staff. [55] In this publication Reid noted how the woman's body was acquired as well as the techniques that were used to convert her into a museum specimen. When this 'well developed muscular female subject', aged about 35, was brought to the Anatomy Department, he wrote, 'the only history I was able to obtain was that the individual was found in an outhouse in this town in an insensible and moribund condition and that she died a few hours afterwards.'[56] From her body, which was 'very well formed' and younger than was usual for a dissecting-room subject, Reid decided to 'make sagittal [vertical] sections of the trunk in the frozen state'.[57] Then from one of the four resulting sections a 'drawing' was produced, in tones of grey watercolour with white outlines for added definition. The preserved sections and the image were placed together in the Anatomy Museum, and the image, labelled with a numerical key, was photographed (illus. 99). Thus the woman's body was sequentially transformed – to demonstrate her anatomy – into dissecting room subject, specimen, drawing and photograph, the latter reduced in scale for publication in the scientific forum of the *PAAS*.

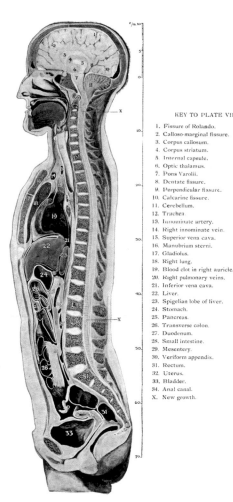

KEY TO PLATE VIII.

1. Fissure of Rolando.
2. Calloso-marginal fissure.
3. Corpus callosum.
4. Corpus striatum.
5. Internal capsule.
6. Optic thalamus.
7. Pons Varolii.
8. Dentate fissure.
9. Perpendicular fissure.
10. Calcarine fissure.
11. Cerebellum.
12. Trachea.
13. Innominate artery.
14. Right innominate vein.
15. Superior vena cava.
16. Manubrium sterni.
17. Gladiolus.
18. Right lung.
19. Blood clot in right auricle.
20. Right pulmonary veins.
21. Inferior vena cava.
22. Liver.
23. Spigelian lobe of liver.
24. Stomach.
25. Pancreas.
26. Transverse colon.
27. Duodenum.
28. Small intestine.
29. Mesentery.
30. Veriform appendix.
31. Rectum.
32. Uterus.
33. Bladder.
34. Anal canal.
X. New growth.

99
Photographed pencil drawing and watercolour of a 'section of female subject aged about thirty-five years', *c.* 1906, 'drawn from' a section prepared by Robert Reid and preserved as a specimen for the Anatomy Museum, University of Aberdeen.

Such transformations then fed back into dissecting-room practices: students studied the resulting specimens and images in order to guide their work when anatomizing further bodies. As Thomas Cooke pointed out, when preparing to dissect, students should firstly study the relevant part in anatomical illustrations and museums so that they could see 'what to look for; where things are, what they look like, how they run; where he is on safe ground and can cut freely, where he may do damage and must be cautious'.[58] Failing to scrutinize museum specimens in this way would result in a student approaching a dissection 'blindly', lacking the foresight to conduct the work according to expected standards.[59] Museum displays, constructed by experts, thus enabled students to see, in advance, versions of the anatomical interiors that they were about to uncover in their own dissections: the displays provided for students the desired parameters of knowledge to be gained through their own material interrogations of bodies.

FOCUS AND PROJECTION

If drawings elucidated dissections, they also offered, like photography, means of adjusting the scale of anatomical objects, thereby encouraging focused, attentive study. While dissected body parts were reduced when drawn on manageable, portable sheets of paper, and specimens were reduced via photography for publication, procedures of enlargement produced absorbing and compelling views of bodily interiors. Study with microscopes, magnifying anatomical parts invisible to the 'naked-eye', was facilitated by the Anatomy Department's expanding collection of slides.[60] Three-dimensional anatomical models enlarged small parts, such as the

100
Wall chart showing a 'schematic representation' of the inner ear, 1899, watercolour on paper, after Léo Testut, *Traité d'anatomie humaine*, vol. III, 4th edition (Paris, 1899), Fig. 483.

101
Illustration of a horizontal section of the right eye, from Léo Testut, *Traité d'anatomie humaine*, vol. III, 4th edition (Paris, 1899), Fig. 258.

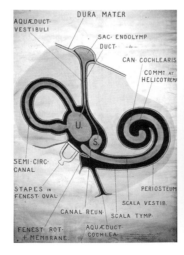
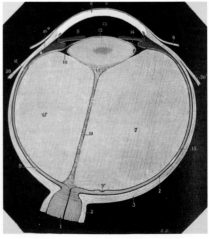

102
Lantern slide of an
unwrapped mummy
held by Nora
Macdonald in the
Archaeological
Museum, King's
College, c. 1900.

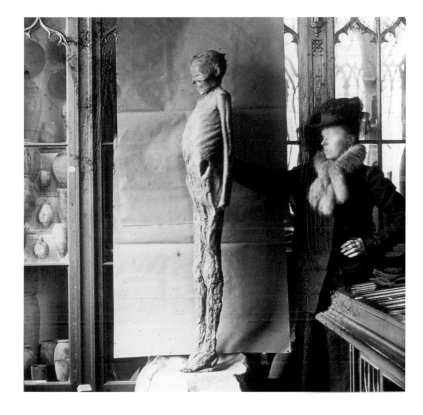

human eye, ear or kidney, to sizes easier to grasp in visual and tactile terms
(see illus. 40, 83). Two-dimensional versions of enlarged body parts were
employed too – for example Robert Reid's anatomical diagrams made
in-house on large-format paper for display on walls.[61] A 'schematic representation' of parts of the inner ear (illus. 100), for instance, was a giant
rendering of an illustration in Léo Testut's textbook *Traité d'anatomie
humaine* (1899), held in the department's collection.[62] The translation
from textbook to wall chart enlarged the diagram to increase its visual
accessibility and strengthen its impact. The book's diagram had already
visually extracted relevant anatomical parts from their surrounding body
and the subsequent removal/transfer to wall chart performed a further
extraction, excising image from book to more effectively focus visual attention upon it. Now scaled up in size, it could be examined by many students
simultaneously when displayed, for example, during lectures; this group
viewing effectively disseminating, and collectively reinforcing the validity
of, the diagram's anatomical insight.

Focusing students' attention was achieved with the use of another convention in anatomical illustration – the masking of background. A diagram
of the eye, for example, again from Testut's textbook, was framed by an

empty blackness which, in visual terms, isolated and decontextualized the part (illus. 101).[63] Selected anatomical features were thus simplified and differentiated with the use of colour, while the dark surround voided pictorial space. Photographic images produced in the department also used the convention of background masking. Among these was that of an unwrapped mummy, from the University of Aberdeen's Archaeological Museum at King's College, photographed in 1900 against a blank backdrop (illus. 102). Nora Macdonald, that museum's conservator (1900 to 1907), held the preserved body at arm's length, but when the image was published (in *PAAS*) the surrounding museum cases, windows and Macdonald herself were cut away. On the printed page the mummy was positioned horizontally,

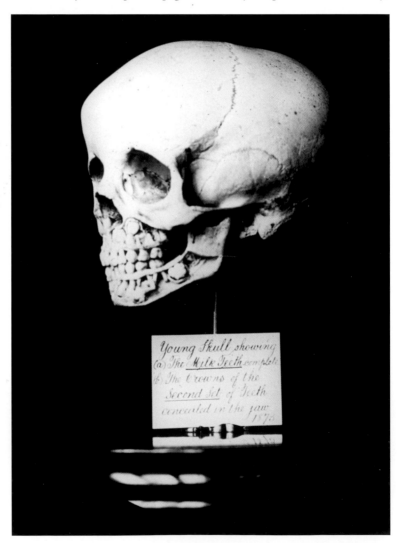

103
Lantern slide of a young skull, 1908, labelled as a specimen in the Anatomy Museum by John Struthers in 1873.

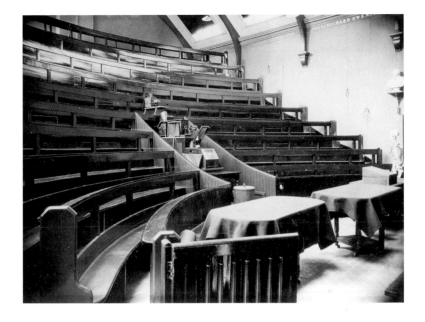

104
Lecture theatre
with seating capacity
of 250, Anatomy
Department,
Marischal College,
University of
Aberdeen, 1929,
photograph.

appearing recumbent, and all surroundings, including shadows, had been effaced. A lantern slide of the mummy, which Macdonald showed in a lecture for anatomy students and staff, received similar treatment, its spatial surround covered with black tape to render it invisible when projected.[64] These masking and deletion procedures produced views of specimens at a remove from their museum context and apparently free of interference from the curator's hands.[65]

Specimens from the Anatomy Museum were routinely photographed in seeming isolation, selectively highlighting them for display, especially in the form of glass lantern slides. An infant's skull on a slide from 1908 (with its 1873 label), for example, was sharply defined against an inky black background (illus. 103). In slide format the Anatomy Museum's specimens were visually amplified, when projected in the department's lecture theatre, for large audiences of students (illus. 104). So Reid would take actual specimens, such as the series of sections of the human head, from museum to theatre to point out anatomical details upon them, then 'by means of the lantern he transferred the section to the screen where the details were viewed on a large scale.'[66] The technology of the slide enabled an apparently seamless transfer from museum shelf to a high-impact big screen that showed images enlarged to virtually fill the observing student's visual field. Projecting in this way provided anatomists with a powerful tool for attuning the observational skills of their students.

Anatomists recognized further advantages of slides. By photographing museum specimens before enclosure in glass jars, 'distortion and reflection' was avoided in the resulting photographs which, when labelled, guided study of the specimens and provided the basis for drawings of the same. Significantly, lantern slides made from these photographs for teaching purposes allowed numerous specimens to be shown speedily during demonstrations, and they could also be easily sent to other appropriate institutions for study.[67] Thus the display of museum specimens within medical schools was enhanced with regard to scale and speed, and wide distribution among educational settings was enabled.[68]

At Marischal College hundreds of lantern slides were made from photographs of anatomical specimens and illustrations during the early 1900s, amounting to a comprehensive collection – maintained in dedicated wooden cases with multiple drawers.[69] Museum specimens in slide format were easily sorted and also transported for viewing in different spaces, without disturbing delicate displays or dismantling massive skeletons. And they could be shown in relation to an array of images either pre-drawn or sketched on the spot by anatomists: besides the lecture theatre's equipment for exhibiting lantern slides (with a magic lantern) and for projecting anatomical specimens (with an epidiascope), there were screens for attaching diagrams and blackboards for sketches in chalk. So, while listening to lectures, students saw aspects of human anatomy displayed in photographic and diagrammatic formats and projected at different levels of magnification.[70] The department had apparatus for making X-rays from 1902, and these images too were shown as slides in lectures, aiding the study of 'movement and anatomical structure [in the living body] as revealed by the X-ray technique'.[71] The Anatomy Museum was viewed, and its value affirmed, by these practices of image production and projection, which encouraged meaningful focus on particular specimens in its collection. Such practices facilitated the display of specimens, and their comprehension, within multiple different visual sequences alongside other current anatomical images.

Photographs were afforded a privileged position within this nexus of image use and specimen interpretation. The epistemological claims of photography were asserted in one of the department's atlases from 1911. Richard Berry, professor of anatomy at the University of Melbourne, Australia – previously lecturer in Edinburgh and examiner in anatomy at the University of Aberdeen (1901 to 1905) – stressed in his *Clinical Atlas of Sectional and Topographical Anatomy* that 'sources of error are entirely eliminated' by the use of photography when making reproductions of anatomical specimens. Hand drawing, tracing and engraving could introduce errors, but he was confident that photography, as a 'medium of recording', 'affords the most faithful reflex of the originals' and therefore produces 'exact . . . representation[s]'.[72] Yet the ideal of mechanical objectivity alluded to here – of making images with methods that minimized the intervention (and therefore subjective influence) of the maker, whether scientist or artist – was met by an approach that valued deliberate manipulation for legitimate pedagogical reasons.[73] Berry's anatomical photographs were evidently accentuated, overlaid with colour and labelled (illus. 105). Internal structures and shapes were made more pronounced when, for example, parts, such as the ribs, were outlined and 'photographic shadows' were strengthened in black. Also, embedded in the photographs were devices designed to guide and aid their use by anatomy teachers and students. Thus images were marked with centimetre scales and lines so that anatomical structures visible in the photographs could be 'projected' – that is, 'transferred' by means of measurement – onto the surface of the 'living subject', thereby enabling identification of those structures within live bodies, such as those of living anatomy models observed by medical students.[74] Berry's atlas suggested further visual formats into which its photographs could be converted: they could be made into lantern slides and, when projected onto a screen, 'greatly enlarged tracings can be constructed suitable for diagrams.'[75] By adopting these methods for reworking photographic images, anatomy teachers could effectively take them from book to lecture-theatre screens for display alongside slides showing relevant museum specimens.

Stereoscopic photographs, furthermore, allowed students to view anatomized bodies in what appeared to be three dimensions, disrupting

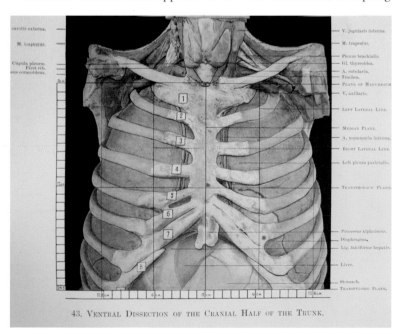

105
Illustration of a dissection of the trunk, from Richard J. A. Berry, *A Clinical Atlas of Sectional and Topographical Anatomy* (Edinburgh, 1911), Fig. 43.

43. Ventral Dissection of the Cranial Half of the Trunk.

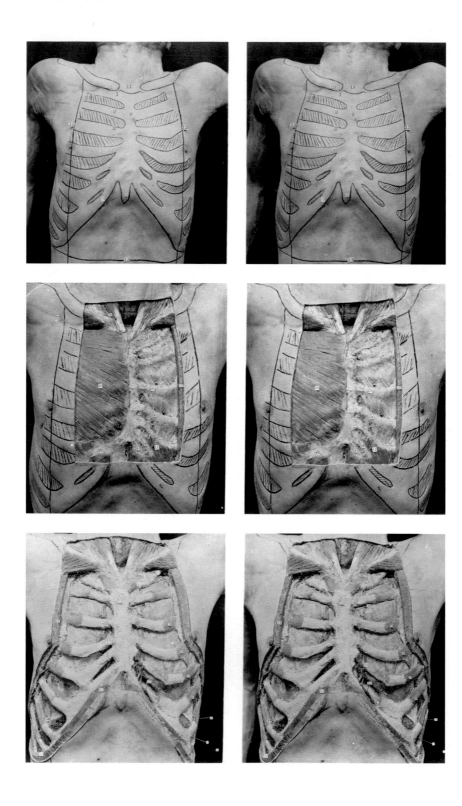

distinctions between three-dimensional specimen and two-dimensional image. Copies of *The Edinburgh Stereoscopic Atlas of Anatomy*, published in 1905–6, were widely utilized in Scotland's medical schools, including at Marischal College (illus. 106).[76] Five boxed sections contained 250 cards on which stereoscopic photographs were mounted with descriptive labels. When viewed in sequence, these images displayed parts of preserved bodies at progressive stages of dissection, guiding the observer seemingly directly into bodily interiors (illus. 107, 108). Photographs of the thorax, for example, staged an excavation of the entire anatomical region which began with the body's surface – where outlines of ribs were drawn on the skin to guide the scalpel – then proceeded inwards through layers of muscle and membrane that were cut away until the deepest levels of dissection were reached. Reviews praised the high-quality photographs of dissections, which had been prepared and 'selected with much judgement'.[77] Another publication, Arthur Thompson's stereoscopic *Anatomy of the Human Eye* of 1912, also acquired by Marischal College's Anatomy Department, allowed students to see enlarged, clarified views of this body part that was difficult to dissect. Such was the perceived efficacy of this kind of image that, during the 1920s, the department purchased its own stereoscopic camera to produce photographs on site.[78]

Stereoscopic images – observed either through devices held to the eyes or via box-shaped cabinet viewers accommodating a number of images for viewing in succession – sought to restore the three-dimensionality of human anatomy that was lost in drawn and printed images. They made bodily interiors strikingly visible in depth, aiding study of the spatial location and relative position of parts, which appeared less like flat images and more akin to anatomical dissections or museum specimens in the flesh. This effect helped students to compare these educational images with their own difficult to discern dissections. In this context of learning, the relations construed between bodies and images were not reducible to a unidirectional translation of the complex three-dimensional into the simplified two-dimensional,[79] especially because the approved conduct of anatomical observation required visual and tactile examination of actual bodies in dissecting rooms and anatomy museums. As Reid insisted, 'representations' such as photographs should not 'pretend' to 'take the place' of 'original specimens' because the latter are 'replete with information which no reproduction can possibly display'.[80] Three-dimensional specimens were not replaced by two-dimensional images; rather, multiple movements between renderings in the flesh and in different media enabled bodily interiors to be explored by eyes and fingers, to become known through the learner's developing 'digital eye'.

106–8
Three pairs of stereoscopic photographs of a dissection of the thorax, from David Waterston, ed., *The Edinburgh Stereoscopic Atlas of Anatomy* (Edinburgh, 1905–6), Section 1, Nos. 1–3.

While images – drawn, painted, photographic and printed – were assembled, the collection of specimens, both human and animal, for the Anatomy Museum, remained a priority at Marischal College. Indeed, acquiring three-dimensional anatomies and, from these, producing two-dimensional versions, were interrelated, mutually reinforcing practices. Bodies and body parts were obtained from local as well as overseas sources – the latter sustained through colonial apparatuses – with Robert Reid, like his predecessor John Struthers, working within his network of social relationships to achieve museum expansion. Many animal parts were obtained from the immediate locality: between 1905 and 1910 skulls of a horse and a lamb, in addition to over twenty skeletons of other small vertebrates, were cleaned and articulated in the department, and the Aberdeen owners of a former prize-winning St Bernard show dog, named Wallace, gave his body for conversion into bony display.[81] With regard to human remains, the department's dissecting room was still a crucial site for specimen gathering/making, receiving as it did bodies from the Aberdeen funeratory – the institution which took in deceased persons (the unclaimed) from the city's Old Machar Poor House, St Nicholas Poor House, the Royal Infirmary, City Hospital and the Royal Lunatic Asylum (later renamed Aberdeen Royal Mental Hospital) and, when numbers diminished in Aberdeen, from poorhouses, asylums, hospitals and prisons in Scotland's northeast between Perth and Inverness.[82]

Extending beyond Scotland, Reid mobilized his contacts to attract acquisitions during the height of the British Empire, so the body parts of paupers, the apparently mentally ill and animals, from domestic sources, were joined by those from colonized territories.[83] Reid's brother, Colonel Alexander Reid, sent two human skulls from India, these taken from a male and female killed during a military expedition in 1895.[84] Relatives of Reid's university colleagues were obliging too. Alexander Ogston, professor of surgery, encouraged his son, a sailor, to look out for interesting animal skeletons for Reid, and a kangaroo was thus gained (it having died onboard ship on being transported from Sydney to a zoological garden in England).[85] Long-distance anatomical collecting was thus conducted via familial ties, just as it was via continuing bonds with alumni of Marischal College. Medical graduates sent animal bones for the purposes of comparative anatomy – such as those of a female rhinoceros arriving in the 1890s from Alfred William Alcock, superintendent of the Indian Museum in Calcutta – and they were equally at pains to forward human body parts (as discussed below).[86]

Reid's professional relationships provided further impetus and means to accrue museum specimens from far and wide. He nurtured contacts

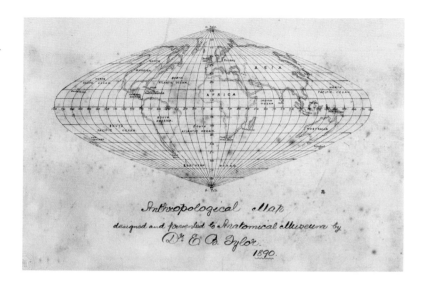

with leading anatomists and anthropologists, especially in Cambridge, Edinburgh, Dublin, London and Oxford.[87] Arthur Keith was keen to assist the Anatomy Department (he was an external examiner of students' work, 1898 to 1901) and Edward Burnett Tylor, anthropologist and keeper of the Oxford University Museum of Natural History, who had visited Aberdeen around 1890, took special interest in Marischal College's Anatomy Museum, presenting it with a drawing, entitled *Anthropological Map*, which he designed (illus. 109).[88] The map gave visual expression to an important aspiration for the Anatomy Museum – to build a collection that enabled the study of human races across the globe. As Tylor asserted, only with 'proper anatomical examination' could differences between races be identified, and anthropologists found these differences 'most clearly in stature and proportions of limbs, conformation of the skull and the brain within, characters of features, skin, eyes, hair . . . mental and moral temperament'.[89] So, on taking a skull down from a museum shelf to properly examine it, Tylor explained, its race should be readily recognized.[90] While William Flower asserted the urgency of collecting and preserving, in large numbers, (parts of) skeletons of races facing 'destruction' – due, he suggested, to the 'rapid extension of maritime discovery and . . . commerce' – hundreds of skulls were routed from across the globe to university collections of anatomy, such as those in Glasgow and Edinburgh.[91]

Instrumental in enlarging the Anatomy Museum's holdings of human skulls, and other body parts at Marischal College, were Reid's contacts with colonial administrators, medical practitioners and missionaries in widespread locations: the 'world' as seen in the Anatomy Museum arose (partly) from the sum total of all these social relationships.[92] Through such relations, numerous skulls traversed considerable distances – many former students, for instance, were employed in the West African Medical Service around 1900, and skulls were duly sent by them from the Gold Coast (Ghana) and from southern Nigeria.[93] Upon arrival, each skull was categorized and labelled according to the geographical region in which it was collected – for example 'European', 'African', 'Melanesian' – and sometimes inscribed directly on bone.[94] A handwritten waxed paper label was attached to each skull with wire or string, providing a record of the date it was received and the name of the person who presented it to the Anatomy Museum. Such information, along with the sender's account of how a skull was obtained (if provided), formed what was termed the specimen's 'history'.[95] Removed from the body of a person, and abstracted from the social context of that life and death, a skull's meaning and value was informed by its 'history' – indeed, this history was regarded as a guarantee of the specimen's legitimacy or, according to Flower, its 'authenticity'.[96]

Yet, although important during the initial incorporation of a specimen into the Anatomy Museum, this history could be subsequently relegated to the background, moved out of focus, when the specimen was displayed and observed. In particular, imaging techniques were used to frame specimens – to cut them out of context, as noted above – and two examples here indicate how this framing upgraded the specimen's visibility while deleting anything regarded as extraneous to that specimen, including textual traces of the social and power relationships that had yielded it. As the following examples suggest, the acquisition of a specimen for the Anatomy Museum was a process that extended well beyond the moment a body part arrived at the department: not only was anatomical work required to assign the part status as a specimen, but images of it were produced – and images formed further acquisitions which then inflected the observation of that specimen.

The first example relates to fourteen human skulls sent to the Anatomy Museum by Allan James Craigen, a former student of Reid's, from Port Moresby, British New Guinea (Papua New Guinea), around 1902, when Craigen was chief medical officer.[97] Craigen explained that the skulls were initially collected by Judge Christopher Robinson, when acting-governor of British New Guinea, and these included nine from Goaribari Island which were 'obtained on a punitive expedition made in 1901 on account of two missionaries having been killed and eaten there'.[98] A lecture on the skulls, given in the department by Robert Haig Spittal, junior assistant to Reid, reiterated the narrative of indigenous people's violence and cannibalism – actions attributed to those represented as 'savage' in contrast to the 'civilised' within this colonial representation.[99] Spittal further noted, from the skulls' documentation, that these people 'have a practice of collecting human skulls, both of friends and of enemies, and they preserve these skulls in their war-houses or "dobus", and also in their dwellings'.[100] This mode of indigenous collecting was clearly made subordinate to that of Western scientists.[101]

Reported details of the social and material setting from which the skulls had been taken were, however, treated as extraneous to the analysis of physical characteristics as prioritized in the Anatomy Department. Although Spittal invoked and interpreted such details when examining 'decorated' skulls as 'works of art' (in this case evaluated as 'primitive'), his predominant concern was with these skulls' 'chief features' observed from an 'anthropometric point of view', and thus a lengthy series of measurements was recorded including internal cubic capacity. Specimens with 'elaborate ornamentation' – such as those from the Bamu River area with 'claylike' coverings and 'protrusions' studded with seeds (illus. 110) – were notably difficult to measure. Ornamentation impeded measuring procedures, anatomists worried; when it 'obscured' anatomical features it lead to incomplete measurements, as Spittal regretted.[102] Direct access to bone was preferred rather than problematic layers of decoration, which were often fragile and difficult to handle without causing damage. Photographic images of skulls were here considered entirely advantageous: although they could not penetrate through surface layers of ornament, they allowed sustained and detailed visual examination of specimens from various angles (see illus. 113a–d), and they enabled the display of specimens to multiple viewers within a common scientific community via lantern slides as well as in publications. In these formats skulls appeared in apparent isolation, having been photographed, then cut out to remove background and shadows, and subsequently rephotographed to frame them in blank space (see illus. 110). By deleting context, this operation accentuated the skulls' status as specimens for intensive visual scrutiny.

A second example of this extended acquisition process – in which visual images further abstracted specimens from the contexts in which they were initially obtained – involved the feet of a Chinese woman, which had been 'distorted' while she was alive through the practice of foot-binding. These were presented by another medical graduate, William Middleton, during his time as medical officer of health for Singapore.[103] From there Middleton had already shipped to the Anatomy Department the skeleton of a Chinese man, secured from the Pauper Hospital with the help of a

110
Photograph of a 'Decorated skull from New Guinea. Side view', c. 1905, preserved as a specimen in the Anatomy Museum, University of Aberdeen.

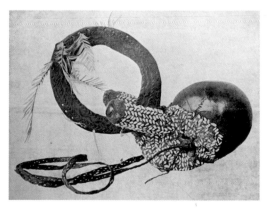

member of staff. As Middleton explained to Reid in a letter, this acquisition had been difficult; he had gone 'warily about' it because the man had already been buried and, from Middleton's perspective, he saw that 'the Chinese [. . . are] very superstitious in the matter of their dead and dread all sorts of visitations from departed spirits should the remains of their dead be disturbed.'[104] But Middleton's awareness of local beliefs and concerns were clearly overridden by his desire to contribute to the Anatomy Museum, and thereby to the 'continued prosperity' of his alma mater. Indeed, this desire prompted a further shipment: the feet of a 31-year-old woman who died of bubonic plague at the Infectious Diseases Hospital in Singapore. Middleton informed Reid that he 'got the feet at the PM [post-mortem], the body in such cases not being returned to her friends', and these body parts arrived in 1904, preserved in fluids and accompanied by the woman's 'disinfected' shoes, 'worn during her life'.[105]

At the Anatomy Department the feet were subjected to a range of observational and imaging techniques. Dissection to reveal the muscles, tendons and nerves of the left foot was followed by measurement, then drawing to render it in clear lines as a diagram. The right foot was X-rayed and the skiagram (radiograph) exhibited to allow analysis of the 'deformity'

111
Photograph of a 'Skiagram of distorted foot of Chinese female. Right foot viewed from inner aspect', c. 1904, preserved as a specimen in the Anatomy Museum, University of Aberdeen.

caused by 'excessive bending' at the joints'.[106] Further framing of the specimen took place when the skiagram was cut out and then photographed for publication in an empty surround (illus. 111), a procedure that evacuated superfluous detail and asserted the power of X-ray vision in revealing the anatomical interior.[107] Modes of visual excision were thus employed to compelling visual effect. However, arguably such frames did not absolutely constrain the specimen's meanings. For interested viewers, if they wished to persue it, could access an imaged specimen's 'history', and thereby retrieve selected aspects of the context from which the specimen was derived, in cases where anatomists' museum practices maintained linkages between images, labelled specimens and their textual records.

ANTHROPOMETRIC LABORATORY /
ANTHROPOLOGICAL MUSEUM

The Anatomy Museum, with its expanding collection of specimens, models and visual images, was integral to the anatomical practices conducted at Marischal College. With the opening of further spaces for collecting and display – namely the anthropometric laboratory in 1896 and the Anthropological Museum in 1907 – the Anatomy Museum's purpose and significance were reiterated and adjusted.[108] The anthropometric laboratory was formed to facilitate the practice of anthropometry. As the influential Paris-based anthropologist Paul Topinard explained, in this mode of enquiry the human body – 'living or upon the dissecting-room table' – is measured

> to determine the respective proportions of its parts: 1st, at different ages, in order to learn the law of relative growth of the parts; [and] 2nd, in the [human] races, so as to distinguish them and establish their relation to each other.[109]

Emphasizing the significance of this research in Aberdeen during the anthropometric laboratory's early years, Robert Reid instructed students that anthropometry, including craniology (involving the measurement of the skull), was an important means to study 'physical characteristics', and accordingly it was carried out at Marischal College with regard to 'groups' and 'races' at home and overseas.[110] And correlation of external physical characteristics with internal attributes, such as degrees of intelligence, was explored.[111]

From the 1870s anthropometry in Britain had been gaining momentum, with growing interest in its techniques and methods. The work of the British Association for the Advancement of Science, including the Ethnographic Survey of the British Isles, produced measurements, tables, reports and collections of photographs – such as those relating to people in 'isolated' districts of Aberdeenshire presumed to be as yet largely unaffected by industrialization.[112] The Anthropological Institute of Great Britain and Ireland, in its publication *Notes and Queries on Anthropology* (second edition), encouraged people who were travelling to systematically record body measurements and physical features, including eye, hair and skin colour, using a standardized guide.[113] Anthropometric laboratories were set up in various locations. Francis Galton's temporary laboratory at the 1884 International Health Exhibition in London attracted over 9,000 visitors, who were measured and tested for height, weight, keenness of sight and other features and capacities.[114] Inspired by Galton in the early 1890s,

Alfred Haddon, then a zoologist at the Royal College of Science in Dublin (later an anthropologist at the University of Cambridge), and Daniel Cunningham, an anatomist at Trinity College, Dublin, established a laboratory at the latter college's Museum of Comparative Anatomy. This anthropometric work in Ireland aimed to measure people from the city, rural areas and islands to investigate 'different types' and 'racial characters'.[115] Haddon, Cunningham, Galton and Charles Hercules Read, co-author of *Notes and Queries* and president of the Anthropological Institute, all gave their support to anthropometric initiatives in Aberdeen.[116]

Marischal College's anthropometric laboratory was initially a room in the Anatomy Department allocated for measuring medical students and compiling records thereof.[117] Installed with display cases, however, it was also referred to as the Anthropometrical Museum and as the Anthropological Museum, signalling its uses as a site for exhibiting (illus. 112).[118] Here, by 1899, were gathered over 3,000 items – such as spears, shields, clothing, canoes, ornaments and utensils from many parts of the world.[119] Prominent among these was a large collection of 'specimens illustrating the arts, customs and folklore of primitive peoples in . . . Fiji, and British New Guinea' lent (and subsequently bequeathed) by William MacGregor, a medical graduate of Marischal College who had held senior colonial posts in these places.[120] Like the Anatomy Museum, the holdings of the anthropometric laboratory grew within a matrix of social relations embracing medical practitioners and colonial officers who, in positions of authority, were keen to contribute to what, by the first decade of the 1900s, was

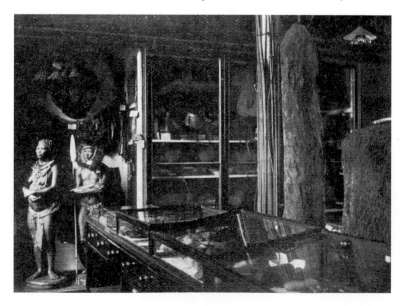

112
Anthropometric laboratory, 1906, Anatomy Department, Marischal College, University of Aberdeen, photograph.

considered a 'large and valuable collection of objects illustrating the habits and customs of different races of mankind'.[121] In this setting, anatomists conducted anthropometric observations of skeletal remains and of living persons, thus moving between bodily interiors and exteriors. Students were trained in these observational practices as well as undergoing anthropometric observation themselves, so students became both objects of enquiry and learning subjects; they were required to focus both on their own bodies and on those of 'other' races, to discern physical differences in ways that were always inflected by value judgements.

To produce reliable knowledge, work in the anthropometric laboratory extended the primary epistemological orientation adopted in the dissecting room and the Anatomy Museum, together with the latter's material resources. Just as learning in these spaces required the focusing of attention on the insides of bodies, where 'trustworthy' knowledge was gained, in anthropometry the skeleton was regarded as a source of 'anatomical truth', the stable point of reference from which 'real' measurements could be taken.[122] Nevertheless, the 'external proportions of the body clothed with its soft parts, muscles and tendons', as Topinard emphasized, had to be considered 'as much as the dry bones'. Furthermore, he argued, because 'large series of subjects' were necessary, and the number of skeletons in museums 'absolutely insufficient', it was from living people that measurements were to be taken in sufficient numbers to provide a 'degree of certainty'.[123] Access to skeletal remains *and* living bodies was thus crucial – and at Marischal College the former was provided by the Anatomy Museum, while the latter was mainly supplied by the annual influx of medical students. By the 1930s Reid could report that the 'physical characters' of some 2,000 students had been 'investigated', systematically measured in the anthropometric laboratory.[124] Medical students' bodies were thus collected in the form of anthropometric data.

With regard to human bones, many of the Anatomy Museum's specimens were temporarily transferred to the anthropometric laboratory for examination, movements which had implications for the status of knowledge production in both spaces. While incorporation into the Anatomy Museum validated specimens, promoting them as legitimate entities for further scientific attention, study of these very specimens in the anthropometric laboratory enhanced their educational value when back in the Anatomy Museum. During the first two decades of the 1900s, for instance, four skulls from Uganda, Nigeria and British New Guinea were moved from museum display to the laboratory for anthropometric study involving close observation, measurement, description and the making of visual images.[125]

When Charles T. Andrew, a junior assistant to Reid, observed four skulls from the Fly River in British New Guinea, for example, he recorded

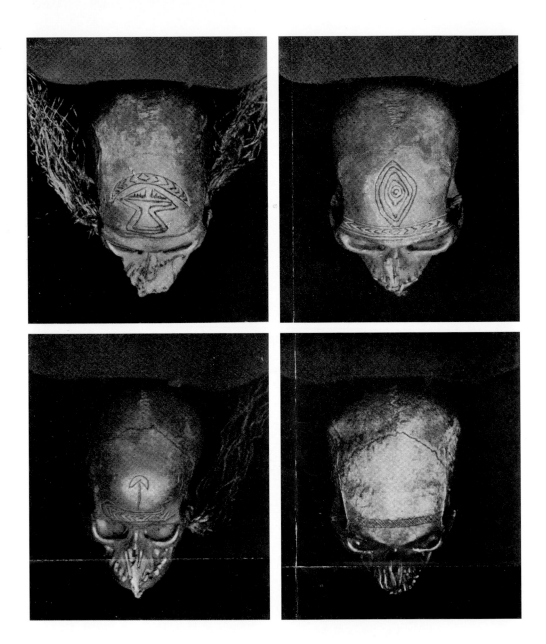

113a–d Photographs
of 'Four decorated
New Guinea skulls',
c.1900, preserved
as specimens in the
Anatomy Museum,
University of
Aberdeen.

their cubic capacity and at least 23 measurements in addition to describing them in a numbered series.[126] Andrew's description, like those produced by his senior colleagues, was based on observational skills and vocabulary learned through anatomical work in the dissecting room. Just as the anatomical description of human bodies undergoing dissection was concerned with the 'exact topography of any organ or structure' and its 'relations' to other parts, as well as the comparison of organs in 'man and other animals', so Andrew's description of the skulls focused on their bony 'features' in their relative locations along with a comparison of the 'design[s]' inscribed upon them with 'specimens of New Guinea art' held in the anthropometric laboratory. This comparative procedure treated organ and design as equivalent.[127] On the basis of these observations Andrew suggested that three of the skulls possessed 'Melanesian characteristics', but No. 4 'appears to be of a higher racial type', with a cranial capacity exceeding that of the others.[128] The description was presented, and the skulls exhibited, at a meeting of the AUAAS held in the Anatomy Department's lecture theatre, and in a subsequent framing and visual dissemination the specimens were photographed for publication in the *PAAS* (illus. 113a–d).

From the Anatomy Museum, the skeleton of a Chinese man sent by William Middleton from Singapore was similarly measured by Reid and Andrew, along with the skull of a man from north China and an 'ordinary European skeleton'; a comparison of the three was seen to generate 'instructive' results.[129] Again there was emphasis on physical differences from which a hierarchy of higher and lower types was discerned, an act of interpretation underpinned by the cultural politics of this knowledge practice. Assigning value according to such a hierarchy, Reid and Andrew noted that

> although the European skull shows a few low racial characteristics, yet when observed as a whole it is superior to either of the two Chinese skulls as regards its cranial capacity, horizontal circumference, development of frontal region and in breadth of face.[130]

The understanding of physical characteristics, however, required shifts in focus from the Anatomy Museum's osteological specimens derived from the deceased, to the exterior of living bodies – and these shifts were promoted via displays in the lecture theatre. On one occasion a living person – a 'native of the East African coast' – was shown at an AUAAS meeting. Ian Rose, who had studied at Marischal College and worked as a medical officer during the construction of the Uganda Railway, addressed the AUAAS in June 1900, giving a lecture on the 'native tribes of Eastern Equatorial Africa', accompanied by 'his Swahili boy' named Hasani.[131] Presumably in

Rose's employment as a servant, Hasani was viewed in terms of his exterior 'physical features', which were seen to indicate his 'race', and was deemed to be from an 'intelligent tribe', as indicated by his ability to deliver a 'graphic account' of how he was once wounded by an arrow during another tribe's hostile 'raid'.[132] Hasani was staged as a specimen, and photographed as such in the department, positioned passively in front of a blank wall, facing the camera (his eyes looking slightly to the right), arms by his sides, bare feet visible below his full-length garment; a living counterpart to the five human skulls that Rose presented to the Anatomy Museum.[133]

Such displays were produced through colonial power relations – and this was also evident in the exhibition of lantern slides which again featured photographs of living bodies. When pathologist (and, later, professor of ethnology at the London School of Economics) Charles Seligman visited Aberdeen in 1907 to give a lecture for the AUAAS on the recent Daniels Expedition to British New Guinea, he reported on measurements of living people, linked with those of skulls collected in the area, and showed photographs of people as 'types'.[134] In Seligman's account people, identified by numbers rather than as named individuals, became representative of racial categories, of tribes and of inhabitants of particular geographical regions.[135] Photographs in this genre had been taken in colonial contexts from around the 1860s onwards for purposes of survey and classification, ranging from images of 'native types' to anthropometric photographs of living people's naked bodies positioned, according to the procedures of science, alongside measuring devices.[136]

Emphasis on the living body as a site of scientific scrutiny was further enacted with the (temporary) removal of plaster casts from the Anatomy Museum to the anthropometric laboratory, as featured in the earliest (surviving) photograph of this room (see illus. 112). These casts, of the live 'Bushwoman' and 'Bushman' purchased over 40 years earlier were, by 1899, displayed in this setting for anthropometric study, dressed with artefacts in a staging of these static figures as though more dynamically – perhaps dramatically – alive.[137] With adornments in the anthropometric laboratory, the plaster bodies seemed to animate 'collections showing his [man's] characteristic customs and methods of living, his arts, arms and costumes'.[138] The casts, stripped of clothing, were returned to the Anatomy Museum, around 1907, to rejoin the 'specimens illustrating the [physical] structure and comparative anatomy of Man, including many skulls of existing races of mankind' along with 'numerous bony . . . remains and casts of skulls of Pre-historic Man' (see illus. 88).[139]

The transit of casts back to the Anatomy Museum was just one of many removals from the anthropometric laboratory as a mass of 'specimens' were relocated to form the basis of the Anthropological Museum in 1907; manoeuvres which had implications for displays of the human body. Specifically, items collected to 'illustrate' the 'culture of the different races of Man' – the myriad 'native cultural objects' from weapons to musical instruments and 'fetishes' containing medicine – were moved to the Anthropological Museum in Marischal College's front quadrangle.[140] Reid acquired this gallery for exhibiting when the library was removed, enabling him to bring together previously 'dispersed' specimens from across the university's buildings – including 'local relics' from northeast Scotland, classical and eastern antiquities, numerous coins and Egyptian artefacts (along with the rest of the Archaeological Museum's collection). Thus constituted, the Anthropological Museum thrived under Reid's curatorship, which extended from 1907 until the late 1930s when Robert Lockhart became curator with his appointment as professor of anatomy.[141]

While this museum initially emerged through anatomists' social relations and working practices, with Reid himself underlining the epistemological kinship of the 'anatomical point of view' and anthropology – the latter developing 'naturally' from the former when the examination of variations in physical characters 'awakens' the 'desire' to explore variations in the 'cultural status of different races' – the spatial separation of specimens used to teach and learn anatomy from those relating primarily to 'culture' constituted a significant material and conceptual differentiation.[142] So although the human skulls situated in the Anatomy Museum were defined as relevant to *both* anatomical and anthropological study, to found the separate Anthropological Museum was to largely distinguish it from the Anatomy Department's displays in terms of content, purpose and audience.[143]

After 1907, then, the anthropometric laboratory was newly configured in a different room furnished with specialized equipment and measuring devices (illus. 114) – and the vacated space reconfigured as the embryological laboratory for collections of specimens, research and teaching relating to embryology. Devoid of 'cultural' artefacts, the anthropometric laboratory was dedicated to observation of the Anatomy Museum's skulls and measurement of living bodies. Anthropometric records of medical students' bodies continued to be compiled in volumes of printed forms completed for each individual by Reid and his assistants. Students were documented with regard to outward appearance (including skin and hair colour), cranial circumference/length/breadth/height, span of arms, weight, breathing capacity, eyesight and hearing. Fingerprints were also taken.[144]

With standardized techniques and instruments, a named person was thus converted into a series of numbers for analysis and comparison.[145] These procedures tended to efface the living person, translating their

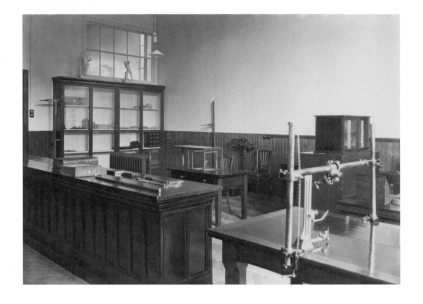

114
Anthropometric
laboratory, *c.* 1920s,
Anatomy Department,
Marischal College,
University of
Aberdeen,
photograph.

living body into numerical data.[146] But portrait photographs, kept alongside each written record and operating as a means to collect 'live' bodies, nevertheless preserved some aspects of individual personhood.[147] As in family albums of the time, specificities of appearance and comportment could be seen in these photographs, many of which were probably supplied by students themselves. For example, Cristina Wilson's record of 1905 was accompanied by a portrait photograph in which her facial features (documented on her adjacent anthropometric record) were clearly visible yet also framed by her distinctive plaited hair, lace blouse and brooch at her throat; with the inclusion of such photographs, the objectifying procedures of the laboratory would not eradicate traces of a person even as they tabulated their physical body.[148]

Furthermore, just as observations of students' bodies were recorded on the anthropometric laboratory forms, biographical notes were also sometimes subsequently added that so specific details of students' lives and deaths would be incorporated. Arthur Kellas's record, with a 1906 photograph, for instance, was later annotated in red ink and a further portrait of him, this time in uniform as a major in the Royal Army Medical Corps, was pasted to the page (illus. 115). The note stated that Kellas was 'killed in action on the Dardanelles, 6th August, 1915, aged 31': he died, like many medical students and alumni of Marischal College, serving in the First World War.[149] Here the anthropometric record of a once-living body also became a memorial for a specific person, a trace of war marking the loss of that individual. This particular textual and visual treatment of students' collected 'bodies' was not, however, applied to those of colonized people

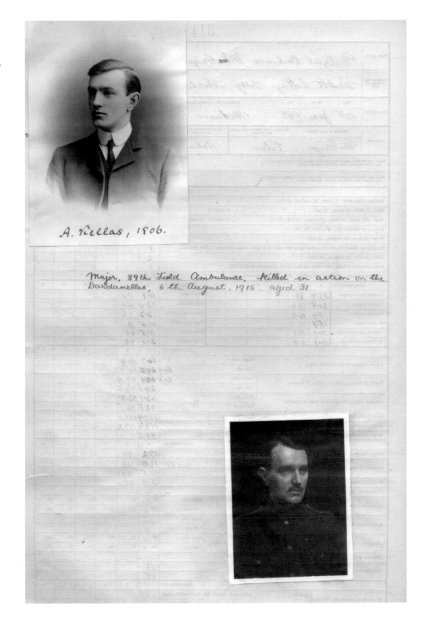

115
Anthropometric
record, taken in the
Anatomy Department,
Marischal College,
University of
Aberdeen, 1906
with supplementary
note c. 1915.

displayed in the department which, as photographs or casts, remained
deindividualized and generalized.

With its anthropological collection relocated, the anthropometric
laboratory was intended for staff and students, not for public admission.
So too the Anatomy Museum was more clearly marked out for professional
educational purposes. Attendees of Reid's popular lectures on anatomy,
given between 1890 and 1902 on Saturday evenings for 'people outside his

profession', had been invited to view the Anatomy Museum, and further groups, including the Aberdeen Branch of the Association of Teachers in the Secondary Schools of Scotland and the Aberdeen Working Men's Natural History and Scientific Society, were also admitted – the attention of these visitors having been drawn especially to skulls and skeletons of humans and other animals.[150] But by 1899, a local newspaper announcing the Saturday afternoon opening of the Anatomy Department's museums to the public emphasized the Anatomy Museum's importance for students while warning that its exhibits were probably less appealing according to the 'general public taste' than the anthropological collection.[151] Although skeletal remains – illustrating evolution, 'various races', 'prehistoric man' and comparative anatomy – were presented by Reid and in the press as of general public interest, the Anatomy Museum's other specimens – of the 'eye, ear, brain, heart, etc.' – were described as 'highly technical', more appropriate for medical students' viewing. So bones might have been considered more widely comprehensible and fitting for an interested public to see, but many preserved soft parts of bodies were deemed more fitting for specialist appreciation.[152]

Perceived degrees of technicality combined with prevalent 'taste', or aesthetic evaluation, thus guided the viewing of bodily interiors during a period when anatomical displays in Britain were increasingly reserved for medical professionals' and students' uses rather than public display. Indeed, by the early years of the 1900s institutionally based anatomy museums were restricting access to their collections, and there were few commercial sites where human anatomy was publicly exhibited.[153] In late nineteenth-century Aberdeen a bookshop-window display of apparently 'indecent' anatomical models was prohibited by law, and the proprietor of a commercial anatomical museum – soon to be renamed the 'Museum of Science' – was charged with distributing obscene advertisements for his aids to health.[154] The Saturday afternoon opening of Marischal College's Anatomy Museum was short-lived and Reid's well-attended popular lectures on this topic ceased, while the Anthropological Museum opened in a more prominent gallery. Here displays of 'cultural' specimens removed from the Anatomy Department's interior and displayed in glass cases according to the parts of the world they were acquired from, whether 'Europe', 'North Africa', 'Asia', 'Polynesia', 'America', 'Australia', 'Melanesia' or 'Africa south of the Sahara', were promoted not only for university members but for 'the public at large'.[155] The strategic division and spatial location of anatomical and anthropological collections was here significant in defining domains of knowledge (disciplines) both in terms of their substance and their social dissemination.[156]

Privileged visual, and, to a certain extent, tactile access to the anatomical interior of bodies, human and animal, was made possible through the strategic expansion of museum collections, in concert with work in dissecting rooms and the production of visual images – processes that were enmeshed in social and power relations extending from the locality out through the empire and back again. Within the Anatomy Museum intermedial displays were installed and beyond its walls, in adjacent spaces of the Anatomy Department, selected museum specimens were closely observed, photographed and projected. While the anatomized deceased were viewed from the inside, techniques for studying the bodily exteriors of the living were developed. Anatomical practices utilized bodies of the departed and of the living, excavating bodily depth and exposing bodily surface from which the interior was deciphered. Through these material practices, however, to make visible – as in drawing, photography and the manufacture of specimens – was also often to extract, frame, mask and delete. The interplay of the dead and the living, of the visible and the invisible, in displays of anatomy are explored in the next chapter during the first half of the twentieth century, a period when anatomists increasingly mobilized living bodies as resources for the constitution of anatomical knowledge, and when anatomy museums – although largely reserved for medical professionals and students – were far from cut off from the outside world.

Six
LIVING ANATOMY

In an unpublished poem – 'The Anatomist's Dream' – written in the winter of 1923 by Robert Lockhart, the anatomist/author falls asleep in the dissecting room with his copy of the classic textbook *Gray's Anatomy*,[1] whereupon an illustration of the nervous system comes alive:

> 'Twas while I was dissecting, about the dusk of day,
> I fell into a slumber, before me lay my 'Gray',
> And out upon its covers stood a figure quaint who said,
> 'I am the nervous system and I've stolen from my bed.'[2]

The animated nervous system proceeds to describe its ailments using precise anatomical terminology with touches of humour before declaring, mock-ominously: ''Twould kill a psycho-analyst to diagnose my dreams.'[3]

As Lockhart's poem goes, the anatomist/author enters a dream and sees the nervous system speaking of its anatomy. The dissected yet living cadaver that participates in its own anatomization was a familiar figure in early modern European images, and Lockhart would certainly have been conversant with this visual convention (see illus. 49). But however much the poem reworked such past images, the jaunty rejuvenated nervous system was also a manifestation of anatomists' interests in *living anatomy* – the anatomical study of living bodies – which underwent significant development through twentieth-century teaching techniques, especially the making and use of images for display in spaces of medical learning.

When Lockhart penned his poem he was lecturing on anatomy at Marischal College, having graduated in 1918; he had enrolled there as a medical student in 1913, but suspended his studies during the First World War when serving in the Royal Navy Volunteer Reserve as a surgeon probationer. After further service as a surgeon lieutenant at sea and ashore (1918–19) he taught at his alma mater until 1931, when he was appointed professor of anatomy at the University of Birmingham. He returned to Aberdeen eight years later to take up the anatomy professorship, remaining in this post until retirement in 1965. Following this, Lockhart continued in his position as curator of the Anthropological Museum for a further fourteen years – so working in that post from 1939 for four decades.[4] As signalled by 'The Anatomist's Dream', Lockhart's professional endeavours were characterized by a pronounced emphasis on animated bodies, living and deceased, human and animal, in the effective teaching and learning of anatomical knowledge. And living anatomy – as a mode of anatomical practice that utilized a wide range of media – was enacted with, and informed perceptions of, collections held by Marischal College's Anatomy Museum.

During the period of Lockhart's professorship the Anatomy Museum was well maintained for professional use, with previously obtained specimens and models rearranged to ensure the continued educational potency of displays, as discussed below. The acquisition of new museum specimens became less pronounced than the production and collection of still and moving images for viewing in the Anatomy Department's teaching rooms and for educational consumption in specialist publications, yet this shift was to enhance (rather than diminish) the perceived significance of the Anatomy Museum and its holdings.[5] As under Reid's and Low's curatorship, the making and pedagogical uses of anatomical displays were intermedial processes taking place within the Anatomy Museum, dissecting room, lecture theatre and other designated spaces. But by the mid-twentieth century a broader range of images was being mobilized in the service of a somewhat differently articulated anatomy. For Lockhart – as anatomist-curator working with colleagues and students in Aberdeen and in his wider social and cultural context – created and utilized interrelated media, especially photographs, slides and films, in innovative ways. Like many of his contemporary university associates in Scotland and England, Lockhart was determined to enliven anatomy by foregrounding the living body, and, in doing so, to invigorate the anatomy of the dead. Lockhart's agenda in this respect was pursued via a distinctive anatomical poetics operating in related visual, material, spoken and written modes, which this chapter goes on to examine.[6] This anatomical poetics, as practised here, augmented the educational value of the Anatomy Museum as displays were reconfigured and activated in relation to freshly produced, vividly composed and compellingly narrated visual images of living anatomy – images that powerfully invoked and co-opted live bodies.

Unlike animated anatomical bodies in the print and wax of centuries past, which appeared to reveal their deepest physical innards, Lockhart's

1923 figure of the lively nervous system was a 'dreamt' version of an illustration which, when conjured in a poem, drew attention to the impenetrability of its innermost psychic recesses; its dreams were undiagnosable, it declared. If the poem's evocation of dreams within a dream perhaps suggested the elusive, or even infinitely receding, nature of knowledge when relentlessly sought from the deceased body on the dissecting table, the poem also countered this image of unobtainable knowledge by presenting the anatomized, enlivened dead as engagingly informative. While Lockhart wrote – in his 1927 manifesto on the art of learning anatomy published in the medical journal *The Lancet* – that dissection of the dead was absolutely necessary, he also emphasized the importance of studying 'the dead upon the living', of relating anatomy as seen in dissections to bodies alive and moving, including students' own bodies; to anatomize in this way thus entailed active exploration of the physical self. Furthermore, anatomical investigation in which dead and living bodies were studied *pari passu* (with equal step, or hand-in-hand) demanded deeply engaged imaginative work, even as it required the observation of 'facts'.[7] In contrast to previous anatomical practices in which the work of the imagination was overtly criticized, by the early 1900s scientists were explicitly embracing it, just as they acknowledged the importance of expert interpretation and judgement.[8] The practice of imagining could now provide a route to scientific insight when stimulated and guided by trained professionals in contexts of disciplined observation. Marischal College's Anatomy Museum became a scene and a resource for this empirically grounded yet avowedly imaginative anatomical learning.

With these developments the Anatomy Museum underwent a process of invigoration during the 1940s to mid-1960s, a time when the medical museums in educational institutions in Britain were on varied trajectories: some were destroyed or dispersed, some were actively maintained and others were newly set up.[9] Critical perspectives on particular kinds of museum holdings did not amount to the wholesale rejection of museum displays. Confidence in visual technologies, especially X-ray apparatus used to view the anatomy of the living, had indeed led some practitioners to condemn museum specimens with claims that 'the day of the description of dead specimens as essentially representing the conditions of life has gone for ever' – but others saw such X-ray images as problematic 'shadows . . . capable of almost infinite distortion', and therefore potentially inferior to museum specimens.[10] In practice, many anatomists remained committed to producing and utilizing specimens in medical-school teaching spaces, alongside X-rays and other relevant visual images and three-dimensional models. In Aberdeen Lockhart's dissection of nerves in the human head and neck (see illus. 136), for instance, was one of many that he crafted and displayed throughout his career. Key here was not only the form that museum specimens and exhibits took, but the manner in which they were used by anatomists in coordination with further favoured media and in line with preferred teaching methods.

During the middle decades of the twentieth century the Anatomy Museum was reconfigured in relation to anatomical work with live bodies, and through pedagogical practices that actively stimulated and engaged students' imagination, as analysed in what follows. The anatomical poetics – or means of making anatomical meaning – developing in this context operated via display strategies that drew upon diverse visual and textual forms, often seemingly unrelated to anatomy such as literary works and magazines, while also appropriating aspects of popular performance, such as circus acts, for professional anatomical training. As Lockhart honed his performative repertoire as skilled anatomist, displaying and disseminating anatomical expertise, students were guided into disciplined yet exploratory bodily learning with their own bodies as well as those of the dead.[11] Anatomical displays were animated by practices that cut across distinctions between the living and the deceased, the mental and the physical, the popular and the professional, and even between what was dreamed and what was empirically observed.

DRY BONES

Although living people had been exhibited and analysed in sites of anatomical practice for some time, and the ability of anatomists to bring 'dry bones' to life was seen as a sign of a skilful teacher in the second half of the nineteenth century, the decisive shift towards living anatomy in the early twentieth century was advocated as a new departure.[12] Significantly, living anatomy came to be partly defined through anatomists' forceful critique of dry bones, both literal and metaphorical, in their teaching – preserved bones often being important components of anatomy museums. As Grafton Elliot Smith, professor of anatomy at the University of Manchester, explained in 1918, it was wholly inadequate for students to learn by examining skeletons separately from the rest of the body, as in 'antiquated' osteology classes. 'The phrase "dry bones"' had become 'a byword for dullness and lifelessness, and all that was dreary in the way of acquiring knowledge', he noted, but for teachers to 'make dry bones live' was to provide students with valuable anatomical lessons.[13]

Thus bones were studied as part of the living body, and the dead were dissected in concert with the examination of active, living bodies. Elliot Smith asserted with regard to the medical student:

It is vitally important that at every stage of his investigation of the corpse he should be forced to picture to himself, and, so far as possible, to study on the living body – by the examination of the surface anatomy of living models, [and] by the use of X-rays . . . – what significance the facts have in the active living body.[14]

It was students' own anatomy and that of live models, therefore, that had to be frequently observed from the skin's surface.[15] Many anatomists concurred with this 'newer attitude', and also underlined the value of visual demonstration through 'pictorial display': this teaching required 'every possible contrivance', including an illuminating box for X-ray plates, an epidiascope, a cinematograph, a lantern [for projecting glass slides], a screen for diagrams and blackboards.[16] This equipment in lecture theatres was used to support and supplement study in dissecting rooms and museums, enabling vivid anatomical demonstrations of living bodies. For although anatomizing deceased bodies was deemed to provide students with a 'solid foundation of fact', corpses were regarded as potentially misleading.[17] To familiarize students with the anatomical structure of the living body and 'modifications in form' resulting from 'functional processes', images – especially X-rays shown on fluorescent screens – were used 'to correct the erroneous impressions created by studies of the cadaver'.[18] With appropriate methods and equipment, the aim was to take anatomy 'from the charnel house [or ossuary] to the realm of the dynamics of the living human body'.[19]

In Aberdeen Robert Lockhart focused on these dynamics with an approach to anatomy that employed a variety of methods and media to coordinate dead and living bodies, embracing movement and colour, and sometimes deliberately provoking surprise and amusement. His investigation and teaching of living anatomy sought to closely relate deceased and live bodies, yet his pedagogical practices still marked differences between them. When he wrote, in the late 1950s, that the 'rigid, bare bones of the macerated skeleton belie the qualities of living bones', he articulated a long-held concern with the distinction between the disheartening display of the skeletal dead and the animated anatomy he wanted to develop.[20] Something of this distinction was apparent to Lockhart in 1919, when, as a surgeon lieutenant in the Royal Navy, he visited an ossuary – the Chapel of Bones in Valletta, Malta.[21] On a souvenir postcard (illus. 116) he copied a translation of the Chapel's Latin inscription which apparently advised visitors to '*Go in peace, remember that thou shalt die.*' This memento mori message was dismissed by Lockhart, who was more concerned with live medical matters and wrote in response to the inscription: 'Rather gloomy conception of life, is it not? The priest [at the Chapel] said he

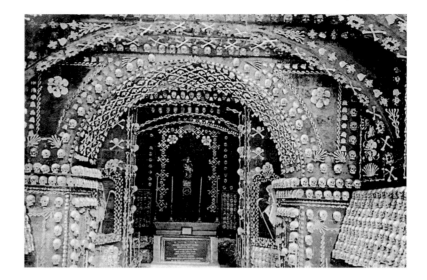

116
Postcard of the
Chapel of Bones,
Valletta, Malta,
c. 1919, collected
by Robert Lockhart.

was suffering from diabetes mellitus so I gave him the name of the latest book on the subject.'[22] Encountering this arrangement of human bones, then, Lockhart preferred not to ponder the prospect of death that it deliberately evoked, and this turning away prefigured his commitment to developing lively forms of anatomical display that directed attention to bodies during life in dedicated medical teaching spaces.

His pedagogical emphasis on the vibrancy of living bodies was, furthermore, inflected by the violent mass death of the First World War and what he saw of its effects on Marischal College's medical students. Interviewed towards the end of his life, Lockhart recalled teaching students who had fought in the horrific 1917 Battle of Passchendaele, near Ypres in Belgium.[23] They had been particularly affected, he said, by German explosives which blasted soldiers' fresh graves to the extent that unearthed bodies were 'hanging from trees'; the remains had to be taken down and reburied – 'it was very sad work'.[24] Such wartime traumas, and reports of them, no doubt fed Lockhart's commitment to living anatomy, with its emphasis on live, functioning bodies, not mutilated, fragmented parts. Lockhart's teaching of anatomy inspired positive enthusiasm for learning from live bodies whose visual appearance countered disturbing images of the war-torn dead. And his working practices remained informed more generally by wartime experiences: his colleagues noted his insistence on discipline, cleanliness and neatness in students' conduct and dress, for instance, linking his approach with his military training.[25]

Throughout the Second World War, debates about the significance of Britain's medical museums intensified. In particular, extensive damage from aerial bombing in May 1941 at the Hunterian Museum of the RCS –

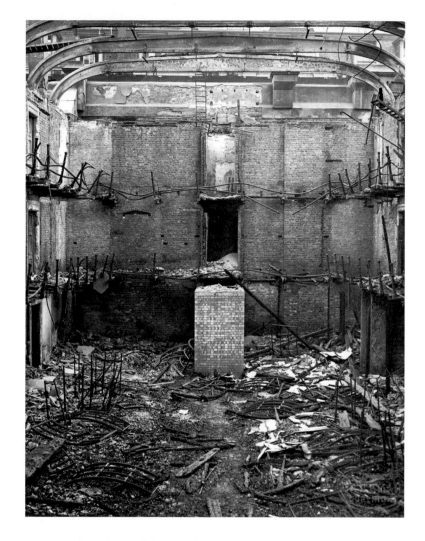

reported as a 'disaster' for the famous 'national collection' – provoked
public commentary on the current condition and future of museums in
medical education.[26] At the RCS, although precautions had been taken with
the move of selected museum holdings to the basement for protection,
entire exhibition galleries were shattered along with thousands of specimens in glass jars (illus. 117).[27] In the aftermath, museum staff and helpers
laboured to retrieve as much as possible from the wreckage. Arthur Keith,
who had retired in 1933, contributed to the salvage effort surrounded by
a 'charred mass' and a damaged, ash-covered bronze bust of Richard Owen,
one of Keith's nineteenth-century predecessors as conservator (illus. 118).[28]
With the building's roof demolished, further havoc was caused by rain,
damp and mould: 'mended crania collapsed into fragments, plasterwork

118
Salvaging remains
after the bombing
at the Hunterian
Museum, Royal
College of Surgeons
of England, 1941,
photograph.

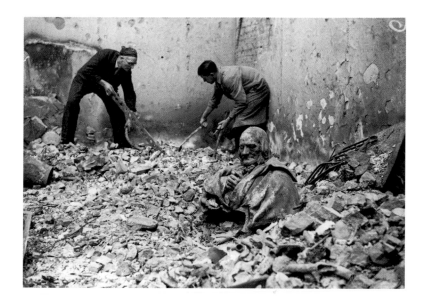

disintegrated in places, and swollen cabinet draws stuck fast; catalogues in
a strong room were soaked.'[29] This daunting mess did not, however, deter
the prolonged effort of recovering specimens, a process of cleaning and
repairing that was doggedly carried out to restore some order.

Following the bombing, medical professionals discussed the utility or
otherwise of museums in their spheres of work. An article in *The Lancet*
quoted an anonymous 'eminent physician' with firm opinions: '"Museums!"
he said. "Do you know what I would do with medical museums? Burn the
lot."'[30] Less radical views were expressed as creeping doubts and suspicions
that once precious collections had begun to resemble neglected, decaying
remnants of an almost-forgotten cabinet of curiosities:

> A visitor to most of these museums must have been depressed
> by what he saw – an apparently endless series of jars containing
> specimens of doubtful value from which every vestige of colour
> had long departed, a few tattered and out-of-date catalogues, derelict
> zoological curios, a few prize dissections, a mouldy collection of
> botanical specimens, some obsolete surgical instruments, one or
> two dangling skeletons, and some wax models of skin diseases.[31]

Despite this melancholy reflection on the recent state of some medical
museums – which were also apparently 'cramped by lack of space' and
starved of staff and finances – the educational value of these institutions
was nevertheless recognized by many teachers and students who were
increasingly seeking to use them. Medical visitors were no doubt encouraged

by those medical museums which had reportedly seen 'progress' both in the 'quality of material displayed' and in methods of arrangement.[32]

The 'reconstruction' of the Hunterian Museum at the RCS, regarded as a 'tribute to the past but also an obligation to the future', was taken as a signal that certain moves were underway to rejuvenate medical museums for educational purposes.[33] Indeed, a 1949–50 survey in Britain recorded 90 such museums, including new ones under construction. While these included museums of pathology and surgery, at least twelve museums dedicated to anatomy were operating in universities and colleges at this time.[34] Displaying museum specimens with visual images, ranging from lantern slides to films, directed students' attention to the living body, while also enabling learning from preserved human and animal remains. In Aberdeen, Lockhart advised students to 'keep your eye on the . . . body', explaining that:

> anatomy is raised from the dead by the study of the living. Apart
> from the ability of the hands to detect the action of muscles, to feel
> the beat of the heart . . . ghostly shadows cast by the X-rays reveal the
> movements of bones and joints and the passage of opaque substances
> through the vessels and the viscera.[35]

This 'raising of the dead', a bringing to life of sorts, was conducted when Lockhart, aided by assistants, coordinated displays for teaching with combinations of bodies undergoing dissection, museum specimens, visual images and students' own bodies. The performative action of the anatomist and an openly imaginative anatomical poetics facilitated students' learning by engaging their bodies in particular ways, promoting a thoroughly internalized understanding of living anatomy as explored in the rest of this chapter.

JOURNEY

Even with the rising importance of living anatomy, deceased bodies were still regarded as 'vitally important' sources of knowledge.[36] Anatomical demonstrations and images of live bodies were therefore spliced into teaching and learning practices that utilized the dead in dissecting rooms and museums. Instructions in manuals on how to dissect, for instance, also encouraged students to study their own surface anatomy to develop a 'practical conception of the intact living body'.[37] The dead were considered indispensable because students needed not only to *see* bodies from the surface of the skin (and below it by means of X-rays) but to *feel* bodies

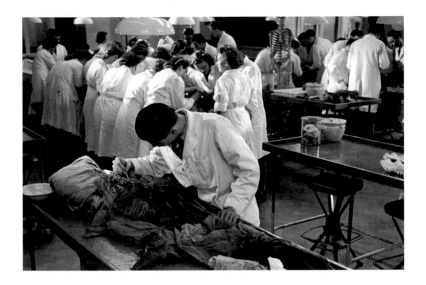

119
Wolfgang Suschitzky,
*Anatomy Class,
University of
Aberdeen,* 1948,
photograph.

from the inside. Lockhart's avid commitment to teaching via active in-depth anatomizing was evident in his requirement that students' hands 'must be trained', they 'must be kept dissecting'. Failing to 'cultivate the use of the hands is to neglect the finest machines ever created', he declared.[38] And students certainly responded: some intensive sessions of manual activity in the Anatomy Department's dissecting room during the late 1940s were captured at Marischal College in Wolfgang Suschitzky's photographs, taken during filming of his documentary *Scottish Universities* (illus. 119).[39]

In the dissecting room, kept 'spotless and gleaming' by cleaners including one Mrs Wood, the old slate-topped wooden tables had been replaced by around 50 new ones in tubular steel with green marbled-glass tops.[40] Bodies (of the unclaimed) dissected here were obtained from hospitals in Aberdeen and further afield in northeast Scotland, but numbers were frequently low in the region and Lockhart arranged for the transportation of supplementary supplies from medical schools and hospitals in England.[41] Students dissected anatomical parts, starting with the limbs, and were required to make appropriate use of 'tools', keeping their scalpels sharp. Maintaining as much cleanliness and tidiness as possible at the dissecting table was necessary for good work and clear thinking, Lockhart advised. Furthermore, students' clothing had to be 'business-like', not fancy, he instructed, because skilful dissecting was impossible 'when one eye is on a new suit and the other on a greasy table'; by the 1940s white coats were routinely worn.[42]

Urging students to improve their dissecting-room skills, Lockhart sometimes complained that learners' feet looked to be more agile than their hands; students were likely to be more accomplished at dancing than dissecting, he teased, and their Charleston would probably put their hands 'to shame'. But with perseverance, Lockhart assured them, dissection offered the 'royal road' to anatomical knowledge, and it was this road that students had to take, even though (and perhaps because) it 'follows a pass through difficult mountains'.[43] Likened to a passage through tough terrain, dissection – a learning process that engaged students' entire bodies, not just their hands – was described as a journey within the human body envisaged as anatomical territory. A 1940s dissecting manual that guided students' practical work explained: 'the student learns to find his way about the body and to appreciate the main features of the landscape', thereby gaining a 'sense of [the body's] topography'.[44] And it was not only male students, as implied by this manual's gender-specific pronouns, who embarked on this learning as women were increasingly admitted for medical training in the first half of the twentieth century, especially during wartime.[45]

The formulation of the bodily interior as land for exploration was not new: during the early modern period anatomical practices had been likened to the mapping of territories; anatomists made internal voyages just as travellers explored the globe.[46] At the end of the nineteenth century Thomas Cooke's anatomy textbook offered a similar metaphor of the body as geographical space. It suggested that 'the surgeon should see his way through its [the body's] various structures much as the somnambulist sees his way in what most people call darkness': just as the sleepwalker sees without light by moving their body through a place, the surgeon sees inside the body by navigating within it.[47] For Cooke, 'thorough practical acquaintance with the human body' was comparable to a person's 'knowledge of the locality in which he lives' – that is, to knowledge of yards, alleyways, paving stones, doorsteps and so on, gained by frequently travelling on foot.[48] Students finding their way within the body were thus aided by key markers – like the familiar trees or lamp posts that guided their walks through London's streets in thick fog.[49]

Such accounts of dissecting to gain anatomical knowledge situated the mobile learner entirely inside the body undergoing exploration as though the learner was moving within a body/cityscape. Early twentieth-century anatomical practices developed the notion of dissection as bodily movement through geographies. Elliot Smith, for instance, emphasized the importance of cultivating the skill of spatial orientation within the body's anatomy, a skill he likened to urban route-taking:

> The primary value of dissection to the student is to enable him to find his way about the body. Much of the knowledge he acquires is

of a subconscious nature, but is none the less real on that account. By a limited experience I have learned to find my way from Princes Street to the University [in Manchester], but I cannot name a single street or landmark; nor give more than the vaguest description of the route; yet I have the essential knowledge which meets my needs [. . . and] knowledge of anatomy is of a similar nature.[50]

According to this view, wayfinding through the body was more important for students to accomplish than remembering all the names of anatomical parts. Nevertheless, in the bodily practice of learning by seeing and touching anatomy, words were significant – an issue to which this chapter returns later. So human anatomy was defined as territory for both travelling within *and* for understanding with words.

This approach was illustrated by one of Marischal College's students of medicine, in a poster announcing a lecture for the Aberdeen University Anatomical and Anthropological Society (AUAAS) run by medical students (illus. 120). The lecture, given at the Anatomy Department in 1957 by surgeon Gordon Gordon Taylor, who had studied classics in Aberdeen, defended the use of eponyms (an eponym in this case being the name of an anatomical part derived from the name of the person credited with first identifying it) at a time when they were being questioned by medical professionals recommending the international use of Latin anatomical terms.[51] On the poster, eponyms were inserted humorously into an imaginary landscape where Rolando's fissure (in the brain, named after Luigi Rolando, 1773–1831) was located in a hill, the Islets of Langerhans (in the pancreas, named after Paul Langerhans, 1847–1888) appeared in a lake, Henle's loop (in the kidney, named after Friedrich Gustav Jakob Henle, 1809–1885) was formed by a river, and the Fallopian tube (leading from ovaries to the uterus, named after Gabriele Falloppio, 1523–1562) featured as a London Underground train line to the city. The lecture was billed as a journey

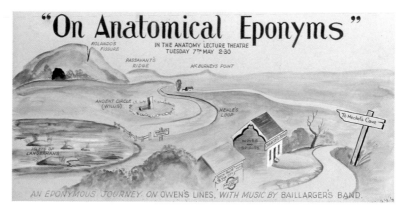

120
Slide of a poster for a lecture 'On Anatomical Eponyms', in the Anatomy Department, Marischal College, University of Aberdeen, 1957.

within this body/landscape accompanied by music from Baillarger's Band, the latter being a play on the anatomical bands of Baillarger composed of nerve fibres in the brain (named after Jules Baillarger, 1809–1890).

Anatomical learning envisaged as movement through spaces – both inside and outside the body, both concrete and imagined – was also practised at Marischal College during demonstrations using the Anatomy Museum's three-dimensional models. For example, from the 1930s to the early 1960s, Robert Lockhart regularly used an enlarged model of the ear, encouraging students to imagine a giddy journey into this body part. The plaster model, with a width of over 2 ft (0.6 m) and an enormous eardrum and stirrup, was easily observed by medical students seated in the lecture theatre. Students would watch as Lockhart showed its inner components while performing an animating narrative, sometimes 'causing great amusement in the audience' (illus. 121, see illus. 131).[52] The 'giant scale ear' became a dramatic focus of attention when he invited students to travel with him 'in our imagination to a strange and unknown world, a world of "Hearing and Equilibration [balancing]"'. Students imagined themselves entering the ear through a channel and a 'pearl grey transparent door' (the eardrum). After climbing onto three staircases (the hammer, anvil and stirrup) and through an 'oval window', they were 'submerged in a Marine cavern' (the fluid-filled semicircular canals) where, in a speedboat, they ventured 'all [a]round with great fear and excitement'.[53]

This imaginative journeying took place in lectures given to students at meetings of the AUAAS when Lockhart would adapt his ear narrative for different cohorts, and it was also encouraged in his routine anatomical teaching. Here dramatic narratives were commonly used as mnemonic devices to help students remember the internal configuration of the human body. Furthermore, aspects of the journey into the ear were worked into

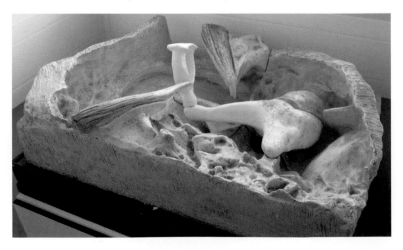

121
Model of the ear, by
Dr Alexander, Vienna,
early 20th century
(with repairs 2014).

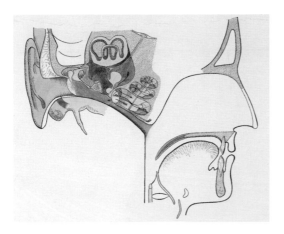

122
Student's (anonymous) drawing of the inner ear, c. 1960, made in the Anatomy Department, Marischal College, University of Aberdeen.

Lockhart's 1959 co-authored textbook *Anatomy of the Human Body*, in which students were guided on an imagined 'tour' inside a giant 'cavern', 'tunnels' and other structures as they read the anatomical description of this organ, travelling 'loop the loop' and 'helter skelter' along the way as though on funfair rides.[54] Anatomical forms, such as the ear – conveyed both through narrative demonstration of models and textbook description – were also recalled and configured in students' own drawings. Lockhart recommended that students should draw as a way of learning: 'it is an excellent habit for students, themselves, to practise sketching the disposition of structures and reproducing diagrams', he advised.[55] So, imagining their route through the ear, students would draw from dissections as well as illustrations in approved textbooks. The 'Diagrammatic Guide to the Mechanisms of the Ear' in *Anatomy of the Human Body*, for example, was used as the basis of further drawn versions produced by students.[56] Referring to descriptions, dissections and printed illustrations, students would map the inner ear in vivid, contrasting colour (illus. 122).

Anatomical knowledge was, therefore, gained in the Anatomy Department through bodily movement – enacted during dissecting, narrated and imagined in lectures and demonstrations, and made vibrant in drawings. Students also memorized aspects of anatomy when going about their daily lives in Aberdeen, especially while in transit when they would think through anatomical parts. Dr Dorothie Younie, for instance, recollected walking from Marischal Quod to College Bounds with her friend and fellow medical student Nellie Jardine, 'and all the way down [this mile-long route] we were recalling the arteries in the lower arm and the ramifications of the ulnar nerve'.[57] Another woman remembered her regular bus ride from home to Marischal College, during her studies in the late 1950s, when she would read anatomical descriptions to herself from a pocket-sized book and imagine those parts inside her own body.[58]

Anatomical wayfinding was thus a bodily and imaginative process that extended from designated teaching spaces into commonplace streets, surprising landscapes and fantastical architectures. Learning anatomy was a journey that worked the learner's mind and body. As each learner explored and came to remember anatomy though disciplined, active study – gaining skills with dissections, specimens, living bodies, visual images and models – she or he would be both imaginatively immersed within that anatomy *and* expected to mentally and physically recognize (or envisage and sense) it inside themselves; the learner travelled inside an all-encompassing anatomy just as they discovered it within their own bodies. This was a journey of visual, tactile and imagined movement through bodily 'terrain', a terrain both outside and inside each student which was made distinctly and dramatically observable and palpable through the process of anatomizing.

But training in anatomy was not just about learning the body's 'geography' because, as Elliot Smith had emphasized, students must also understand the 'meaning of its structure' and the factors that influenced its growth and form.[59] Learning to 'think anatomically' about the living body was achieved when the meaning of its internal structures was appreciated in terms of their functions and with regard to the implications of injury or disease.[60] To comprehend the functional purpose of anatomical structures was to 'realise' their meaning, and to help students accomplish this, anatomists had to 'interpret' those structures and communicate those interpretations successfully.[61] Rather than attempting to teach every anatomical detail – the study of which could 'last a life-time' – anatomists directed students' efforts towards those areas deemed most educationally important, and in doing so they encouraged students to 'correlate structure and function'.[62] The skilled anatomist now acted not so much as a master of detail, as John Struthers had done in the nineteenth century, but as an expert in coordination.[63] If students acquired knowledge of anatomy in 'scattered fragments' during their practical work – as when they dissected bodies in 'parts' – anatomists' teaching was concerned with 'linking up' that knowledge, promoting comprehension of the whole functioning body while highlighting salient aspects.[64] Inspiring students' interest and enthusiasm was 'at the root of all real training', insisted anatomists, and key to this was teaching not with the 'lifeless tissue' of the dead alone but by incorporating living, moving bodies into anatomical displays.[65]

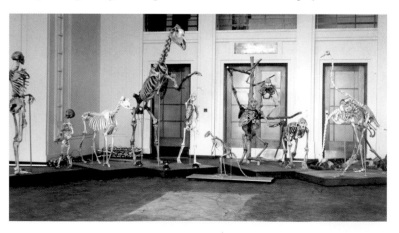

123
Displays in the Museum, Medical School, University of Birmingham, 1938, photograph.

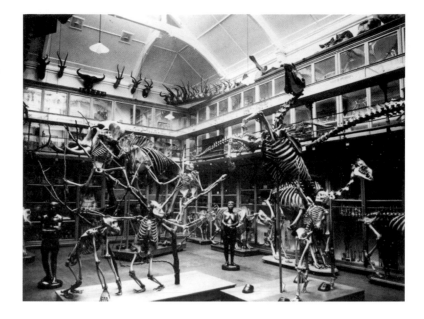

124
Anatomy Museum,
Marischal College,
University of
Aberdeen, 1942–64,
photograph.

Lockhart became proficient in this coordination of the living and the dead, managing displays in flesh and bone, curating and teaching with visual images and texts. To coordinate was a matter of making linkages and associations, and when this was achieved in displays that were striking and stimulating, anatomy was made meaningful as well as memorable. This anatomical poetics developed through practices that, by the 1940s, were termed the 'new anatomy', at the centre of which was the study of anatomical structure in terms of the body's 'living processes', such as growth and repair.[66]

CIRCUS OF LIFE

Identifying the Anatomy Museum as 'a most important practical reference room', Lockhart modified and coordinated displays to promote the study of living anatomy at Marischal College.[67] Upon his return to Aberdeen in 1938 he had planned to develop an anatomy department in the new 'modern style' medical school at Foresterhill – the site of Aberdeen's recently built hospitals where the majority of medical subjects, including pathology, surgery and bacteriology, were to be taught. But when Lockhart's requirements for rooms and equipment could not be met, the only solution was to remain at the college, in its 'magnificent Victorian designed accommodation'.[68] Here the anatomical collections acquired over the past century were retained and augmented as valuable resources, occupying space that was free from the threat of encroachment by the other medical departments, which had departed to Foresterhill with their respective museum collections.[69]

'Economy' or frugality in museums was a wartime necessity, continuing to a certain extent with rationing into the 1950s, so that prudent preservation of collections combined with strategies for obtaining further acquisitions were important in Lockhart's curatorial approach.[70] He arranged for a 'well tooled' workshop to be installed in the Anatomy Department for tasks such as articulating skeletons and mounting specimens, and museum maintenance work was carried out by several technicians, among them William Anderson, who was in post from 1945 to 1972.[71] Lockhart was accustomed to overseeing, and participating in, the preservation of selected specimens from human bodies anatomized in the dissecting room. Some skeletal parts, as well as some dissections of soft issue, appear to have been retained for the museum during the mid-twentieth century, but there was also a move towards the purchase of commercially available human skeletons supplied to many of Britain's medical schools by the leading London-based firm Adam,Rouilly (which imported from Calcutta [Kolkata]).[72]

Purchases of this kind were deemed important for medical teaching at Marischal College, especially with the decline in the Anatomy Department's intake of human remains via anatomists' connections with former students and medical practitioners across the empire: with post-1945 decolonization, these former sources of museum acquisition were, progressively, no longer operating.[73] There was also growing recognition that to ship indigenous peoples' remains to Britain's medical schools and museums, as gifts sent by medical professionals to anatomists, was not unproblematic. When a doctor had sent Lockhart the skeleton of an 'Australian aboriginal' in 1939, for instance, the anatomist had recorded that to the best of his knowledge such specimens were 'not to be got out of Australia, by official request, except with the greatest difficulty', a statement that perhaps indicated awareness of the indigenous prohibitions and sensitivities surrounding this traffic in the dead. He advised that details of the acquisition should not be released to Aberdeen's newspapers.[74]

The arrival of non-human remains at the Anatomy Museum from overseas also became far less frequent. An exception to this trend – again a material trace of colonial practices, though not a direct shipment – came in 1941 when the locally resident Viscountess Stonehaven offered numerous items including some 'very fine African heads which were [hunting] trophies' belonging to her recently deceased husband.[75] John Baird, later Lord Stonehaven, had collected extensively during the early 1900s on expeditions in East Africa, and the Viscountess suggested that these possessions could be removed from her home (Ury House) to the university's museums for many to enjoy.[76] Lockhart accepted, and temporarily stored in the Anatomy Museum, 'specimens' such as weapons and musical instruments from Abyssinia (Ethiopia) and Sudan, which were destined for the Anthropological Museum, and animal remains, for example turtle shells and snake skin, which were to be passed on to the Natural History Museum – these latter two museums being located nearby in Marischal College's front quadrangle. Antelope heads from the Viscountess were assimilated into the Anatomy Museum's displays along the gallery and, Lockhart informed her, the lioness and cubs in their glass case were exhibited in the Anatomy Department's vestibule 'beside the mounted skeletons of our elephant, rhinoceros, hippopotamus, giraffe, camel, etc. etc.'[77]

These skeletons of comparative anatomy were being diligently preserved as part of the Anatomy Museum's collections, with the whale skeleton obtained under John Struthers's direction remaining suspended in the department's entrance corridor (see illus. 89). Lockhart continued to honour Struthers's collecting efforts when he gladly received the crocodile skeleton (see illus. 71) – so keenly sought by the professor during the 1860s – from the Aberdeen Medico-Chirurgical Society in 1956.[78] The Anatomy Museum was not, however, treated primarily as a repository for the preservation of the past, as it was actively made to yield anatomical knowledge of (then) current interest. Although part of this museum was used as short-term storage during the early 1940s, it was not a space for sedimentation for it was subsequently rearranged and the floor cases removed to stage animated displays of living anatomy.

Lockhart had been impressed by Robert Reid's displays of apes in the Anatomy Museum, which showed articulated skeletons arranged in the branches of trees as though alive – indeed, Lockhart had emulated these in the anatomy museum at the University of Birmingham, where he had been involved in designing the new medical school (illus. 123).[79] So, when back at Marischal College, Lockhart kept Reid's lively specimens, releasing them from their glass cabinets, and adding the skeleton of a racehorse (obtained from George v), which was posed in a 'lifelike', 'prancing' position with a 'female human skeleton at its head, poised holding its bridle'.[80] Transferred from Birmingham to Aberdeen with the anatomy professor, the horse joined further animal skeletons, which were moved into the Anatomy Museum from the department's vestibule (illus. 124).[81] Styles of articulation from the late nineteenth century were thus incorporated into an amplified living anatomy scheme, and to prevent the interpretation of such specimens as mere 'dry bones' further strategies were developed to bring them to life. These display strategies linked the Anatomy Museum with aspects of popular performance and entertainment to energize exhibits and enhance their educational potential.

Transactions between museums and other performative sites have a deep history. As discussed in Chapter Four, anatomists in the second half of the 1800s elevated their educational displays above commercial anatomy exhibited for the public, even as they drew on a wide spectrum of popular shows, especially when sourcing specimens, and as they cultivated their own modes of performance. But if during that period fairgrounds, entertainment halls and the like were often defined as low and inferior in contrast to instructional museums,[82] by the mid-twentieth century aspects of the vibrant world of public performance – including theatrical, musical and choreographed shows that were widely disseminated in a variety of media – were appropriated and displayed as educational resources for professional training using museum collections. Thus in the Anatomy Museum the plaster figures of African people commissioned by Struthers in 1860 and cast from a living woman and man were joined by many further participants curated by Lockhart as anatomical performers in the flesh and in visual images. Anatomical displays could be staged as dramatic acts without diminishing their capacity to disclose apparently observable facts about bodies, just as dissection could be legitimately envisaged and narrated as a journey moving between the mundane and the fantastical.

Lockhart became adept at recruiting and assimilating popular performers and visual images thereof into his anatomical practices. In one of his lectures, 'The Circus of Life' – which he modified and refined from the 1930s onwards for medical audiences, especially student societies and meetings of practitioners such as nurses – he would declare: 'the circus with paper hoops and spangled limbs and clowns and prancing ponies is not exactly foreign to Anatomy.'[83] Observe, he suggested by way of historical examples, the work of anatomists Rudolf Virchow (1821–1902), who studied the 'contortions of the famous Marinelli', and of Karl von Bardeleben (1849–1919), whose book captured in photographs 'the antics of this acrobatic clown'.[84] The drama and excitement of the circus were not lost on Lockhart, whose childhood memories of being taken by his mother and father to the famous Hengler's Circus in Glasgow remained vivid for him: in later life he still recalled the equestrian acts with 'horses coming flying onto the stage'.[85] In the early decades of the twentieth century circus arenas featuring human and animal performances, such as clowns, aerialists, elephants and lions, were potentially interesting for anatomists seeking to develop engaging displays of living anatomy.[86] Lockhart employed acrobats to make anatomical images, and he showed photographs of circus and other performers in lectures to illuminate museum specimens by encouraging visual comparison of the latter with bodies in action (illus. 125).[87]

125
Slide of a magazine
clipping of a
photograph of a
circus performance,
collected by
Robert Lockhart,
c. 1930s–'50s.

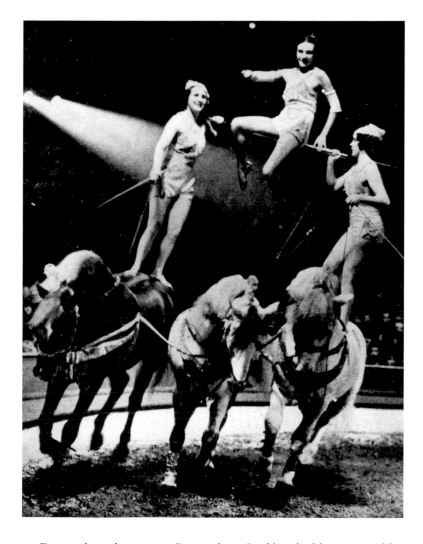

125
Slide of a magazine clipping of a photograph of a circus performance, collected by Robert Lockhart, c. 1930s–'50s.

During the early 1930s in Birmingham, Lockhart had been assisted by acrobats from two troupes known as the Mid-Air Girls and the Hindustans who were appearing at the Theatre Royal in the pantomime *Dick Whittington*. He recruited them for his 'scientific investigation into the movements of joints and the actions of muscles . . . carried out by X-ray, cinematograph and anatomical experiment'.[88] Photographs, radiographs and films were made to reveal the skeletal structure of the acrobats and their muscles during movement. As Lockhart would announce at the start of his 'Circus of Life' lecture, such anatomical images allowed him to present 'the glamour of the footlights in the cold shadow of the radiogram'.[89]

By replacing stage or show lights with the X-ray and other imaging technologies, Lockhart displayed performing acrobats as anatomical images that converted theatrical bodily acts into educational exhibits. Directed by the anatomist, two artistes from the Mid-Air Girls – Doris Smart and Babette, both with expertise in bending and balancing – 'faced the cinematograph camera' as described in a press article, and the Hindustan Troupe of 'young men of fine physique' were also filmed with special attention to 'the flexing and relaxing of their muscles'. The resulting images were expected to provide anatomy students with an instructive 'demonstration of muscle play'.[90] Such an approach to bodily display was also employed in other medical schools: professor of anatomy David Rutherford Dow, in Dundee, invited a 'lady contortionist' from her local stage venue to his lecture theatre to demonstrate her muscular anatomy; professor Thomas Yeates displayed a heavyweight boxer's muscles to an anatomy class at the Middlesex Hospital Medical School; and anatomy lecturer Dr A.J.E. Cave took X-ray photographs of Babette, from the Mid-Air Girls, to aid his teaching on the muscles of the neck and back at the University of Leeds.[91] Lockhart continued to display images derived from acrobatic performance so that, for instance, a photograph of a young woman performing a 'perfect high kick' was included in his 1948 photographic atlas, *Living Anatomy*, to demonstrate the 'relaxation of the hamstring muscles'.[92] Images of 'muscle play', then, were shown in lectures and in book format to stimulate students' study of living bodies and to provide visual material that they could use to better interpret museum specimens.

The visual analogies that Lockhart set up between photographs of popular body displays and skeletal anatomical exhibits were particularly instructive. While his anatomical practices drew performers – from acrobats to ballet dancers – into his research, especially on the movements of joints and the 'mechanism of walking', he also collected images of catwalk fashion models, music hall dancers, gymnasts, athletes and aerialists from newspapers, magazines and journals to project as slides in lectures.[93] By displaying photographs of trained, muscular bodies in action Lockhart encouraged students to view human and animal skeletons in terms of how they worked during life, and so to imagine bones 'clothed in their related structures'.[94] Just as photographs of circus horses in rearing motion were projected and described in parallel with the Anatomy Museum's skeleton articulated in a similar position, for example, images of gymnastic and athletic performance were viewed as living versions of the human skeletons on display. Such connections were reinforced in Lockhart's *Living Anatomy*, which prompted the observation of preserved human skeletal parts in direct relation to relevant muscles and bones in living bodies (see below).[95]

Learning anatomy in this way was facilitated by visual linkage, coordinated by the expert anatomist. In this intermedial process, museum exhibits were brought to life through their association with images projected in the lecture theatre or shown on a book's page. In anatomical displays the circus of life was kept in motion by animated acts calculated to attract attention and to inspire amazement. Yet Lockhart's appropriation of circus tended to translate the extraordinary into the everyday. When dramatizing bodily differences – as he did when displaying two contrasting human skeletons referred to as a 'giant' and a 'dwarf' (see illus. 123, far left) – he would explain physical conditions and actions in routine, seemingly demystifying anatomical terms, in this case with reference to the activity of the pituitary gland and processes of growth.[96] Similarly the extremes of human physical capacity – as shown in unusual acrobatic feats, for example – were rendered comprehensible and somewhat less remarkable through anatomical explanation. The oscillation between popular and scientific domains, and the movement of medical audiences from amazement to comprehension (and sometimes back again), were persistent features in Lockhart's display strategies. In *Anatomy of the Human Body*, the section on the lower jaw stated, for example, that 'The bite in man is powerful – witness the "iron-jaw" acts of the circus ring where the performer hangs his or her weight rotating from a clenched mouthpiece.'[97] And in lectures Lockhart would illustrate this point, explaining anatomical structure and strength while showing a slide of Edgar Degas' painting *Miss Lola, au Cirque Fernando* (1879), in which an acrobat hangs from a height by her teeth.[98] Co opted for anatomical display, amazing circus performance provided insights into the routine workings of living bodies just as seemingly ordinary parts of human anatomy could be made to seem astonishing.

STILL AND MOVING IMAGES

The coordinated display of visual images, museum specimens, dissections and living bodies facilitated the imaginative yet empirically rigorous study of anatomy as alive and dynamic. Lockhart's collecting practices yielded many images for this purpose, many reproduced or clipped from publications ranging from anatomy textbooks to weekly magazines. The dedicated production of images in Marischal College's Anatomy Department during the mid-twentieth century, mainly for publication in *Living Anatomy* and *Anatomy of the Human Body*, also boosted capacity for the communication of anatomical knowledge. Lockhart referred to the potency of images, especially X-rays, in teaching living anatomy as 'graphic power'; he saw that images could grip and persuade viewers, as did other medical educators who, by the 1940s, were utilizing a widening array of 'visual aids' including motion pictures, posters, cartoons and comic strips.[99] It was in this context, where considerable resources and staff time in the Anatomy Department were devoted to the production of heavily illustrated anatomy books, that the Anatomy Museum was maintained and used: it provided specimens to be photographed, drawn and painted, and formed a site for the display of the resulting images. And following publication, Lockhart expected students to study his books' two-dimensional printed images in relation to the Anatomy Museum's three-dimensional exhibits, whether displayed in the museum's space or elsewhere in the Anatomy Department. A nineteenth-century plaster cast, for instance, which was adapted on-site to display nerves in the 1950s, carried a label requesting viewers to compare the 'statue' with several corresponding illustrations in *Anatomy of the Human Body* (see illus. 154).[100]

This textbook – which Lockhart wrote/produced with his colleagues, lecturers Gilbert Frewin Hamilton and Forest William Fyfe – underlined the centrality of images. It opens with a quotation from Lewis Carroll's *Alice's Adventures in Wonderland* – 'What is the use of a book without pictures?' – the question posed by Alice, in the novel, just before she drops into a dream world and follows the White Rabbit.[101] *Anatomy of the Human Body* boasted double the number of 'illustrations' in standard textbooks, and the authors underlined the relative advantages of images – specifically drawings – compared with words:

> different students are more likely to start with the same impression from a drawing than from words, and in reverse, a rough sketch by a student will at once reveal knowledge or betray error when both might be obscured in verbal description.[102]

From this point of view, drawings were considered less open to different interpretations than words and therefore clearer, or more direct, in the communication of knowledge. While drawings might be revelatory in anatomy, words were, by contrast, given to opacity. Nevertheless, textual description and labelling were considered essential in anatomical exposition so that careful management of text vis-à-vis image was paramount. Text was arranged on the same page as the relevant image and the two were linked with pointers – lines – that led from the names of parts to the illustration of the same (illus. 126). In this way the textbook guided the reader/viewer's eyes between detailed illustration and textual description, movement that clarified and sharpened observation, helped to define anatomical parts and make them appear more distinct.

Anatomy of the Human Body was initiated by Lockhart in 1942, and its production was a collaborative effort involving over 30 lecturers and assistants in the Anatomy Department. With his co-authors, anatomists

Hamilton and Fyfe, Lockhart employed several artists to execute the book's 965 illustrations. Edinburgh artist R. W. Matthews began the task, followed by the artists Gordon S. Cameron, Donald J. Stephen and Alberto Morrocco, who were colleagues teaching at Gray's School of Art in Aberdeen, and William Cruickshank, a technician in the Anatomy Department.[103] Photographs and X-rays were taken in-house for the book, and the majority of the illustrations were drawn, then painted in watercolour, from bodies that had been embalmed and dissected on site by the anatomists and their assistants.[104] In addition to the newly made dissections, specimens from the Anatomy Museum were also used as the basis for drawings. Lockhart's 1925 dissection of the head (see illus. 136), for instance, was drawn to illustrate the cranial nerves.[105] Here particular nerves were shown in colour to enhance their visibility, a technique used in many illustrations throughout the publication to accentuate relevant parts.

Colour, according to Fyfe, gave the illustrations a three-dimensional appearance that heightened their efficacy as educational images, and the three-dimensionality of diagrams in the book was certainly praised by readers of this 'stimulating' and 'remarkable' publication.[106] If the three-dimensional understanding of anatomy was partly facilitated by viewing coloured illustrations, it was also advanced through a range of further related teaching methods. Fyfe was reportedly a 'skilled sketch artist, sculptor [and] photographer', making many 'props' and models for his anatomy lectures, including a human larynx, sculpted at twenty times its usual size from wood with rubber tissues and muscles attached.[107] Lockhart, too, constructed enlarged anatomical models for museum display and also performed models in his classes by making 'reconstruction[s]' of anatomical parts with wax and Plasticine (a soft modelling material); he regarded this modelling as 'akin to drawing' and encouraged students to do it themselves as a helpful method for 'impressing [anatomical structures] on the mind'.[108] Illustrations for *Anatomy of the Human Body* were developed within this broader context of materially based, action-oriented pedagogical practices in the Anatomy Department. The original illustrations were mounted in frames and arranged like giant pages of a book, hinged on a wall of the general laboratory (illus. 127). Such arrangements were evident in medical displays elsewhere in Britain where a variety of interrelated images formed an effective 'graphic method of museum demonstration'.[109] In the Anatomy Department students could leaf through the wall 'book' while they also studied specimens from the Anatomy Museum's collections together with photographs of dissections.

In *Anatomy of the Human Body* combinations of visual images were arranged so as to guide observation of the illustrations, corresponding diagrams, X-rays and photographs of living people acting as anatomical models. The latter images, especially those showing muscles, were selected from Lockhart's *Living Anatomy*, of which five editions were published between 1948 and 1960. This photographic atlas aimed 'to awaken' students' interest in observing 'muscles in action' as 'demonstrated [by . . .] living subject[s]' or living models which students could also study 'first hand' in their anatomy classes.[110] Lockhart recruited 50 medical students for his atlas, mostly men but also several women, directing them as models and carefully selecting the final 187 images for publication. Students were

---

274   CUTANEOUS NERVES OF THE NECK

Posterior Primary Rami

The GREATER OCCIPITAL NERVE (C2) is the large medial branch arising from the posterior primary ramus of the **second cervical nerve** as it emerges below the posterior arch of the atlas. The nerve curves round the lower border of **obliquus capitis inferior**, ascends deep to **semispinalis capitis**, first pierces that muscle and then trapezius and, now accompanying the **occipital artery**, supplies the skin of the back of the head as far forwards as the vertex. Muscular twigs supply the deep muscles of the back of the neck (p. 280) The

THIRD OCCIPITAL NERVE (C3), from the medial branch of the posterior primary ramus of the third cervical nerve (p. 273), pierces **trapezius** to supply the skin of the lower part of the back of the head medial to the greater occipital nerve.

The posterior primary ramus of the fourth cervical nerve has a **cutaneous branch** to the skin of the neck, as has the fifth and sometimes the sixth nerve.

Anterior Primary Rami
(Branches of the cervical plexus)

The LESSER OCCIPITAL NERVE (C2), variable in size and sometimes double, curves from behind round the **accessory nerve** and ascends along the posterior border of sternomastoid, sending some twigs to the skin over trapezius. Becoming superficial near the skull, it supplies the scalp behind and above the ear, sending an **auricular branch** to the skin of the upper third of the cranial aspect of the auricle.

The GREAT AURICULAR NERVE (C2,3), the largest ascending branch of the cervical plexus, passes at first a little downwards behind sternomastoid, curves round the posterior border of the muscle and, sweeping upwards deep to **platysma**, pierces the deep fascia and accompanies the external jugular vein towards the angle of the jaw. It divides into an **anterior branch** to the skin of the lower cranial surface of the auricle from which a twig pierces the auricle to innervate the lateral surface of the lobe and lower part of the concha, a **posterior branch** supplying the scalp behind the ear, and a leash of small **parotid branches** which are entangled in the superficial part of the gland and supply the skin over it and over the angle of the jaw.

The ANTERIOR CUTANEOUS NERVE OF NECK (C2,3) hooks round the posterior border of **sternomastoid**, then pierces the deep fascia and, crossing the muscle obliquely, superficial or deep to the **external jugular vein**, divides under platysma into ascending and descending branches. The **ascending branches**, directed toward the submandibular region, are distributed, after piercing platysma, to the skin of the upper anterior part of the neck. The **descending branches** supply, by fine filaments through platysma, the skin of the front and side of the neck as low as the sternum.

The SUPRACLAVICULAR NERVES (C 3, 4) are three groups of branches arising from a common trunk which emerges from the posterior border of **sternomastoid** and divides, deep to platysma, into divergent medial, intermediate and lateral branches. These descend to pierce the deep fascia above the clavicle. The **medial supraclavicular nerves** cross sternomastoid and the external jugular vein, send twigs to the sternoclavicular joint and supply the skin to the midline.

The **intermediate supraclavicular nerves** cross the clavicle, sometimes grooving it slightly, to supply the skin over pectoralis major and deltoid, as far down as the third rib, where they communicate with cutaneous twigs from the upper intercostal nerves.

The **lateral supraclavicular nerves** reach and supply the skin of the upper and posterior part of the shoulder, over trapezius and the acromion.

FIG. **398**. SIDE OF NECK. Platysma and the upper part of sternomastoid are removed and the suboccipital triangle is exposed by a deep dissection.

The nerves described on this page, particularly the lesser occipital, are all liable to considerable variations in size, as might be expected from their numerous communications. The great auricular nerve communicates with the auricular branch of the vagus nerve and with the lesser occipital nerve and its auricular branch. The lesser occipital nerve communicates, in addition, with the greater occipital nerve and the latter with the third occipital nerve. Moreover, all these nerves (like the branches of the trigeminal nerve on the face) communicate peripherally with terminal branches of the facial nerve.

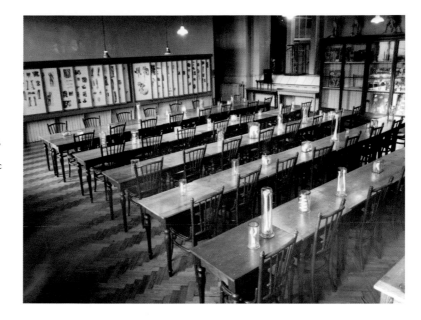

127
General laboratory, with museum specimens (human skeletal) on study tables, original illustrations for R. D. Lockhart, G. F. Hamilton and F. W. Fyfe, *Anatomy of the Human Body* (London, 1959) mounted in frames, a stereoscopic viewer and display cases containing osteological specimens, *c.* 1960, photograph.

chosen for 'leanness', rather than 'a high state of physical development'; from this perspective lean bodies tended to yield better photographs for observing muscles and surface contours.[111] Even so, if muscles were to be made sufficiently visible for anatomical examination, particular positions and poses were required of, and achieved with, the models. The photographs were thus records of coordinated anatomical performance by the collective involved in producing the atlas – the anatomist, models, assistants and photographer.

To allow muscles to 'speak for themselves', as physicians do with patients, Lockhart explained in the atlas, a person's movements had to be resisted 'so that the muscles act more powerfully' and are hence more readily observable. Using this clinical method the anatomist choreographed the partially dressed and naked models, requiring them to adopt specific postures, and applying 'resistance' by physically counteracting their movements so that the anatomy of their muscles became more pronounced and therefore accessible for visual study (illus. 128). Muscles of the back, chest, neck, arms, legs and hands were performed in this way. This staging of living anatomy required careful costuming: the models only revealed those parts necessary for a particular demonstration and when pictured naked, to provide 'comparison of male and female forms', masks were printed over the eyes of female models to prevent identification.[112]

Lockhart appeared in several photographs with the models, orchestrating the show of muscular anatomy, and sometimes an assistant in a white laboratory coat was present within the frame acting as an 'operator' to

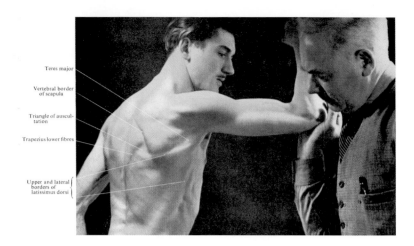

128
Labelled photograph of a living anatomical model showing muscles in the back demonstrated by Robert Lockhart, from R. D. Lockhart, *Living Anatomy: A Photographic Atlas of Muscles in Action and Surface Contours*, 5th edition (London, 1960), Fig. 41.

similarly reveal the models' musculature.[113] And the anatomist himself modelled the muscles of the hand and wrist, the resulting close-up photograph capturing his shirt, cufflinks and jacket sleeve. With a key role in the project, Alexander Cain, who had begun as a cabinetmaker and became senior technician in the Anatomy Department, undertook the photography, which Lockhart acknowledged as work that required 'enthusiasm as well as judgement, skill and patience'.[114] According to Fyfe, Cain's photographic skills were especially apparent when he was 'lighting muscle, tendon and bone contours and "bringing them out" in his prints from soft negatives'.[115] Readers of the atlas appreciated the 'beauty' of the surface musculature that was so 'convincingly demonstrated'.[116]

Along with images produced for *Anatomy of the Human Body*, original photographs for *Living Anatomy* were displayed in the general laboratory's wall-mounted 'book' (see illus. 127, top left). They were also projected as slides in lectures and copies were made for showing in the Anatomy Museum. The photographs were therefore viewed as components within wider intermedial displays. Indeed, some images in *Living Anatomy* aided viewers' navigation of anatomies rendered in different media and materials, potentially encouraging observation of parallels between living bodies and the Anatomy Museum's preserved and articulated bones. In photographs of a live model's leg, for instance, the lower limbs were positioned alongside articulated bones of the same. This invited close visual comparison of living and skeletal legs so that each was understood anatomically in relation to the other.[117] By learning this relational viewing, students' anatomical observations in the Anatomy Museum would have been directed from preserved specimens to living bodies and back again.

Lockhart's hope for the atlas was that 'these pictures may play a little part in the quickening task of raising anatomy from the dead'.[118] And to bring anatomy to life, students' own bodies became important points of reference for both visual and tactile examination. Like his predecessor, Alexander Low, Lockhart insisted on the importance of the 'living model' in anatomy classes, directing students to conduct regular anatomical studies of their own bodies through disciplined self-observation.[119] This involved locating structures (such as bones) by sight and touch, and drawing outlines or surface markings of these on limbs that could then be studied in motion.[120] Thus the student was positioned as both mobile anatomical model for observation *and* a body deeply engaged in that very learning: he/she was to study their own anatomy from the outside while living that very anatomy from within. When students entered the Anatomy Museum, therefore, they could envisage themselves as live specimens moving among the many exhibits that the practice of living anatomy sought to animate.

Lockhart's *Living Anatomy* atlas was reviewed as a successful 'representation by still photography of a dynamic subject'.[121] But he also produced and exhibited films to enhance the study of bodies during life. Made in the early 1930s with acrobats, Lockhart's motion pictures focusing on the action of muscles and movement of joints were published by the Kodak Medical Film Library of London and screened by university departments of anatomy.[122] In silent black and white, often before a dark, curtained backdrop, 'living anatomical model[s]' demonstrated their muscles by tensing their bodies or performing bends and lifts.[123] As in his later photographs for *Living Anatomy*, Lockhart appeared – sometimes visible only as hands with neat cuffs or as feet in shoes with smart spats – moving into the frame to position the model or to reinforce and define their moving muscles for the camera. The models were directed to reveal their surface anatomy by hopping on one leg, lifting limbs into the air and flexing muscles in the arms, back and chest. Male acrobats, dressed in briefs, demonstrated muscles in action by performing somersaults shot from front, side and back views, which were shown in slow motion for ease of observation. A human pyramid formed by five acrobats became a lesson in balance and the contraction of muscles. Female acrobats, sporting sequinned bikinis, demonstrated the anatomy of the hip joint and vertebral column by performing high kicks, back bends and handstands while rotating their legs in the splits.

The films were edited to include anatomical descriptions and X-rays of bones so that, given the appearance and actions of the models, the movies oscillated between popular show and educational display.[124] Furthermore, by repeatedly and easily shifting from views of surface anatomy to images of internal skeletal structures, these medical films tended to interrelate bodily exterior and interior so that the latter appeared as a deeper manifestation of the former.[125] In the Anatomy Department during the early twentieth century anatomical practices had entailed observational movement between the insides and outsides of bodies, and medical films now offered insights into living anatomy that alternated between views of bodily exteriors and interiors (especially X-rays) when the moving images were projected on-screen.

Lockhart's films attempted to visually capture the 'fluid anatomy' of living processes, the motion of (and within) bodies in space and time, which was of wide interest within his professional community, and he took inspiration from diverse sources to create his compelling films – from late nineteenth-century photographic studies of motion, as in Eadweard Muybridge's work, which Lockhart viewed as relevant in anatomical study (illus. 129), to (then) present-day entertainment and medical practices.[126] In Aberdeen during the 1940s and '50s Lockhart screened his films for students, including a production he made at a physical training college to display the clavicle when the arm was raised. He also showed films on thoracic (chest) surgery at a London hospital, on the physiology of the kidney and on the functions of the heart shown by X-ray cinematography. Students noted that the moving images left a 'lasting impression on all who saw them', and aspects of anatomy that were difficult for a teacher to explain in words were 'made clear through the medium of film'.[127] For students, therefore, these films provoked strong responses, providing impressive clarifications of anatomy. Indeed, film affected viewers by 'creating bodily sensations' not just visual reactions, as studies of early twentieth-century cinema have suggested.[128] When medical students saw the movement of live anatomy on screen, their reception of those filmed bodies – what they learned from them – would have been shaped by such bodily sensations as well as by students' deepening anatomical awareness of their own bodies developed through disciplined self-examination as living models.

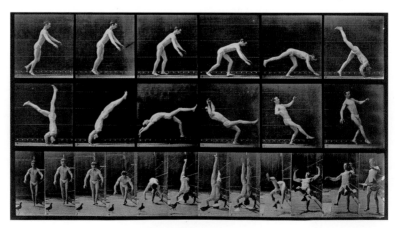

129
Eadweard Muybridge and University of Pennsylvania, a man performing a forward flip, 1887, collotype.

Film became widely recognized as a potent 'stimulus' for learning, as noted by a 1950 government advisory committee on education in Scotland which remarked on film's 'power to capture the stir and rhythm of the living world'. Yet, as long queues at cinemas indicated, there was avid 'fascination' with film as a form of entertainment and this generated concerns regarding the medium's genuine pedagogical value.[129] To underline the legitimacy of anatomical films as educational tools, they were framed, edited, captioned and screened in lecture theatres of medical schools, so that cues indicating what students should observe and how they should appropriately respond were built into films and supplied in contexts of viewing.[130] Nevertheless the 'dramatic effect' of moving images was certainly harnessed to enhance the communication of anatomical knowledge in such settings.[131] And drama was generated on screen not only by film but by novel methods of visual demonstration. For instance, the Aberdeen anatomist Gilbert Hamilton gave lectures on the nervous system in which 'with the aid of a spiral drawn on a plate of Perspex, and an epidiascope, he would send kaleidoscopic dots along the nerve tracts', creating an 'exposition which so electrified the audience' it received standing ovations.[132]

These compelling visual images brought anatomy to life through movement projected onto screens, so that films were just one medium among many creatively employed as part of 'composite' sets of devices and methods for displaying dynamic anatomies.[133] In Marischal College's Anatomy Department 'flowing, moving diagrams' were drawn on the lecture theatre's blackboard by one teacher of embryology to show students the growth of embryos in sequences of chalk images.[134] While the display of living anatomy with visual images highlighted movement in time, anatomists also emphasized that students must learn to 'think in three dimensions'.[135] To achieve this, students learned to link and synthesize visual images, bodies in the Anatomy Museum and the dissecting room, and their own anatomy.

The use of stereoscopic devices aided this movement between two and three dimensions. With the publication of one exceptionally detailed colour stereoscopic atlas during the 1950s and early '60s, for instance, students could observe photographs of dissected regions of the human body – such as the head and neck – on sequences of reels, while also reading the associated anatomical labels in accompanying illustrated books.[136] Purchased in sets by the Anatomy Department, reels or discs devised for commercial production by David L. Bassett each comprised seven pairs of stereoscopic photographs of dissected parts. When observed through the appropriate viewing apparatus, these photographs appeared as vivid three-dimensional dissections which could be studied at progressively deeper levels as the viewer rotated from image to image on each reel and then worked through the series of reels, identifying anatomical parts in the relevant volume of two-dimensional labelled diagrams. And here again, a technique for displaying anatomy moved between popular and professional domains. As one medical journal enthused, the 1954 set of reels – displaying the head and neck – modified for 'anatomical use' the 'new type of stereoscopic view-boxes through which school children of the present day [. . . see] colour views of areas around the world', just as a 1905 precursor (see illus. 106) had adapted for teaching anatomy the 'home stereoscope' used on 'parlour tables . . . for viewing scenic wonders'.[137] The ingenuity of this mid-twentieth-century appropriation was praised, and its wide take-up by medical students and physicians was predicted.

ANATOMICAL POETICS

Developing displays in two and three dimensions, Robert Lockhart was explicit about the relative weakness of words in the teaching and thorough understanding of anatomy. Like his contemporaries, Lockhart doubted the value of dense anatomical vocabularies and 'dreary descriptions', leaning in favour of learning through vision and touch.[138] This view was critical of words as a means to describe the body, and its earlier manifestations can be seen in mid-nineteenth-century anatomists' practices that rejected so called 'word-knowledge' while promoting learning through observation and practical work. Around the start of the twentieth century Thomas Cooke had condemned medical students' habit of trying to learn anatomy by memorizing the names of body parts through 'book-work' without adequate 'practical knowledge'. Such a 'scaffolding of words' was nothing more than a flimsy 'house of cards', he wrote. From this perspective important 'facts' would always be lost in the 'wreckage' of a memory 'over-burdened' with bookish details.[139]

Of course, not all words were rejected. Rather, their uses and importance in relation to other methods for teaching and learning were debated and shifting. Appropriate anatomical labelling was considered necessary, as noted above, and the value of description was also evident in international efforts to establish a standardized anatomical terminology, which was published and revised from the 1890s onwards.[140] In practice anatomical terminology was, during the mid-twentieth century at Marischal College, written and spoken as part of a poetics in which vivid metaphors were also used to convey knowledge. The text in *Anatomy of the Human Body* is indicative of this approach, which combined apparently 'familiar' (among anatomists) and 'accepted' or officially recommended nomenclature with striking metaphor.[141] Indeed, the book was so packed with metaphors associating bodily parts with seemingly unlikely items that the body began to resemble a Surrealist assemblage.

Upon reading it, students would discover that the skin is more amazing than a 'magician's mantle', acting as 'waterproof, overcoat, sunshade, suit of armour and refrigerator' while also 'hold[ing] the mirror to age and health'. Certain bones in the skull are 'light as eggshell and more delicate', while the lower jaw is 'arched in Gothic form'. Body parts appear in a multitude of shapes: a section of the shoulder blade is 'pear shaped', the hip bone is 'like the figure 8', one bone in the hand resembles a boat and another is like a 'large pea'. The system of blood and lymph vessels is likened to rail transport, and the nerves to a telephone system with wires, transmitters and receivers in the 'country' of the body. Some nerves form chains like a 'necklace' with 'beads' but others are like 'unskilled crochet work'. Anatomical parts in the book thus accumulated as architectural excerpts, fruit, numbers, vehicles, mechanical contraptions, vegetables and letters of the alphabet. In some instances disparate items are gathered in clusters to convey the complexity of a bodily structure. Features of the ear, for instance, are likened to jellyfish, a coiled serpent, a spiral staircase, a xylophone and a porthole.[142] Here verbal images, metaphors and analogies inhabited anatomical description.[143] They were intended to convey anatomical form, to trigger and propel the imagining of the bodily interior in three dimensions. The textbook utilized the movement of metaphor – its capacity for linkage – associating anatomical parts with objects that shared their shape. To imaginatively draw together such entities was to animate anatomy, inspiring medical students and enhancing their ability to visualize and understand internal bodily components.

The human body constructed in the play of metaphors throughout the book comprised a multitude of juxtaposed objects. This dissonant internal geometry of the body resembled Surrealists' imagery, especially their often referred to 'chance juxtaposition of a sewing machine and an umbrella on a dissecting table'.[144] In its entirety this textbook body was a bizarre and surprising hybrid, disrupting distinctions between the human form, artefacts, plants and living creatures. Yet each verbal anatomical image – or 'each line of the book' – read one by one, as Lockhart recommended, would come to make sense when 'verified' in relation to dissections, museum specimens and students' own bodies.[145] Students' readings of such metaphors would therefore have moved between the extraordinary and the ordinary or familiar. Indeed, however unusual such metaphors might initially have seemed to students, their comprehension of them would have been, according to anthropological analysis of metaphors, very much 'grounded in bodily perception and action'.[146] Like Surrealists' works, this anatomical poetics subverted boundaries between the exceptional and the everyday, the animate and the inanimate, and between what was internal and external to the human body, yet Lockhart developed this poetics not as an avant-garde practitioner but as an authoritative and somewhat conservative professor who was respected and promoted within his profession.[147]

Just as metaphors have been used to conceptualize museums in various ways, so those in *Anatomy of the Human Body* produced particular understandings of the body. The textbook made anatomy vivid and memorable, as did Lockhart's lectures for students, which were delivered, they enthused, in 'language which pleased us with its blend of poetic fancy and anatomical fact'.[148] Drawing on texts from literary works to fairy tales, Lockhart's talks were full of vibrant verbal images – images that shaped perceptions of the Anatomy Museum's holdings. At meetings of the AUAAS during the 1950s, for example, the anatomist's lectures on the human ear (see above) thoroughly exercised his powers of allusion. As one student reported, Lockhart

> reduced us to Lilliputian stature, to lead us with Snow White and the Seven Dwarfs in a tour of the Ogre's Ear, which was portrayed on a large wall map . . . He introduced us to Long John Silver, Alexander's Ragtime Band and Jimmy Durante who was looking for the last chord in the inner ear.[149]

Here Lockhart conjured characters from a fairy tale (collected and published by the Brothers Grimm in the early nineteenth century) and drew on an image of tiny people from Lilliput in Jonathan Swift's *Gulliver's Travels* of 1726; he made a pirate from Robert Louis Stevenson's 1883 *Treasure Island* meet with a 'ragtime band' (featured in an early twentieth-century popular song) and a vaudeville star; and he performed this composite narrative before an enlarged diagram displaying the anatomy of the inner ear while also demonstrating museum specimens and models of the skull and ear (see illus. 121).[150]

Diverse references to popular and literary culture were characteristic of Lockhart's anatomical compositions, which, in his own words, 'stretch[ed] from the literal to the metaphorical . . . from the scientific to the popular, from the romance of bones to the majestic, trivial and tragic romances of life'.[151] Literature cited by the anatomist included Edgar Allan Poe's macabre (posthumously entitled collection) *Tales of Mystery and Imagination*, Jules Verne's science fiction, Byron's poetry and Samuel Taylor Coleridge's *The Rime of the Ancient Mariner*. In one of Lockhart's animating narratives, the 'mariner' adapted from the latter poem was the largest museum specimen in the Anatomy Department – the whale skeleton displayed in the entrance corridor.[152]

130
Slide of a
rhododendron display
in Robert Lockhart's
sitting room at his
house in Rubislaw
Den, Aberdeen,
c. 1950s.

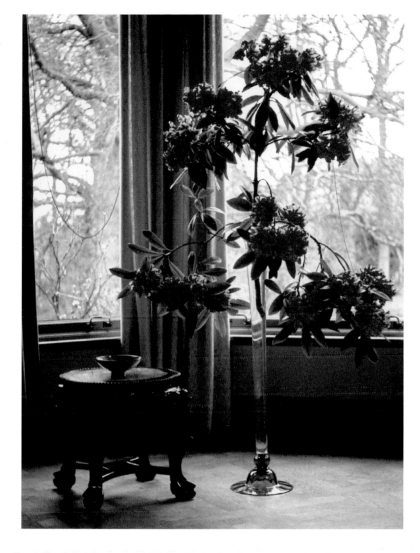

Significantly, the use of metaphor infused anatomy with colour, imparting life to dissections and faded museum specimens.[153] Lockhart would assert, for instance, that 'the colour in muscles of rapid motion [is] the honey bee's rosy red layer in the Himalaya hybrid' – this being a rhododendron that Lockhart grew in his garden and often photographed to show during lectures in slide format (illus. 130).[154] This poetic, visual linkage of body and flower conveyed the colour of living muscles within the moving human body. At Lockhart's last anatomy lecture for medical students before he retired – in which he once more demonstrated the model of the ear (see illus. 121) – the students wore rhododendron flowers, scattering them at its close (illus. 131). Students had filled his dove-grey Daimler,

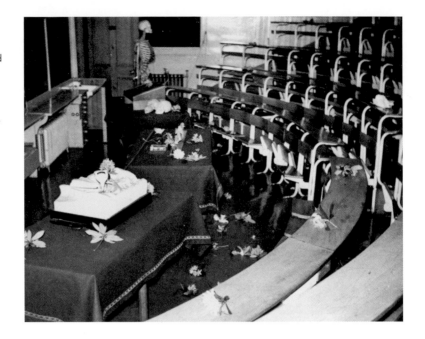

parked in Marischal College's front quadrangle, with the blooms and in the lecture theatre they 'silently threw down rhododendron flowers until the old Anatomy Theatre was deep with their colour and beauty'.[155] For the anatomist the rhododendron had personal memorial significance: he had grown in his garden a new variant, with 'black-red' flowers, which he named after his late mother Elizabeth Lockhart.[156]

JUXTAPOSITION

Seemingly disparate entities – from plants to aeroplanes – were linked and associated with parts of the human body to communicate the colour as well as the form and function of living anatomy.[157] Operating through interrelated textual, visual and material modes, the anatomical poetics in this context generated meaning through linkage and juxtaposition. Among Lockhart's favoured collecting and display practices was the taking of clippings from magazines, newspapers and journals, which he sorted and selected for exhibiting in combination with photographs of dissections and museum specimens. Compiling such clippings was not an unusual activity for scientists as well as artists in the first half of the twentieth century,[158] and this activity with scissors produced images that were, for Lockhart, very useful alongside specimens produced with scalpels. Amassing diverse compelling (often) colour images, he had many converted into slides,

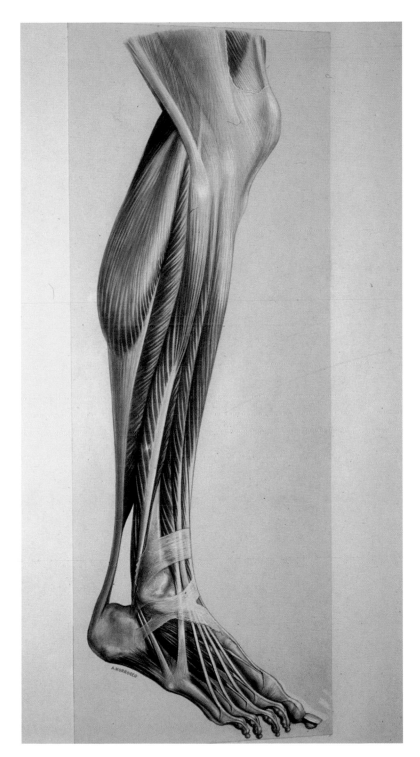

132
Alberto Morrocco, illustration of the muscles of the lower leg, *c.* 1949, watercolour, commissioned for R. D. Lockhart, G. F. Hamilton and F. W. Fyfe, *Anatomy of the Human Body* (London, 1959), Fig. 372.

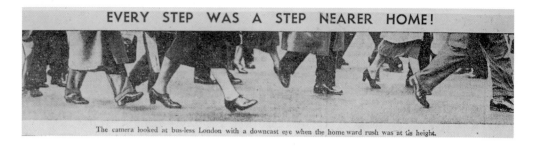

EVERY STEP WAS A STEP NEARER HOME!

The camera looked at bus-less London with a downcast eye when the home ward rush was at its height.

133 Slide of a newspaper clipping: 'Every step was a step nearer home!', c. 1958, collected by Robert Lockhart.

which he then assembled as series for showing in lectures for medical students. Working with clippings-as-slides was a display strategy that created surprising visual alignments and contrasts in order to communicate anatomical knowledge.

In the lecture theatre, then, Lockhart would explain aspects of living anatomy with sequences of projected images arranged in unexpected and visually arresting ways. For example, an illustration of dissected lower leg muscles, made for *Anatomy of the Human Body* by Alberto Morrocco (illus. 132), was displayed after a photograph of legs in the act of walking (illus. 133).[159] Clipped from a newspaper, the original caption for this photograph read: 'The camera looked at bus-less London with a downcast eye when the home ward rush was at its height'. Probably snapped during the 1958 London bus strike, the photograph was put to use in anatomical display as an image of live, moving legs. Students were thus, again, prompted to associate the dissected leg with animate limbs, so that the dead body part was understood in terms of its living function in action.

The range of clippings drawn from print media into the slide display of living anatomy was wide, as one further example indicates. Lockhart showed a 1954 cover of *Woman's Own* magazine featuring an active smiling face (illus. 134), Pablo Picasso's 1939 *Head of a Woman* (illus. 135) and a photograph of his own 1925 dissection of the human head (illus. 136).[160] The sequence of slides thus juxtaposed images of the head firstly viewed from the surface, then painted by a Cubist from several angles, then dissected to reveal the deep interior. In the Anatomy Museum this latter photograph served to label the specimen displayed adjacent to it. In the lecture theatre, via slide projection, the specimen was linked with colour images of living heads, prompting viewers to imagine the head's functions and mobility in life. Observation of museum specimens, and therefore human anatomy, was invigorated through visual association with body parts in art and popular print.

If juxtaposition brought the popular into the domain of professional medical training, it was also an organizing principle in Lockhart's temporary exhibitions which he produced for the wider public in his capacity as

134
Slide of *Woman's
Own* magazine cover,
2 December 1954,
collected by Robert
Lockhart.

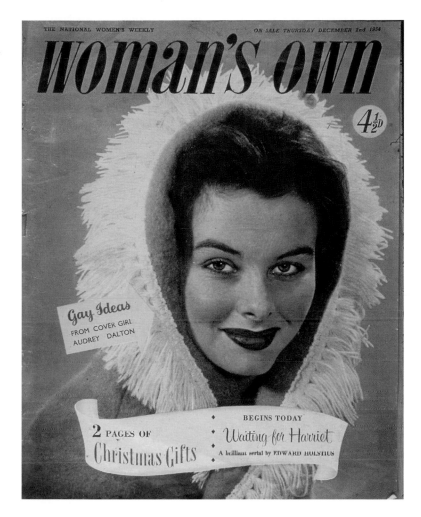

honorary curator of the Anthropological Museum at Marischal College. One 1970s display featured specimens once in the Anatomy Museum – including a preserved and dissected foot of a Chinese woman, a Maori tattooed head and a human skull from British New Guinea (Papua New Guinea) – positioned alongside an array of artefacts including hats and headdresses from different parts of the world (illus. 137; see illus. 110, 111).[161] Placed in proximity to the human remains was a plastic female mannequin head, like those in shop windows, 'alive' and gazing back at exhibition visitors; the dead again shared display space with the living, and the museum gallery was made to intersect with the everyday space of the high street to draw viewers in. Chapter Eight discusses the relocation of such preserved body parts, especially skulls, to the Anthropological Museum as just one shift among many in the post-1965 transformation of

135
Pablo Picasso,
Head of a Woman,
1939, oil on canvas.

136
Photograph of a
museum specimen
labelled: 'Dissection
to show cerebral,
spinal and
sympathetic nerves
in human head and
neck. See adjacent
dissection', dissected
by Robert Lockhart,
1925.

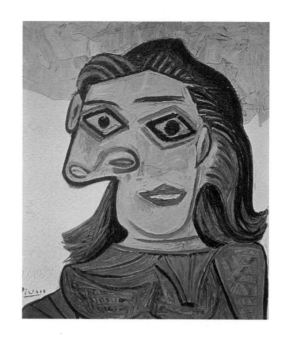

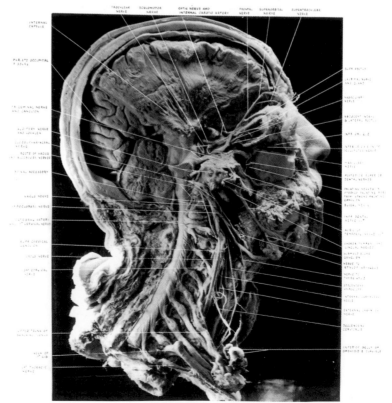

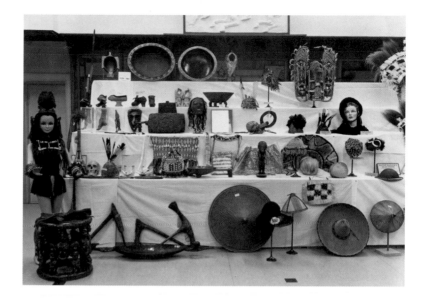

137
Temporary display,
c. 1970, in the
Anthropological
Museum, Marischal
College, University
of Aberdeen,
photograph.

the Anatomy Museum – a transformation that fashioned the entire display as an anatomical body that students entered and learned to navigate.

The dynamic displays explored in this chapter sought to make the human body meaningful to medical students as living anatomy. Deceased bodies in the dissecting room and Anatomy Museum were therefore animated through visual, textual and performative strategies that engaged medical students' own bodies. This poetics brought anatomy to life, taking students on journeys within the body when they conducted dissections, watched slide displays and films, absorbed anatomical narratives and examined museum exhibits. Learning was an imaginative process grounded in students' bodily action, especially disciplined observation. In a twentieth-century context where medical museums were debated and reconstructed, the Anatomy Museum was invigorated in the movement between the popular and the professional, between fact and fantasy, between science and art. The next chapter turns to the material and visual aspects of anatomical displays as well as the multiple interrelated methods employed to exhibit bodies so that their effects on medical students were deep and lasting.

Seven
PAPER, WAX AND PLASTIC

Human anatomy has been displayed in the flesh itself and in manifold materials including ivory, plaster, leather, glass, wool, wood, calico, velvet, Plasticine, paper, wax and plastic (or plastics).[1] These are just a few of the materials employed in attempts to make anatomy 'visible and tangible' in two and three dimensions.[2] The significance of substance as well as form in aspects of anatomical display are explored in this chapter from the nineteenth to the mid-twentieth century in contexts of medical-school teaching and learning in Britain. Displays composed of human bodies, illustrations and 'fabricated' models were produced by anatomists and their assistants to be used, manipulated and sometimes co-produced by medical students. The emphasis placed on active (rather than passive) involvement of medical students in learning anatomy from around the 1850s onwards was such that anatomical methods and teaching 'aids' were designed to guide the users' bodily and conceptual participation in particular ways.[3] Furthermore, the materials involved in anatomical display, and the forms that these materials took, had implications for the knowledge and skills that were learned. How human anatomy has materialized in processes of knowledge-making is analysed in what follows, with attention to the interactive and interrelated practices of cutting, (dis)assembling, layering, outlining, threading and shaping.

Such material practices were devised and disseminated for exploring and communicating anatomy. Their development was complex, but three overlapping factors can be highlighted here. First is the growing importance of students' engagement in practical anatomical study and the perceived necessity of embodied modes of learning for gaining medical knowledge. As one medical commentator explained in 1851, the 'time and labour' involved in dissecting an anatomical part was crucial if students were to form a lasting 'mental picture' of that part.[4] The influential comparative anatomist Thomas Henry Huxley, speaking as rector of the University of Aberdeen in 1874, advocated that medical students should gain 'practical, familiar, finger-end knowledge' of anatomy – like that of a watchmaker – in the dissecting room and laboratory rather than the lecture room or library. He advised students that by concentrating on the 'complexities of organ and function' for six or seven hours a day, month after month, the 'greater truths' of anatomy and physiology would 'become an organic part of your minds', to the extent that 'you . . . know them . . . as a man knows the geography of his native place and the daily life of his home' (a potent and resilient analogy discussed in the previous chapter). To study in this way was to obtain knowledge which was regarded as a valuable, 'life-long possession'.[5]

By the 1890s students were expected to

> display with knife and forceps, and such manipulative skill as he can acquire, the constituent parts of the human frame, until he knows how they are arranged and what their relative position is, the one to the other.[6]

Displaying anatomical parts to deepen knowledge of bodily structures and their functions was, therefore, regarded as a student's 'duty'. As the Edinburgh anatomist William Turner enthused at the opening of the University of Oxford's new anatomy buildings in 1893, students' 'personal work', conducted 'over a period of time sufficient to allow the multitude of details to slowly but surely penetrate the mind and imprint themselves deeply in the memory', equipped those students with an essential 'body of facts'. This would then allow a student to 'call up at will a mental picture of the objects and structures seen in the course of his practical work' and so 'utilise with safety and confidence' this essential knowledge.[7] Anatomical practices thus co-opted the active learning bodies of students whose disciplined work was directed towards the cultivation of bodily and mental capacities – and in particular towards what was deemed an almost physically embedded mental picture of anatomical parts, their relations and growth from 'fertilized ovum' to adult.[8] This embodied engagement was compelled by powerful discourses of both self-reliance and personal responsibility towards future patients.

While strong commitment to practical methods of learning through hands-on dissection was maintained in medical schools during the first half of the twentieth century and beyond, there was also re-evaluation of the dead as a source of anatomical knowledge relative to other means of learning. This second factor was intimately connected with the rise of living anatomy, in which the live bodies of medical students were also enlisted for study. And thirdly, developments in materials and techniques for the visual representation and three-dimensional modelling of anatomy were significant, such as the availability and uptake of new plastics. These interrelated factors were implicated in emerging approaches to, and devices for, teaching and learning, and they informed medical students' embodied perceptions and conceptualizations of anatomy.

Teaching aimed to stimulate students' active involvement so that knowledge could be imparted and deepened, and skills enhanced. Rather than being situated as passive observers of anatomical displays, then, students were required to participate in them.[9] This participation panned out in different ways, depending on the material and form of the educational resources and teaching devices deployed in medical-school teaching situations. Material entities for anatomical display – bodies, illustrations and models – were made available to students as open objects; they were designed and arranged in sites of learning so that they would stimulate students' interactions with them.

While late nineteenth- and early twentieth-century innovations in pedagogical strategies and tools have been identified by historians as instrumental in shifting the work of science students from passive listening to active training,[10] analysis of the material culture of anatomy suggests that stimulating and sustaining student participation had already become important in medical schools from at least the 1850s onwards – as when dissection was undertaken, and when drawings based on dissections and textbook illustrations were made (see illus. 96, 122). Such active study was not solitary: it was collective in that each student was aware that fellow students in their medical school cohort were learning according to the expectations and standards communicated to them by their teachers. So processes of anatomical display ideally came to require engaged work – and reflexive awareness of that work – on the part of every student within the social contexts of medical education. The visual and material practices through which participation in display was encouraged as a mode of learning are analysed in what follows, alongside changes in requirements for the attainment of anatomical knowledge that moved away from what was regarded as excessive, burdensome detail which deadened the interest of the learner.

(IM)POSSIBLE ANATOMIES

Critical examination of how anatomy comes to be known, and creative efforts aimed at solving perceived problems in attaining that knowledge, have been important aspects of anatomical practices. In the early decades of the twentieth century anatomists were concerned that medical students could be misled by 'errors' in books, just as they could potentially derive 'erroneous impressions' of anatomy from studies of cadavers in dissecting rooms.[11] Therefore dissection of the dead – although regarded by medical educators as a necessity – had to be 'supplemented by every available method which will reveal the conditions [of the body] during life'. The development of such methods, using a wide range of media, was part of a shift in emphasis from 'pure descriptive anatomy', associated with the memorizing of fine detail observed in dead bodies, to the anatomical study of bodily structures in the living, associated with gaining ability to understand the functional 'meaning and significance' of those structures by attending to *both* deceased and live bodies.[12]

Absolute exactitude in anatomical description of the living body was deemed, from some points of view, to be an impossible undertaking. Thomas Cooke, for instance, wrote: 'it is as impossible – and were it possible, it would be useless – to describe the exact shape of an organ at a given time, as to describe the exact shape of the palm of the hand when grasped . . . in friendship.'[13] He highlighted the acute difficulty in obtaining adequate anatomical impressions of the living body, when the viscera or '*soft* and *yielding masses*' were subject to transitory actions, reactions and modifications from hour to hour – many bodily parts had 'no more settled shape than a pocket-handkerchief crumpled up in the pocket'. How could the shapes of muscles be described, asked Cooke, when they alter, contract and relax according to the body's ongoing, altering positions? How could these 'shifting scenes of organic life' be adequately captured for anatomical study?[14]

With an awareness of such difficulties, anatomists remained committed to investigating and demonstrating bodily interiors by utilizing and adapting an array of methods and media, each of which was critically evaluated to weigh up relative advantages and inadequacies, and to combine and navigate between them in ways deemed most educationally effective. Cooke, for instance, explicitly rejected 'paper anatomy', understood as a mode of learning in which students' attention was directed towards reading words so that it was 'riveted to the page of the book and turned away from the page of Nature'; this 'bookism', he insisted, was 'a very ogre gnawing out the brains of our young men'.[15] Instead Cooke provided a comprehensive list of practical tasks to be performed, tasks that would produce 'delightfully lucid' conceptions of the body which 'result from seeing' and handling bodies during dissection – a process which he considered to be the 'nearest approach to the living body'.[16] Students were instructed to 'feel' ligaments, 'explore' and 'name' muscles; to 'trace the course of' and 'map out' veins; to 'examine' joints; to 'point out', 'indicate', 'demonstrate' and 'show in action' anatomical parts as well as the relations between them. They were also advised to 'mark the outline' of structures such as bones and tendons, and to 'draw the lines' of nerves and arteries.[17] Marking, conducted with the finger on dissected bodies, could shift easily into drawing with pencil on paper, so interchangeable were these practices. Through the act of drawing, conducted alongside dissection, body and page were intimately related and therefore this form of paper anatomy, unlike bookism, was deemed productive rather than destructive.

In the late 1890s Cooke reflected on a recent pedagogical shift away from encouraging students to dissect bodies in order to see 'everything'. Now, according to Cooke, parts of the body that were 'easy' to dissect, such as the limbs, were explored in this way, but with regard to those areas that were more difficult to dissect – especially the 'deeper parts' of the head and neck and the visceral cavities – the corpse or dissecting-room subject was sometimes no longer considered the 'most convenient illustration'.[18] These body parts were often examined, then, with the aid of anatomical images and three-dimensional models. Other anatomists, too, recognized that many anatomical structures were often not 'fully examined or completely demonstrable' in dissecting rooms so that museum collections were therefore necessary 'to enable the student to extend and amplify his observations on the cadaver'.[19] Nevertheless three-dimensional models were carefully appraised within medical-school settings, where they were utilized and also compared either with bodies undergoing dissection, living models (including students' own bodies) or live patients seen in clinical cases. Depending on their reception, then, certain models could be dismissed as 'unrealities' from which students should not be encouraged to learn.[20]

The relations between dissection, visual images and three-dimensional models as construed in strategies of anatomical display and learning change and vary over time; their relative value, potential and drawbacks within teaching and learning are contextually debated and negotiated. Historical studies based in Continental Europe have suggested that models were displaced by dissection throughout the nineteenth century, so that by around 1900 commercially produced models of what was defined as 'normal' adult anatomy were largely deemed subordinate to learning by dissecting, although models were widely employed in the study of fields such as obstetrics, embryology and pathology.[21] However, the relative uses of, and value assigned to, both models and images in medical schools during this period were perhaps not so clear-cut and during the first half of the twentieth century there were continued investments in anatomical teaching tools of diverse sorts in Britain, as we have seen in previous chapters.

There were many factors involved here, among them the fluctuating numbers of deceased bodies that anatomists obtained for dissection (which also varied according to region), even following the 1832 Anatomy Act, which was intended to strengthen the legal acquisition of corpses for medical education.[22] Anatomists in Aberdeen were constantly alert to potential and actual shortages in body supplies, as they were elsewhere in Scotland and England. Yet practical work in anatomical study – that is, learning by 'seeing and doing' to develop 'visual and manual familiarity' with the body – was maintained as a priority.[23] Gaining sufficiently skilled, in-depth knowledge of the body would enable the medical practitioner to see the body, as Cooke asserted using the 'metaphor of the day', as though it were 'like glass, transparent'.[24] From this perspective, thorough knowledge manifested as the ability to see through the body, to visually reach into its deep anatomical structures.[25]

In Aberdeen, John Arthur Thomson, professor of natural history at Marischal College, also couched expertise in science in similar terms. He wrote in 1911:

> when we work at a thing and come to know it up and down, in and out, through and through, it becomes in a quite remarkable way translucent. The botanist can see through his tree, see wood and bast . . . The zoologist can in the same way see through the snail on the thorn, seeing as in a glass model everything in its place, the nerve-centres, the muscles, the stomach, the beating heart, the coursing blood, and the filtering kidney. So the human body becomes translucent to the skilled anatomist, and the globe to the skilled geographer.[26]

The body envisaged as glass, a transparent material, allows those knowledgeable and skilled in anatomy to 'see' into its interior, into its very depths with striking clarity. In Thomson's account this way of seeing 'reality' was like the 'X-rays that penetrate through superficial obscurities'. 'Clearness of vision' was attained through precision in working methods, which guarded against seeing only a 'blurred tangle of lines'. Furthermore, practising science involved 'continual protest' against lack of accuracy and disciplined avoidance of ambiguity. Diligent study with anatomized bodies as well as approved visual images and models could cultivate the necessary clear sight, but Thomson was certain – like many teachers of anatomy – that this ability to see could not be 'acquired passively': it could only be 'engendered by our being actively and energetically scientific'.[27]

Reaching towards the ideal of clarity, an anatomical model produced in Germany with clear plastics and displayed during the 1930s to wide international audiences was a compelling material manifestation of the principle of transparency. The last section of this chapter discusses this model in the context of developments in new plastics that fed into the shaping of anatomy in medical education. But first, analysis of the inter-related and changing material practices entailing particular kinds of bodily and conceptual work on the part of anatomists and medical students, from *c.* 1820s to the 1960s, begins with the cut.

CUTTING

The importance of tools in the execution of anatomy had been apparent in anatomical works since the early modern period. Following Vesalius' 1543 *Fabrica* (the Latin term *fabrica* referring to craft or art as well as a skilful production),[28] the physician Helkiah Crooke's 1615 publication, *Mikrokosmographia*, reiterated the anatomist's illustrated inventory of necessary instruments (illus. 138):

> Razors of all sortes, great, small, meane, sharpe, blunt, straight, crooked, and edged on both sides; sheares or sizers . . . long probes of brasse, silver, lead; a knife of box or of ivory, pincers of all sorts; hooks, needels . . . reeds, quils, glasse-trunkes or hollow bugles to blowe up the parts, threds and strings, sawes, bodkins . . . basons and sponges . . . with a table whereon to lay the dead.[29]

Noting the etymology of the word 'anatomy', Crooke explained that 'thom is a Greeke word, and signifieth section or cutting . . . undertaken to get knowledge or skil by.' This could only be accomplished with 'convenient Instruments' for dissection: those on the anatomist's table, along with his

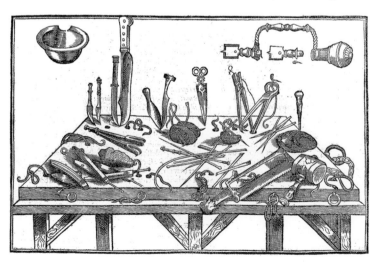

138
Illustration of instruments (after Vesalius) for practising anatomy, woodcut from Helkiah Crooke, *Mikrokosmographia: A Description of the Body of Man* (London, 1615).

hand. Anatomy was conceived as action both of the intellect and of the hand, the latter defined as the 'first instrument . . . the framer, yea and the imployer of all other instruments'. Without the sense of touch, Crooke explained, physicians would be blind and forced to 'grope uncertainlie in darke and palpable ignorance'. And just as the capable hand writes and builds, so it becomes skilled in the labour of dissection.[30] This alignment of dissection, or at least cutting, and writing was also suggested in early modern illustrated manuals, which provided guidance on the conduct of handwriting and instructions on how to make tools for inscription: the knife would cut the quill and then the quill could cut like the knife, albeit metaphorically, when inscribing calfskin vellum or paper.[31]

Instruments that cut and those that write and draw were granted a certain equivalence in nineteenth-century manuals that guided medical students' labour in dissecting rooms. The surgeon James Scratchley's 1826 publication, for instance, advised students on the digital dexterity required in the practice of anatomy:

> the position of the hand in dissecting should be the same, as in writing or drawing; and the knife, held, like the pen or pencil, by the thumb and the two first fingers, should be moved by means of them only; while the hand rests firmly on the two other fingers bent inwards as in writing, and on the wrist.[32]

Dissecting was akin to mark-making just as skin was to paper, and these associations were made visually apparent in Richard Quain's 1844 *Anatomy of the Arteries*.[33] In one of a series of life-size prints or 'lithographic drawings', a dissection of the lower leg shows the artery, highlighted in red (illus. 139). To the left of the dissected leg there is an arrangement of quill, scalpel and open pot of ink, while a roll of paper echoes the peeling away of skin from the limb. The lower hook pulls anatomical parts aside and, on a line indicated by the diagonal direction of this instrument, the shape made by these parts appears again as a corner of paper. This corner overlays the scalpel, reiterating the layering of tissues where the skin opens and folds over the foot.

The tools in *Anatomy of the Arteries* recall those visible on Vesalius' dissecting table in the title page of the *Fabrica* (see illus. 48), but now they played a much more active role in enhancing the visibility of the bodies undergoing dissection on paper. Further plates in the series show ropes and strips of cloth holding up limbs, and bodies propped up by wooden blocks, a chair and a book by Charles Bell. Here tools used to dissect enter the frame of paper anatomies as devices that aid composition and comprehension. Instruments are positioned as guides for viewers' eyes: while fabric wraps,

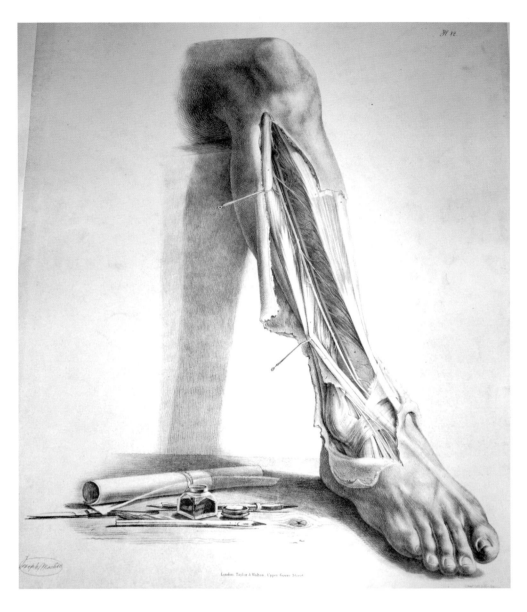

139
Joseph Maclise,
illustration of blood
vessels and tendons in
the leg, lithographic
drawing from Richard
Quain, *The Anatomy
of the Arteries of the
Human Body* (London,
1844), Plate 82.

drapes and frames dissections, hooks, pins, forceps, a probe and a needle point to the parts requiring particular attention. In Quain's Plate 26 a pair of scissors, resting with the arm on a hinged wooden bench, follows the exposed sweep of the artery across the page (see illus. 68). Furthermore, to include this apparatus was to link these images with the spaces in which they had originated and were intended for display: the drawings were based on studies of over a thousand deceased bodies at University College London, where Quain was professor of anatomy; unbound and mounted

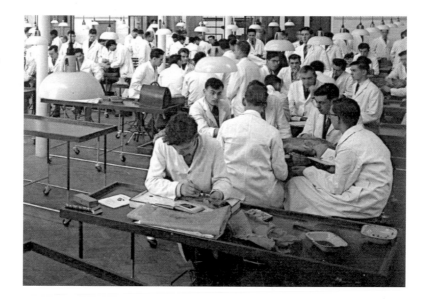

on heavy paper, they were prepared for hanging on dissecting-room walls. The paraphernalia of dissection thus visually placed or located the anatomical image, and the assertion that the images were 'from nature' also reinforced the authority of these paper anatomies.[34] Demonstrating legitimacy was important, especially as there had been criticism of certain forms of 'pictorial anatomy'. In Edinburgh during the 1830s, for example, anatomist Robert Knox satirized and rejected anatomists' use of this 'mural art', with its 'gaudy colours'. Such pictures, he claimed, were 'misrepresentations of nature', some so gigantic – as was one of a human heart the size of a whale's – that they smacked of the country fairs where pictures of large people were displayed to the 'multitude'.[35] Quain's lithographic drawings could deflect such potential criticism, produced in life-size with careful use of colour.

The size of paper anatomies was again an issue in the design of printed books to be utilized by students in dissecting rooms. Large-format anatomical atlases, such as John Lizars's *System of Anatomical Plates* (1822–6) and Sibson's *Medical Anatomy* (1869), were authoritative and prestigious but heavy and unwieldy (see illus. 69, 72). Produced with high-quality paper and ink, using laborious techniques, atlases aimed to be definitive, enduring works.[36] But these were not books for the messy dissecting table and hence smaller books affordable to medical students were also in demand during the nineteenth century.[37] Scratchley's volume, at a handy 4 × 7 in. (10 × 17.75 cm), provided instructions to be read while dissecting, and *Cunningham's Manual of Practical Anatomy*, first published in 1889 and currently still in (revised) print, was only marginally larger in its 1950s version so that it was easily accommodated on work surfaces. In the dissecting room at Marischal College, during the mid-twentieth century, manuals were propped open on dissecting trays or stacked for reference with students' small cases of dissecting instruments (illus. 140). These books continued to advise on the requisite tools – either improvised and adapted using objects readily to hand or purchased from commercial suppliers. Manuals suggested that handy hooks were easily made from thick bent pins and fine waxed string while indispensable probes could be usefully obtained in the form of 'homely articles, such as knitting-needles, crochet-hooks, &c.' If recycled items of anatomical haberdashery stocked the student's 'box of apparatus', this tool set had also always to include, according to *Cunningham's Manual*, scissors, scalpels and forceps.[38]

This manual issued guidance on how to cut as part of an entire range of manual procedures entailed in the process of dissection, providing an 'education of the sense of touch' as much as a training in the dextrous handling of tools.[39] How to position the cadaver; what to examine and trace; which parts to push, pull and stretch; which parts were bony, fibrous, tough, dense, soft or smooth; where the student should feel, grasp or press. In addition to making incisions, snipping and slitting, students were guided in separating, folding back, removing, pinning or stitching parts, cleaning and defining areas (by scraping away fat and connective tissue), inflating parts with a blowpipe, revealing structures such as nerves by extricating them with blunt hooks, and dividing bone with a saw, chisel and mallet. Marks made in pencil sometimes prefigured the cut – to dissect the skull, string was used to encircle it; a pencil line followed this and then the saw.[40]

The operations promoted by the dissecting manual were also turned upon the book itself. Students would often annotate, underline and sketch in anatomy textbooks, but Thomas Cooke advised more radical intervention: taking his anatomy textbook apart for more convenient 'carrying in the coat pocket' and use in the dissecting room. As the subjects were arranged in sections, they could easily be divided 'by simply cutting the bookbinder's threads or tapes'. If Cooke's volume could be cut into sections 'without falling to pieces', the anatomist Edward Bald Jamieson's multi-volume set *Illustrations of Regional Anatomy*, first published in 1934, further developed the principle of the divisible book.[41] This was originally designed as a compilation of pages on 'loose-leaf pillars' that could be unhooked to release individual leaves from the spine; this provided portable illustrations that could be 'arranged into any sequence'.[42] A distinct advantage of this shuffleable paper anatomy was that it allowed the many illustrations to be conveniently rearranged so that their order was synchronized with the order in which bodies were dissected – a very useful feature that helped students to relate book to body during their learning.

Anatomy on the page was made to closely relate to bodies undergoing dissection, such that a material equivalence was suggested between paper and body. While authoritative images could clarify observation of bodies, approved text provided instructions on how to interact with those bodies. In such ways paper and flesh were intercut.

(DIS)ASSEMBLING

Closely connected with techniques of cutting in anatomical practices are those involved in disassembling and then – in reverse – assembling 'artificial' bodies.[43] Models that could be repeatedly taken apart and fitted back together were to gain advantage during the nineteenth century. Those devised by Louis Auzoux (1797–1880) were widely distributed to medical schools in Britain, Europe, North America and Australia, as well as India, Egypt and Japan, forming influential precursors of anatomical models manufactured in plastics with detachable parts from the mid-twentieth century onwards (see illus. 156, 32).[44] Having studied anatomy in Paris, Auzoux developed what he termed 'anatomie clastique', or clastic anatomy, from the Greek *klao* meaning to break, so that his models were composed of multiple components that could be removed and opened to show internal parts – as in a 'real dissection', Auzoux's product catalogues claimed – and then neatly reassembled.[45] In the 1820s Auzoux presented his life-size constructions – a leg, abdomen, head and upper torso – to the Académie royale de médecine, where they received high praise. Further enthusiastic responses to the modelled body parts followed: even the thinnest, softest and most delicate were considered to be 'represented with strict exactitude in their forms, colors, relations and connections'.[46]

Auzoux's models went into production at his factory in Saint-Aubin-d'Écrosville, Normandy, and he opened his Paris shop in 1833, which became a successful commercial enterprise. By the 1850s Auzoux's productions included over 50 models of human, mammal, fish, insect and mollusc anatomy (see illus. 83). His marketing strategies led to the take-up of his models for medical-school education and for promoting the study of anatomy outside the medical profession. Profitable exposure of his models came with their display at international exhibitions, and by the 1880s the models were well known enough to appear in Gustave Flaubert's unfinished novel *Bouvard et Pécuchet*.[47] In the early decades of the twentieth century the Auzoux firm's catalogue had further expanded to embrace anatomical, zoological and botanical models.[48]

Auzoux's creations stimulated interest in Britain when his life-size model of the human body was first presented at the Westminster Medical

141
Anatomical model,
1879, by Auzoux,
Paris.

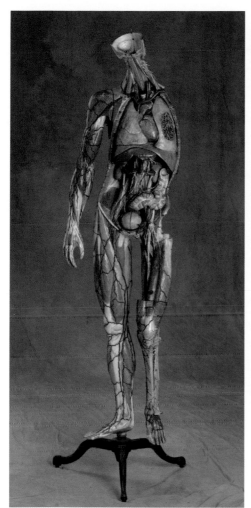
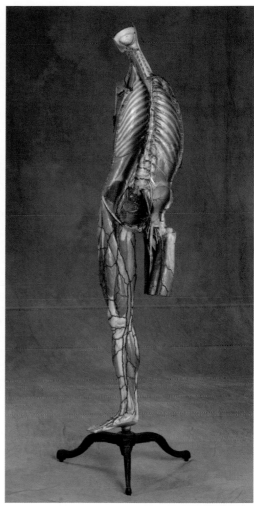

142
Anatomical model
with some detachable
parts removed, 1879,
by Auzoux, Paris.

143
Anatomical model
with all detachable
parts removed, 1879,
by Auzoux, Paris.

Society in London in 1832, an event reported in medical journals and newspapers. The male figure – described as an 'extraordinary anatomical machine' and an 'ingenious apparatus' – was commended for its 'astonishing truth to nature'. Its multitude of parts separated and reunited, and this action of 'analysis and synthesis' was applauded as a means to gain knowledge of the body's 'whole structure' and its fine 'details'.[49] The mannikin comprised muscles, organs, arteries, veins, nerves, lymphatic vessels and bones, allowing students to learn the form and position of parts much faster, it was reported, than in a dissecting room.[50] The model had its limits, however. Although it was considered useful at the start of anatomical studies, and as a means to later 'reimpress the memory', it was regarded as less appropriate for advanced instruction.[51] Medical reviewers suggested that when anatomists needed to show the 'texture of complicated organs' or the 'minute arteries', for instance,

> imitative anatomy must be abandoned, shadows however true to their originals will prove insufficient, fac-similes however striking must lead to error. The portrait must give place to its prototype. The actual, natural, animal body must be seen, studied, and understood.[52]

The definition of models as imitations placed them in a subordinate relation to deceased bodies as pedagogical tools. Evaluated in relation to human flesh, even Auzoux's meticulously detailed models could not 'teach the structures of the membranes, nor communicate any notion of the feel, the palp, the consistence and resistance of tissues'.[53]

While models were deemed auxiliary devices, the drawbacks of dissection were nevertheless also acknowledged. So-called 'artificial anatomy' was not expected to 'supersede the use of the human subject', but it was considered especially beneficial when bodies acquired for dissection were scarce. Even in situations of adequate supply, models had purpose. They were largely resistant to decay (bodies were not), they could be exhibited indefinitely (bodies had to be buried), and they were useful in demonstrating organs and tissues that could not be preserved from dissected bodies as well as very small anatomical parts that required display on a larger scale.[54] Studying with models could also help reduce the time students spent in dissecting rooms 'from which so many injurious consequences arise', including wounds from sharp instruments and a 'foul atmosphere' inhaled for weeks on end.[55] According to a former student at King's College London, at every medical school a number of students were 'knocked up' every year and some apparently died from dissecting injuries.[56] Other undesirable physical effects of dissecting rooms were complained of, such as students' disrupted eating habits: according to one former medical student, morning dissections made them 'feel ravenous' but once at the chop-house the vapour from hot food took away all appetite so that they could 'scarcely eat'; and if they did 'the meat seem[ed] to taste of the body [they] were dissecting' and they felt 'utterly wretched'. This distressing sensation of ingesting human flesh – of cannibalism, no less – was swiftly remedied by tobacco, a 'few whiffs' of a cigarette.[57]

So although some students eagerly seized the opportunity to dissect, others recoiled and battled with feelings of disgust. Even some members of the medical profession, although convinced of its importance, also regarded it as distasteful.[58] It was a 'painful and noisome necessity', as one mid-nineteenth-century medical journal explained, and it was managed through adherence to particular codes of conduct. Students were to maintain cleanliness – of themselves, their instruments and manuals – protecting their clothes from 'filth' by wearing a dissecting gown or long apron.[59] Those delighting in dirt were considered 'rude, untutored, and brutal', while a man who allowed 'charnel-house accumulation' to remain about him, carrying traces of the dead beyond the dissecting room and into the company of others, was said to be 'no more civilised than savages'.[60] Medical students were expected to observe ritualized rules through their own bodily comportment and attitude – showing respect for the dead, displaying decorum and dignity, avoiding levity as at a funeral and refraining from 'unseemly ribaldry or idle jest'. To properly perform duties as a student, he had to control his feelings, not permitting his 'reserve to degenerate into repugnance, nor his caution into cowardice'; he had to 'dissipate all unmanly fears and idle fancies', overcoming 'personal antipathies' with 'reason and habit'. Dissecting with the appropriate action and in the approved manner was thus associated with the attainment of both manhood and professional medical identity; working with perseverance, each student would, then, gain 'steadiness, courage . . . and decision of touch', qualities and skills deemed necessary in the treatment of the sick.[61]

Auzoux's models were also designed to engage the hands and their manufacture in robust materials facilitated this. Many were purchased for anatomy teaching at Marischal College during the 1860s and '70s, including a life-size male figure in over 90 pieces detailing around 2,000 anatomical parts (illus. 141). The model can be rotated on its stand for viewing in the round while its disassembly progressively reveals the body's depths (illus. 142, 143). To display the model's inner structures the operator had to become familiar with its system of articulation, for which Auzoux issued printed instructions (illus. 144). The pieces were numbered consecutively to indicate the order in which they should be detached, starting with number one, and then reattached, beginning with the highest number and proceeding in reverse. These numbers were accompanied by a small printed sign of a pointing hand (far left, centre). This pointing hand – a manicule – was an established instructional convention in printed publications for drawing attention to a particular section of a text, and it was used on Auzoux's models to show the precise point at which a piece of a model should be removed and rejoined.[62] (With this use of the manicule, Auzoux's models borrowed from visual conventions of printed texts, so that model was related to book.) Sequences of numbers and letters of the alphabet, fully affixed to models on small labels, functioned as a key to link model parts with anatomical terms printed on a separate sheet; this avoided cluttering the surfaces of models with too much text. A series of small metal fittings, especially sturdy yet discreet hooks and eyes, provided means to reconnect each model's pieces, to hold its component parts securely

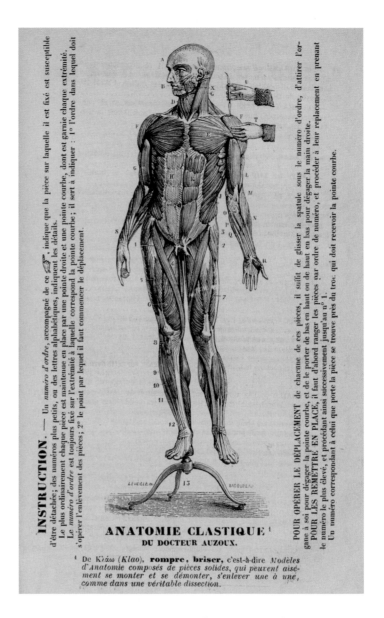

together. These articulations were characteristic of all models from Auzoux's firm, whether the model was of a whole organism, such as a life-size woman, or of selected enlarged parts, such as 'Ovologie', which displayed the vagina, uterus and ovaries, ovulation and vertebrate embryo formation (illus. 145).[63]

Auzoux devised his models with reference to several sources. He was inspired by Felice Fontana's life-size wooden anatomical model at the Faculté de médecine de Paris, which Fontana built in the 1790s so that it could be frequently (dis)assembled. Fontana had argued that anatomy was learned more efficiently with durable wax models than with disintegrating deceased bodies because in no single cadaver could all anatomical parts be simultaneously displayed, given that some parts had to be cut to make others visible – and he had come to view models in wood as even more advantageous than those in wax, which was less amenable to extensive handling.[64] But wood was not suitable for Auzoux's clastic anatomy: it could not be moulded easily, required time-consuming careful carving and could warp. So Auzoux developed a more suitable material, learning from techniques for the manufacture of papier mâché dolls. He concocted a secret compound – a paper paste, like papier mâché, with powdered cork added for suppleness – which could be moulded into any shape and which, when dried, was hard, light and somewhat pliable.[65]

At Auzoux's factory the models were hand-made by skilled workers who produced multiple copies from prototypes. Reusable moulds were used to form each piece of a model from layers of paper and paper paste. When pieces were dry they were fitted together, shaped and smoothed. For full-figure models metal armatures were used to compose and support the pieces. Surface details were affixed to the pieces as appropriate: arteries and veins made from metal threads bound with red or blue ribbon, nerves of textile thread and membranes of cattle peritoneum. Further details were also painted on each piece. The visual and textural effects required by particular anatomical parts were created with materials such as ground mother-of-pearl, semolina and lichen, all protected with a coat of glue.[66]

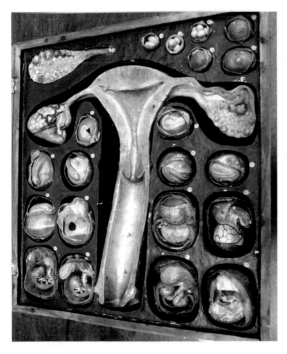

145
Model of 'Ovologie', by Établissements du Docteur Auzoux, Paris, undated, in the Anatomical Museum, University of Edinburgh, 2008.

Fabric and form, designed to facilitate tactile interaction, counted for much in the success of Auzoux's models. From their first launch in London they were evaluated favourably in relation to wax anatomical models. A newspaper in 1832 reported, for instance, that even those in Florence, Bologna and Paris were 'merely wax-work' in comparison to Auzoux's constructions. This was an unfavourable reference to waxwork figures produced for entertainment rather than learning which echoed the negative association of wax anatomical models with toys apparent at the turn of the nineteenth century.[67] Moreover, although some waxes had a few detachable components to allow examination of bodily depth (see illus. 57), many offered only one view from a fixed surface so were restricted to 'the representation of a single layer of parts'.[68] As a consequence, a costly and space-consuming number of models was required to achieve a comprehensive anatomical display. Auzoux's models answered this problem by guiding their users towards deepening structures compacted within each fabricated body or body part.

In the early 1850s the utility of models made only to be viewed and not touched was assessed in a review of medical and surgical objects exhibited at London's Great Exhibition that featured waxes by Joseph Towne, modeller for the museum at Guy's Hospital.[69] Although Towne's work was celebrated for its 'fidelity to nature', still this commentator for a medical readership asserted that such models were most valuable when used to 'revivify the mental pictures that he [the student] has previously acquired by actual dissection'. Also, because it was difficult for models to command 'long continued attention when nothing more is required than to fix the eyes on the object', learning from them was deemed limited, just as 'little would be really learned by looking at an already completed dissection'. What made dissection effective as a mode of learning, this review continued, was the 'time and labour expended before the parts are clearly and definitely exhibited to the eye': 'while this process of clearing and isolating the organs is going on, the mind is making a mental picture of the parts [. . .] which may be recalled for years after the object has been absent from the vision.'[70] From this perspective productive anatomical observation was also participatory action, a process of revealing an organ over time rather than just an immediate looking at it. If a model was like an 'already completed dissection', offering instant visual access to the bodily interior without any work on the part of the student, its efficacy was therefore curtailed. Auzoux's models would not suffer from this critique, for they invited not passive looking but manual and visual interactivity; they were built to be unbuilt and rebuilt. The extent of students' regular manipulation of these models in specific teaching situations is difficult to establish, but the potential for this use was evidently embedded in the models' very design.

Yet wax anatomies for observation but not handling continued to be developed and sold to medical schools by commercial firms during the second half of the nineteenth and the early decades of the twentieth century.[71] They were seen to possess a high degree of anatomical verisimilitude with convincing shapes and subtle colours – properties very difficult to retain in preserved specimens. Large, expensive figures were considered impressively detailed, and could boost the prestige of institutions with the funds to purchase and exhibit them (see illus. 84). Waxes by the well-reputed Maison Tramond, and its successor firm N. Rouppert in Paris, dealers in

146
Wax anatomical model, c. 1921, by N. Rouppert (successor to Maison Tramond), Paris.

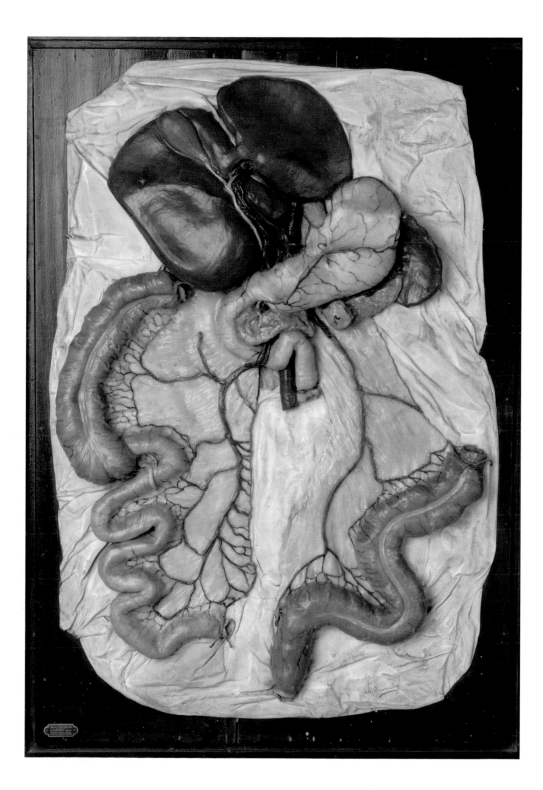

osteological specimens (see illus. 2), modelled difficult-to-dissect body parts, such as nerves and blood vessels in the skull. These they modelled over human bone – a technique that in applying wax components to bone enhanced the models' claims to actuality. Viscera were displayed in life-size wax compositions showing the liver, gall bladder, stomach, pancreas, spleen, sections of intestines and blood vessels, all laid out with intact membranes that were easily damaged during dissection (illus. 146).[72] Here the impression that wax was flesh, with the capacity to properly educate, was augmented by dissecting-room apparatus that staged model as body (just as Quain's lithographic drawings had incorporated such tools): hooks position the stomach for viewing and string ties the ends of intestines that have been 'cut'. Such models were employed in medical school teaching as contributing elements within wider collections of bodies in a variety of media, all of which were assembled, rearranged and replaced as required.

LAYERING

When Auzoux's clastic anatomy was put into action, anatomical parts were taken off (and reattached) 'layer by layer', according to some of the models' medical users in the 1830s.[73] The appreciation of the human body as a composite of layers has been remarkably persistent in Western anatomical practices, variously manifesting in many materials: on paper, in plaster and the flesh itself. Sixteenth-century drawings by Leonardo da Vinci showed the underlying structures of organs; Vesalius' series of live cadavers in the *Fabrica* had muscles peeling away to reveal inner parts (see illus. 49); in early modern 'flap' anatomy male and female paper bodies comprised several printed layers of paper; early twentieth-century stereoscopic atlases displayed the body at deepening stages of dissection (see illus. 106, 107, 108); and specimens were preserved in sections that were also rendered in watercolours and shown in photographs (see illus. 98, 99).[74] The 'Visible Human Project', begun in the 1980s at the u.s. National Library of Medicine, continued to build on such layerings with new technologies: a preserved man and woman were translated into digital images by taking MRI and CT scans of millimetre or less slices through those bodies.[75] Layering has thus provided an organizing principle in anatomical explorations, a means of structuring visual images and a conceptual apparatus for analysing the three-dimensional human body.[76]

In the late nineteenth century not only was dissection envisaged as a movement through 'strata' – from the surface of the skin and 'superficial structures' into the body's 'deep structures' such as the internal organs and bones – but medical schools utilized paper anatomies constructed with

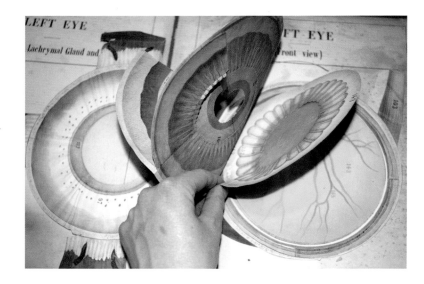

147
Anatomy of the eye shown in layers of paper, from Gustave Joseph Witkowski, *Human Anatomy and Physiology. Part IV. A Movable Atlas Showing the Mechanism of Vision; The Eye; The Organs of Vision* (London, 1880–89).

layers of printed plates that alluded to the process of dissection when put into action.[77] 'Movable' atlases, designed by the Paris physician Gustave Joseph Witkowski and published in the 1880s, represented body parts as coloured paper layers attached together in sequences so that the viewer could easily move from one to the next and back again. In doing so they would gain a sense of the inner composition of the brain, eye, ear, teeth and reproductive organs. The large-scale eye, for instance, comprised fourteen paper discs, colour-printed on both sides and hinged together at the left like a booklet. Some discs had additional flaps to reveal further inner details or tissue-paper inserts to represent the vitreous components (illus. 147).[78] Just as the eye was labelled the 'mechanism of vision', and the ear was the 'mechanism of hearing', so the machinery of flap anatomy allowed each organ to open out, hinge and unfold.[79] The degree of detail in the multiple layers of Witkowski's atlas, considered comprehensive enough to aid medical students, is apparent in comparison to the simplified versions produced for less specialized users. *Philips' Popular Mannikin*, published *c.* 1900, represented the male human body in five main layers: the skin, muscles, blood vessels, nervous system and skeleton. The latter was fitted with paper ribs, forming sub-layers that were hinged to reveal the internal organs, and a section of the skull opened like a miniature book for the brain to be browsed (illus. 148).[80]

In the 1920s and '30s *Baillière's Synthetic Anatomy*, aimed primarily at medical students, divided into fourteen sections, each dedicated to an anatomical region, such as the thorax, or a part, such as the eye and the brain. Offering students sequences of coloured 'drawings' printed on a 'transparent medium' like sheets of paper, this layered anatomy intensified

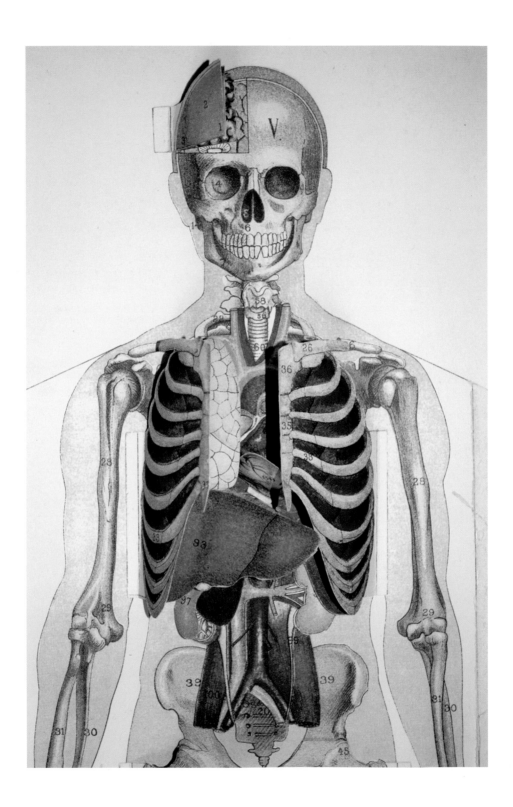

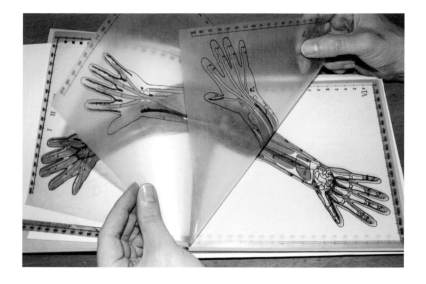

149
Anatomy of the forearm in layers, from John E. Cheesman, *Baillière's Synthetic Anatomy: A Series of Drawings on Transparent Sheets for Facilitating the Reconstruction of Mental Pictures of the Human Body, Part 2. The Forearm* (London, 1926–36).

the involvement of the user in putting it to work. It was designed by a medical officer of health in London, Dr John Eric Cheesman – for study *pari passu* with dissection and 'other instruction oral, visual and manual' – to reduce students' 'blind spots', to help them see inside the body from many 'points of view' at once, and to improve their 'pictorial memory' or the ways in which three-dimensional anatomical structures and their relations were mentally 'visualised'. [81] Within each section (illus. 149), twelve printed pages represented six slices through the anatomical part as seen from the front and six from the back with colour coding throughout: bones and cartilages in white; arteries in red; veins in blue; nerves in yellow; muscles in brown; tendons, ligaments and fascia (connective tissue and fat) in green. Black outlines and vivid colour enhanced the visibility of deeper structures when looking at several transparent pages at once.

Enabling navigation of the atlas, which Cheesman likened to a map, the coordinates of anatomical structures were given in an accompanying index. To locate an anatomical part students followed two intersecting lines leading from two specified numbers, one on the vertical centimetre scale and one on the horizontal scale at the edges of each page. As Cheesman explained, 'the logical corollary to dissection' was the 'reconstruction of the soft parts from their bony foundation' and this could be 'performed with the aid of these drawings'. This reconstruction was akin to reassembling an anatomical model, and it was devised to help the student build a 'composite and stereoscopic mental picture' of each part being studied. To achieve this, students were advised on how to interact with this synthetic body: insert a blank white sheet of paper underneath a single page to 'show it up more clearly' and to focus on it; hold pages up to the light to

148
Anatomy of the skeleton and organs shown in layers of paper, from William S. Furneaux, ed., *Philips' Popular Manikin* (London, c. 1900).

see through several at once; repeatedly reproduce anatomical parts by laying tracing paper over a page and tracing outlines in pencil, then transfer these to paper for colouring in; enlarge parts to life-size by re-drawing them; and make 'diagrammatic copies' to better commit them to memory.[82] This atlas, like Richard Berry's before it (see illus. 105), explicitly invited modes of interactive use that produced further iterations of images adapted to specific contexts of study.

Baillière's Synthetic Anatomy thus prompted students to make their own additions and amendments to the pages, and also encouraged them to perform 'dissociation' – a careful removal of the 'wire stitches' at the spine of each section which would release pages from their binding and allow alternative groupings to be assembled and comparisons made. Exercising the atlas in these ways would, according to Cheesman, 'liberate' its 'latent energy' and thereby improve students' knowledge of the human body.[83] Many responses to the atlas were favourable: medical journals confirmed students' appreciation of it, that it complemented learning through dissection, and that it was welcomed as an aid to studying the surface anatomy of living bodies. The atlas's distribution of over 100,000 copies in several languages was seen as ample 'evidence of its proved value' in teaching anatomy.[84]

OUTLINING

Layering to promote comprehension of anatomy in material and conceptual terms has also been complemented by outlining – a means to simplify and clarify the perceived complexity of the bodily interior. As Thomas Cooke claimed with reference to outlines in anatomical illustrations and textual descriptions, 'when once main lines are well grasped, details are easily filled in.'[85] Here the anatomical outline was both visual and verbal, to be grasped manually and mentally. The overview was prioritized as that which would facilitate the understanding of minutiae; subsidiary elements were marshalled by broader contours. Developments in outlining were consistent with a shifting emphasis in teaching practices from absolute anatomical detail to efficient understanding of living function.

During the 1930s and '40s the anatomist Edward Bald Jamieson (1876–1956) at the University of Edinburgh developed a series of illustrations, using an effective outlining technique for a publication that ran to numerous editions. Jamieson's *Illustrations of Regional Anatomy*, first published in 1934, as noted above, in loose-leaf form, was divided into sections, each depicting an anatomical region – head and neck, abdomen, pelvis, thorax, upper limb and lower limb – in addition to a further section on the central nervous system. The anatomist described these illustrations as outlines or summaries, formulating the visual in terms of the textual. Jamieson explained that 'these illustrations are "paraphrases" of the backboard diagrams that have illustrated my lectures for many years.' Moving from his lectures for medical students, through his diagrams to printed illustrations, Jamieson placed these images under the rubric of the paraphrase, formulating and using them as 'schematic or diagrammatic representations' in his teaching.[86]

The anatomist was open about the usual 'liberties' he had taken when making the images, asserting his authority in the purposeful interpretation of the dissected bodies upon which the images were based. Rather than claiming to have recorded every observable feature of a dissected specimen, Jamieson explained that 'depth and realism have been sacrificed in order that the parts in shadow might stand out more clearly': clarity was produced with the reduction of detail.[87] Outlines of anatomical parts imposed visual order – they were explicitly selective and judiciously kept to a minimum to ensure that they were appropriately visually pronounced. As Jamieson asserted with regard to 'crowded regions', for example the armpit, he had

> not shown in one plate all of the things that can be seen in a dissection but have distributed them over two or more drawings in order to avoid the obscurity and confusion that arise from having numerous outlines and pointers in one small-scale diagram.[88]

Outlining – with a few strategic bold lines, rather than a confusing many – made the bodily interior more distinct and further simplification was achieved with colour in solid blocks. The 1944 edition of *Illustrations of Regional Anatomy* utilized seven coloured inks in addition to black, including purple, emerald green, ruby red, cyclamen and yellow (illus. 150).[89] Bold and striking in their combinations, they were intended to attract the eyes of students and to help them distinguish anatomical parts: operating in concert with outlines, colour was a means to make boundaries more distinct, somewhat akin to cutting out a body part during dissection. Jamieson drew blackboard diagrams in chalk and also made large-scale versions in durable paint where, again, his outlining technique came into play and colour was crucial in displaying anatomical shapes, positions and relations between parts (illus. 151). Although the blackboards were of a size for viewing in a large lecture theatre and could therefore accommodate more colour combinations than those in print, there was consistent colour coding across both formats, creating connections between parts of the same type (for example, all arteries in red), promoting

150
Edward B. Jamieson, illustration of 'Cross-section through kidneys and renal vessels', from Edward B. Jamieson, *Illustrations of Regional Anatomy*, 5th edition, Section 3: Abdomen (Edinburgh, 1944), Fig. 154.

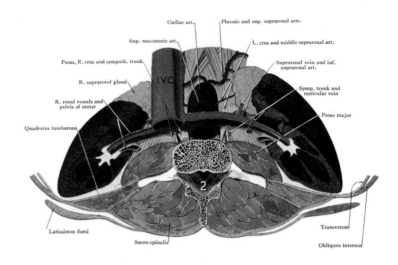

151
Edward B. Jamieson, large-scale blackboard illustration of 'Sagittal section of head', *c*. 1930s, made in the Anatomy Department, University of Edinburgh.

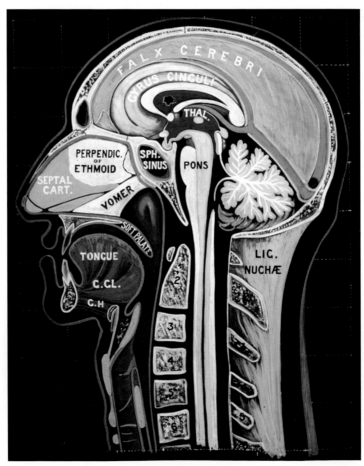

rapid recognition of these structures and thus facilitating the communication of anatomical knowledge.[90]

Each one of the images in Jamieson's publication was initially drawn from observations not of one specimen but of several – some permanently preserved (in the University of Edinburgh's Anatomical Museum), some in progress in the dissecting room, some dissected by Jamieson himself and some specially prepared for him by assistants. So here the visual image acted not only as a summary but as a synthesis. Just as a dissector would approach a body part, Jamieson explained, the images were produced by 'looking round the margin and bringing more structures into view than can be seen from one fixed view-point'.[91] Here he drew attention to one of the main limitations in the capacity of images to convey anatomical knowledge – they are flat and the human body is not. Hence Jamieson described his movement around the edge of the anatomical part, looking at it from different points of view, rotating it, to bring what was around the corner into the illustration. These were composite images for a book to which many contributed (in addition, of course, to those whose bodies were dissected). Although Jamieson drew many of the illustrations himself, he also collaborated with the artists Charles E. Pierce and J. M. Philip, as well as R. W. Matthews, who had worked on the textbook *Anatomy of the Human Body* during the 1940s in Aberdeen. Dissectors who helped prepare specimens, block-makers, printers and publishers in Edinburgh – in an office located near the medical school – all participated in the process.

Jamieson, like Cheesman, instructed students to actively use his illustrations, not to merely look at them but to visually and manually engage with them. To encourage this, illustrations were only printed on one side of the page so that they could be taken out and pasted into students' own notebooks, as though compiling an anatomical scrapbook. Where outlines of anatomical parts had been printed in black lines only, students were advised to apply coloured chalks: those 'who colour their copy will find that they are, at the same time, fixing the relative positions of structures in their memory', Jamieson advised.[92] He also suggested that where bones were indicated with dotted outlines to show their deep locations, these dots could be joined up by students.[93] Such images therefore opened the way for students to participate in the co-creation of anatomical images and in doing so to transfer the image from page to mind.

Learning to interpret outlines in anatomical representations would serve medical students well, for they would work with outlines as medical practitioners. For instance, in doctors' medical assessments, patients' surface physical signs, the indicators of their afflictions, were recorded and communicated with the use of outlines. Clinical stencil plates enabled rapid drawing of standardized outlines within which the practitioner could

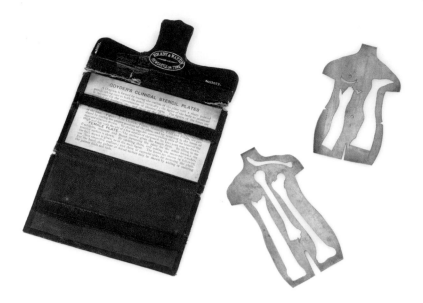

mark those signs (illus. 152). Scientific instrument-makers Brady and
Martin in Newcastle-upon-Tyne, during the late nineteenth and early
twentieth century, produced stencils from which outlines of male and
female bodies could be drawn. Instructions explained that 'a diagram is
formed by tracing the outline of the plate with a sharp pointed pencil,
taking care to hold the pencil vertically.' Male and female body shapes were
traced, the latter with breasts, and the front was marked with a dot for the
belly-button. Outlines of bones could be drawn to indicate the position of
fractures, and outlines of limbs to note the position of tumours or, when
surgery was required, to show the recommended 'line of incision'.[94] The
stencils were intended to be carried about in a pocket, conveniently ready
to hand when required, and protected by a leather case. Just as anatomical
interiors were defined by outlines so were bodily surfaces in medical
encounters where human bodies were translated via medical encounters
into lines, strokes, dots and cuts.

THREADING

'Connective tissue' is an elastic tissue, which serves to bind down the
skin to the parts beneath, thus making our 'suit of buff' fit us far
better than clothes made by the best tailor or dressmaker in the
world; it also surrounds muscles, vessels, and viscera, and binds
them together.[95]

This description of skin as cloth, written in the 1860s, was not unusual as understandings of the body in terms of thread or fibre and fabric had developed through the very vocabulary of anatomy in which metaphors from textiles, weaving, knitting, needlework and embroidery were employed. Since the sixteenth century, the body's fibres – variously formulated – have constituted not only skin but nerves, bones, muscles and organs in bundles, weavings, networks and lace-works.[96] The interwoven, or even bonded, nature of the body's structures was emphasized by Thomas Cooke, who maintained that 'practical anatomy is a question of unravelling the felt-work of the human body' and of reaching an understanding of the 'mesh'.[97] He proposed that anatomists as well as students find their way through the complexities of the body by following threads in the process of dissection. Cooke observed what he considered to be a key 'proverbial expression', '"From thread to needle" . . . "Keep a thread in the eye of your needle;" and if you loose sight of the needle, the thread, which you may rely upon seeing, will at any time lead you up to it.'[98] Thus the body's threads, such as the nerve fibres and blood vessels, were to be traced as a means to navigate from one anatomical part to the next. In this way the structure and relationships between parts would be readily grasped.

Mid-twentieth-century works on paper and other materials made the human body's fibrous composition pronounced with colour and texture. Medical students at Marischal College could study the fibres of the brain stem in a polychrome atlas purchased for this purpose. The brain stem appeared as a sequence of ten sliced sections or layers (labelled A to K). With two half-sections on each page, the nerves were shown as 'analytical fiber drawings' printed in red, orange, light green, violet, blue, deep green,

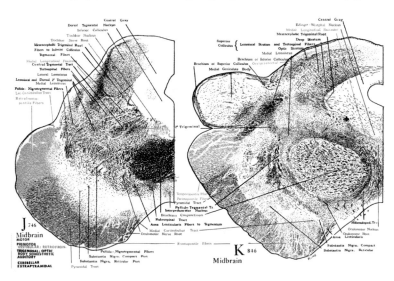

153
Fibre drawings of the brain stem (one half of two sections), from Wendell J. S. Krieg, *A Polychrome Atlas of the Brain Stem* (Evanston, IL, 1960).

brown and black – one colour for each functional system (for example fibres of the auditory system were shown in violet, those of the visual system in deep green; illus. 153).[99] So committed to the use of brilliant colour in these publications was professor of anatomy Wendell J. S. Krieg, at Northwestern University in Illinois, that he formed his own press, Brain Books, in the service of neuroanatomy.[100]

Rendering the body's fibres in coded colours was, in Krieg's view, an ideal way to examine and analyse them. This approach did not, however, go undisputed: one medical review claimed that

> in teaching, colour should be used sparingly in the representation of structural detail. An eye-catching profusion of bright colours tends to defeat its own purpose by distracting attention from the basic structures illustrated.[101]

The pedagogic value of colour was thus debated by professionals concerned with the look and feel of apparatus for medical education. Some complained when it faded from preserved museum specimens; others explored and accentuated it in the making of vibrantly hued three-dimensional models.[102] Colour was deemed crucial for teaching and learning about the nervous system when, in the 1950s at Marischal College, a late nineteenth-century white plaster cast of a classical figure was recycled for teaching by painting dermatomes on its left side while on its right side the distribution of cutaneous nerves was displayed with gold paint which threaded across the surface (illus. 154, see illus. 29).[103]

Three-dimensional textile anatomy in the mid-twentieth century combined colour and texture in models formed from particular fibres. Wool yarns and other threads were employed to create anatomical parts and systems that were displayed for medical students in the Anatomical Museum at the University of Edinburgh. A museum label explained that the set of models was an anonymous gift to the Anatomy Department, a collection of 'knitted, crocheted and embroidered items inspired by Figures in an early Anatomy Textbook'.[104] This knitted anatomy divided the body into about eleven sections, each held in a cotton drawstring bag labelled, for example, 'Renal Apparatus', 'Nerves', 'Muscles', 'Eye', 'Blood vessels', and the enigmatic 'Implications of Physiology'. When removed from the bags and laid out, these soft anatomies displayed selected anatomical parts and systems. The grey knitted stomach (illus. 155) was part of the 'Gastro-intestinal system', which also included the colour-coded liver (brown), pancreas (yellow), gall bladder (green), duodenum (lilac), intestines (purple) and colon (beige), as well as red and blue blood vessels which had been stitched into place. Although they were distinguished by colour,

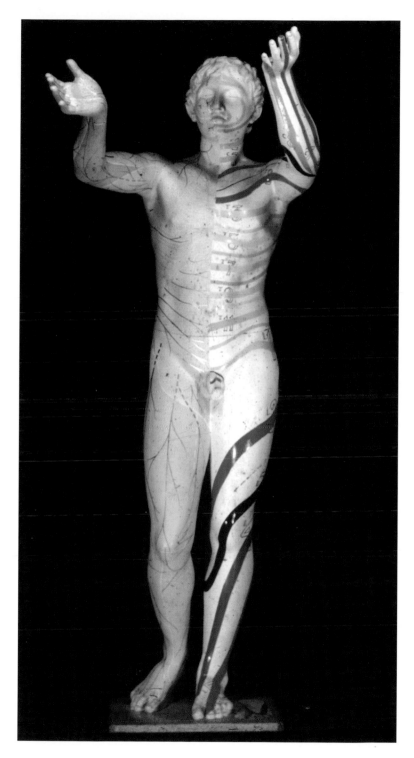

154
Slide of a plaster cast of the Berlin Adorante (cast *c.* 1880), painted to form a model of dermatomes, *c.* 1950s, in the Anatomy Department, Marischal College, University of Aberdeen.

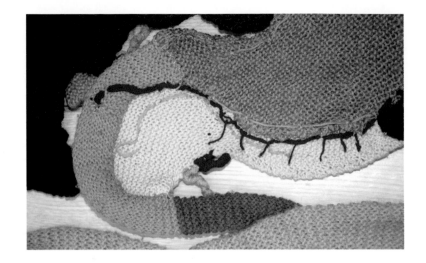

these anatomical parts were also interwoven, continuous and fibrous. Different stitches were used to create textures with a look and feel deemed appropriate for particular aspects of the body, so that the lungs in the 'Respiratory and cardiovascular system' were spongy and elastic, there was a silk uterus with knitted Fallopian tubes and ovaries, and the bag of 'Nerves' contained models crocheted to form the circular and spiky shape of neurons.

SHAPING

Using renderings of anatomy in different materials and media, educators aimed to facilitate particular modes of learning on the part of medical students, to assist in developing their competences and capacities especially with regard to the visual and manual skills required for professional medical work. Just as dissection demanded sustained embodied effort, so anatomical books and models – especially from the second half of the nineteenth century onwards – were designed to invite active tactile and visual interaction. Indeed the perceived efficacy of these aids was rooted in their capacity to physically and mentally engage students. As anatomy took shape through modelling, so engagement with those models informed and shaped learners.

Many successful three-dimensional models were produced by commercial companies based in Continental Europe, but such apparatus purchased for learning anatomy in Britain's medical schools was also complemented by models designed and purpose made in-house by anatomists and their associates. Just as they prepared specimens from dissected bodies and devised anatomical images, so they constructed models. These practices have been many and varied, with models improvised and fashioned using unexpected or seemingly unlikely materials that, nevertheless, have made sense in contexts of anatomical demonstration. Furthermore, while anatomists have made models in order to teach, students have similarly done so in order to learn. For instance, around 1860 in London, one student used a dinner napkin which he rolled and packed into a glass tumbler to model the general form of the human brain: the 'crumpled' fabric with 'elevations and depressions' provided a memorable impression of the 'convolutions' and 'fissures' of this organ.[105] In Edinburgh another student shaped sheets of newspaper into a cone to better comprehend the arrangement of 'muscular fibres' of the heart: the lines of print stood for the fibres and the sheets of paper for the 'layers' of fibres.[106] The involved embodied act of making in these instances of improvised modelling brought improved understanding of anatomy.[107]

Materials readily available or inexpensive for anatomists and students were thus pressed into service for model-making. In pathology teaching, too, during the late nineteenth century, purpose-made models of body parts were constructed, such as those of the human brain fabricated in cardboard and wood by D. J. Hamilton, professor of pathology at Marischal College. Medical visitors to the college praised these highly, along with Hamilton's preparations of the brain in thin slices which, when varnished, became transparent so the direction of the fibres could be seen. Looking 'something like sheets of glue', these preparations were impressively 'indestructible' and could be 'shuffled' or rearranged into different sequences as required.[108] At other medical schools in the early twentieth century brain anatomy was modelled in paper and coloured string; blotting paper was a favoured material for ease of construction.[109] Working with a range of materials, therefore, university teachers in the sciences, and their assistants, developed models of bodily parts that were unavailable from commercial manufacturers, and thereby upgraded the educational capacity of their departments' museum collections and displays.[110]

The materials available and deemed suitable for projects of anatomical modelling changed over time and in relation to teaching requirements. In Robert Lockhart's classes students were taught how to shape anatomical structures in Plasticine from the 1920s onwards, 'fashioning the soft parts upon the dry skeleton', for example. In these instances it was the experience of the modelling *process* that was deemed important in that it was seen to advance students' own learning and to built their 'self confidence'. Such temporary models were made for the student's self rather than for longer-term display for others in Marischal College's Anatomy Museum.[111]

Developments in plastics – perceived as 'modern materials' – offered further possibilities for encouraging users' visual and tactile engagement with models.[112] In the 1930s life-size male and female figures composed in a new plastic, Cellon, gave material form to the notion of a transparent human body which, like a 'glass model', revealed inner anatomical structures. Standing upright with bones, organs, blood and lymphatic vessels visible beneath transparent skin, these models were produced by the Deutsches Hygiene Museum in Dresden and were widely shown at exhibitions in Europe and the USA.[113] Admired for their 'scientific exactitude', the models also attracted interest in terms of their material composition. Their plastic was celebrated for its impressive malleability with which, for example, the models' clean surface contours were achieved.[114] Although not displayed to invite the direct touch of viewers, the models were designed to be interactive: visitors were invited to press buttons that would then illuminate selected organs and thereby highlight their location and shape in the body.[115]

While such interactivity and tactile participation in dynamic exhibits of science, and of art, were promoted among the exhibition-going public,[116] educators in medical schools during the mid-twentieth century promoted the use of plastic anatomical models that elicited medical students' interaction for more specialist purposes. Anatomy lecturer L. H. Hamlyn at University College London and collaborating artist Patricia Thilesen described several types of model used in medical teaching. Although they acknowledged the value of models produced by commercial firms, they also required models specially designed and made in-house for specific teaching purposes. Constructed in a variety of materials – but often cast in plastics (for example, cold-setting Fibrenyle) that were light as well as strong and therefore suited to frequent handling – such models would 'supplement the study of natural material' (that is, human bodies and dissected specimens), and were especially helpful in developing students' appreciation of 'three-dimensional structure' in areas where learning with specimens was difficult and time-consuming. Considered especially useful were enlarged models of small structures, such as those in the ear or eye, and models of embryo development. 'Simplified' models, with detail 'deliberately omitted', were also used as three-dimensional 'diagram[s] intended to focus attention on some principle of structure or function'. In the case of the latter, Hamlyn and Thilesen noted that 'colour plays an important part in focusing attention on the essential points.'[117]

These teachers recognized that most models tended to simplify human bodies, and those manufactured in plastics by commercial firms were no exception. Somso, based in Germany and producing anatomical models since 1876 in plaster, papier mâché and wax, brought models with plastic

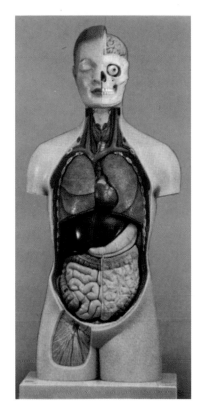

156
Plastic model,
'Trunk of a Young
Man with Head',
c. 1960s, by
Somso models
from Adam,Rouilly,
photograph from
*Somso Models:
Anatomy*, commercial
catalogue, 1970.

components to the market in the 1950s, highlighting the newness and durability of their materials formulated in consultation with the plastics industry.[118] Compared with earlier creations devised by Auzoux's firm, Somso's products had cleaner lines, fewer pieces in uncomplicated designs and an unobtrusive key to indicate names of anatomical parts rather than printed labels that cluttered the models' surfaces. Unlike Maison Tramond's waxes, Somso's models were vertically rather than horizontally oriented, presented in upright position as though (in) a living body rather than lying down like the dead, and this vertical spatial orientation was deemed advantageous for learning (illus. 156).[119] Furthermore each model's clearly defined, smooth-surfaced anatomical parts in vibrant colours were robust and readily (dis)assembled for tactile inspection by students. Widely marketed and distributed for medical education by the company Adam,Rouilly, these models became established as instructive, reliable aids for learning, acquiring a reputation for high-quality products that is still sustained in current teaching practices.[120]

In post-war Britain coloured plastics acquired positive meanings that anatomical models also carried with them; they came to be associated with modern science and technology, hygiene, brightness and shiny newness in an environment recovering from traumatic conflict and extensive bomb damage.[121] Writing in the late 1950s, the cultural critic Roland Barthes was alert to the appeal of this material:

more than a substance, plastic is the very idea of its infinite transformation; as its everyday name indicates, it is this, in fact, which makes it a miraculous substance . . . Plastic remains impregnated throughout with this wonder: it is less a thing than the trace of a movement.[122]

Here the property of plasticity was salient, the capacity for fluid movement prior to setting into a stabilized form. In the context of anatomical modelling, plastics readily took the form they were moulded into, adopting robust shapes that nevertheless yielded to handling by slightly bending then bouncing back. In Barthes' commentary, this material was all the more compelling for its widespread distribution in the form of household objects: 'it is the first magical substance which consents to be prosaic . . . for the first time artifice aims at something common, not rare.'[123] The increasing familiarity of the material, its association with objects of utility rather than rarity, contributed to the appeal and tactility of anatomical models composed of it.

The commercial manufacturing and distribution of affordable three-dimensional models in plastics opened the way for more sustained hands-on learning with artificial anatomies among larger numbers of medical students. These models, like those developed by Auzoux, were explicitly open objects – that is, objects designed to invite interaction through which their capacities (in this case educational capacities) would be potentially more fully realized. Students' active, embodied participation in the display of anatomy was enlisted, prompted and guided not only by models but by printed books whose images elicited interactive engagement and in some cases the making of further modified iterations. Writing in the early 1960s with regard to works of art, Umberto Eco suggested that all are open – they are unfinished as they rely on viewers', readers' and listeners' responses to realize them, to afford them meaning and in some cases to enable the works' potential to be fulfilled by making material interventions.[124] Yet artworks provoke different modes and degrees of involvement on the part of viewers so that, for example, sculptures and installations in public galleries during the 1950s and '60s – in Europe and the USA – made explicit moves towards intensive spectator input and the foregrounding of participants' sensory experiences.[125]

Within medical schools in Britain, students' physical and conceptual participation was mobilized by anatomical models and books; as these objects were put into action they became dynamic through multiple acts of intervention aimed at the development of anatomical knowledge. But within these contexts of learning, the openness of such objects was to a certain extent constrained in so far as students' interactions with and interpretations of them were guided by requirements as laid out by teachers in positions of institutional authority. Designed for use in close association with the practice of dissection, such models and books were also used alongside preserved museum specimens and the study of living anatomy in which students became their own live models. Engagement with models and books as participatory learning aids, then, was always informed by the relations posited between those objects and bodies in the flesh, whether living or dead.

Gaining knowledge of anatomy through practices of shaping, threading, outlining, layering, (dis)assembling and cutting took medical students, and their teachers, through embodied explorations of different materials from flesh to paper, wax, plastic and many more. To make anatomy visible and tangible was to promote conceptual understanding via bodily action, so that these materials and the anatomical forms they came to take fed into each student's so called 'mental picture', or mental visualization, generated from memorable sensory impressions gained and assimilated through disciplined study of anatomy. Training sight and touch, the practices explored above were intermedial; they worked across a range of media, from dissected bodies to printed images and three-dimensional models, that were brought into specific relations with one another in sites of medical learning.

Emerging from these practices, anatomy came to be materially and visually constituted in shifting ways; for instance, intense detail in visual images and in models of the nineteenth century gave way to the simplified lines and shapes that were becoming more pronounced by the mid-1900s. In the years following the Second World War, anatomists debated and recommended medical-school curriculum changes, especially the 'drastic elimination' of 'detailed information' about anatomy that had become 'indigestible' now that the 'advance in medical science' was constantly expanding what medical students were expected to learn and remember.[126] In order to train and equip future medical professionals, many argued that when learning anatomy students' focus should be on the knowledge required by general practitioners for the effective treatment of patients. From this perspective a mass of unnecessary anatomical detail presented for memorizing was problematic, for it 'clutter[ed] up the student's mind and deaden[ed] his interest in subjects that . . . should make the liveliest appeal to him'.[127] Illustrations and models designed and built to simplify human anatomy, some verging on the diagrammatic, were thus developed by anatomists as well as commercial firms.[128] The mental impressions that students gained from these renderings were expected to be correspondingly honed and unencumbered by burdensome, redundant detail.

Something of this simplification, this decluttering or paring down of anatomy, began to manifest in the very fabric of the Anatomy Museum at Marischal College during the late 1960s. So too did pedagogical strategies to engage students in displays: while plastic models invited active manual exploration as a mode of learning, in the Anatomy Museum exhibits once protected by glass were transformed and installed on open shelves to motivate students' use of exhibits. This transformation is the concern of the next chapter, which examines changing anatomical displays in relation to museum and memorial inscriptions – materialized words that informed the display of the dead as well as the ways in which the anatomized deceased have been remembered and memorialized.

Eight
RELOCATIONS AND MEMORIALS

'I wonder if your memories will be like mine? In the stillness of the night
let us look upon the grey walls of the quadrangle where flutter the shadows and memories of many years.'[1] In an interview two years before his
death in 1987, the anatomist Robert Lockhart posed this question – musing
about the possibility of experiencing shared memories at a time when he
was prompted to reflect on his own life. Here he associated the act of
remembering with seeing quivering shadows in the stilled quiet of the
night. Forty years earlier, Lockhart had been interested in the 'ghostly shadows' cast by X-rays, shapes that also featured in his flickering
black-and-white films of human bodies in movement.[2] By the 1980s he
saw shadows as time's accumulated traces, insubstantial against solid grey
walls. The anatomist's memories occupied a place both metaphorical and
real – for him, remembering entailed an imagined gazing upon walls of a
granite quadrangle, walls that he passed on his way to and from work at
Marischal College each day for most of his professional life.

Remembering, in the image conjured by Lockhart, was associated with
the act of looking within a particular architectural space.[3] Taking up the
theme of located remembering, this final chapter explores the transformation of the Anatomy Museum at Marischal College during the late 1960s,
when anatomists were redevising schemes for displaying anatomy while
also creating memorials for the anatomized dead and increasingly participating in ritualized practices of burial, cremation and remembrance for the
people they dissected.[4] In Aberdeen, substantial alterations in anatomical
exhibiting developed in parallel with the emergence of particular memorial
forms: a service, a book of memory and a cemetery memorial. This chapter
focuses on the spatial location and relocation of human remains, within and
beyond the Anatomy Museum, and the implications of these placements
and removals for processes of remembering and memorializing. While

Chapter One examined how the Anatomy Museum was used (*c.* 1999–2009) within an architecture of interconnecting rooms, corridors and staircases, subsequent chapters discussed this museum's formation within a shifting matrix of social and material relations (between people, objects, museums and other sites of display) from the mid-nineteenth to the mid-twentieth century. This last chapter turns to the local ritual complex in which the Anatomy Museum has developed, situating the changing anatomical displays of the late 1960s within an urban 'necro-topography' – taken to encompass the locations in which the dead have been anatomized, then interred, cremated and memorialized, in Aberdeen from the mid-twentieth century to the present.[5]

During this period there was an important shift from the acquisition of unclaimed bodies to the growth in donations of people bequeathing their own bodies to medical schools for dissection prior to burial or cremation. Integral to this shift was the involvement of anatomists in ritualized practices for memorializing body donors. Within this nexus of developments the 1960s transformation of the Anatomy Museum was carried out, involving considerable structural and organizational alterations designed to refocus and reorder the collection and to facilitate particular uses of displays on the part of medical students. Significantly, changes in the Anatomy Museum entailed an increased use of inscriptions, an emphasis that also characterized the memorials that anatomists established for those whose bodies they dissected. Words were materially crafted for purposes of anatomical display and for remembering the dead.

Just as shifting forms of human anatomy have been rendered in a plethora of materials and media, they have also been described and re-described in written texts, narrated and explained through the spoken word. Words – often regarded as insufficient and even potentially detrimental in the learning of anatomy – have nevertheless been worked into anatomical vocabularies comprising names for many body parts, and they have also been elaborated in the performance of anatomical poetics. Material inscriptions within the reorganized Anatomy Museum of the late 1960s and '70s had particular functions and effects. Along with the spatial, material and visual reworking of this museum, textual inscriptions helped to configure it as though it were the inside of the human body composed of anatomical regions. While Lockhart's dramatic anatomical narratives had guided students through the inside of an imagined body, so that each student envisaged themselves *within* the very bodies they were studying, the Anatomy Museum now invited students to physically enter the 'body' as part of their routine studies; entirely immersed in this body/museum, they would walk around, interact with and read about its constituent tissues, bones and organs.

Crafting the Anatomy Museum as a human body entailed selective emphasis on those parts of the collection deemed most relevant; so some specimens, models and visual images were highlighted, and others were removed. Through such an operation this museum became a site of preservation and remembering but also of eradication and forgetting. Parallel to these dual effects are those of memorials, which also participate in social and cultural processes of both remembering and forgetting in that they perform exclusions and stimulate selective remembrance.[6] Words and their materialization in anatomical and memorial displays are analysed in what follows. Here, as throughout this book, the social connections that sustained anatomists' work in reconstructing a museum and establishing memorials are as important as the materials that comprised these interrelated forms.

ANATOMICAL LISTS

The inscriptions perhaps most closely associated with museums are catalogues. At Marischal College's Anatomy Museum, however, the collection was not catalogued until the late 1960s – more than a century after it was founded – when a set of typescript descriptions of objects on display was made available for study in relation to the exhibits. These descriptions were compiled in several loose-leaf binders which medical students read while observing the corresponding specimens, models and visual images in the Anatomy Museum.[7] This cataloguing seems a late development, given the emphasis placed on published catalogues as indicators of a museum's order, durability and prestige.[8] In the nineteenth century, catalogues were regarded as central to museums' classificatory practices. Objects were sorted, assigned to categories and translated into written and visual summaries when linked with labels, numbers, synoptic descriptions and drawings; this was a process of (attempted) 'archival systematization'.[9] Bruno Latour has argued that such inscriptions reduce three-dimensional objects to flat paper surfaces, thereby extending control over them.[10] But practices of inscription in museums have been much more uneven and incomplete than this would suggest, and inscriptions, as argued below, do not necessarily reduce three-dimensional objects to two dimensions – rather, material inscriptive practices entail an interplay of media in two and three dimensions.

The first (currently extant) list of the Anatomy Museum's holdings was published in 1899 by John Struthers in a footnote to his account of the progress of the medical school at the University of Aberdeen.[11] Struthers wrote: 'as there is no record as to when and by whom the museum was formed, it may be well here to mention some at least of the things in the comparative part of the collection.'[12] His avowedly partial list included animal skeletons, wax models and plaster casts, 'the specimens of human anatomy . . . too numerous to be indicated'.[13] Noting the (animal) skeletons' places of origin and the people who donated or helped in their acquisition, Struthers indicated his impressive social connections, boosting the Anatomy Museum's prestige and indicating the geographical reach of its collection. Struthers's successor, Robert Reid, kept a manuscript acquisitions book from 1908, which was used as an internal record of museum additions rather than as a public statement of the Anatomy Museum's holdings and progress.[14] After 1938 Lockhart noted that this book was 'discontinued', as all museum donations and purchases were recorded in the 'inventory' and an annual report to the university.[15]

Many of these annual inventories are no longer currently extant in archives but there is chance survival of a few. The earliest of these is a partly handwritten, partly typewritten document dating from 1959 to 1969, and it is suggestive of the difficulty involved in keeping track of thousands of material objects within a working environment.[16] The list was most probably prepared by technicians who recorded equipment and collections in the Anatomy Department according to their location in each room. The drafted, apparently unfinished list is overlaid with pencil deletions, corrections, underlinings, ticks, circles, crosses and question marks. Many items were listed as present but others were 'not yet found' and gaps in series of models were noted, for example the ten missing from a series illustrating the development of the human heart. The list documented what was preserved and what was destroyed – the latter including, in 1969, fragments of skeletal remains from an archaeological site in Scotland, which were no longer useful in teaching and were thus transferred to the incinerating room.[17]

This 1959/1969 listing took place during a period of transition when the curatorship of the Anatomy Museum passed from Lockhart to David Sinclair (1915–2013) as the latter became professor of anatomy in 1965. Since the late 1930s Lockhart had attempted to preserve the collection, taking inspiration from displays devised by his Aberdeen predecessors (and teachers) but also innovating with the production, collection and display of new visual images in a range of media. Sinclair had trained at the University of St Andrews in the 1930s and Oxford in the late 1940s, and had worked as a professor of anatomy at the University of Western Australia where there was a new medical school from the mid-1950s.[18] And he developed a different approach within the Anatomy Museum; less concerned than Lockhart to keep the entire collection intact, he reduced rather than enlarged it and oversaw extensive changes that would mark a certain discontinuity with previous displays. These changes removed some, but not all, historical traces of the Anatomy Museum's past, for the new display was necessarily composed of the specimens gathering at this site over the previous century.

This reconfiguring of the Anatomy Museum was partly achieved with the strategic use of material inscriptions, such as signs, labels and the object descriptions or catalogue held in loose-leaf binders noted above. Material inscriptions were used to clearly structure the display space, to explain the relevance of exhibits and to prompt students to productively interact with them. Rendering a museum productive for learning purposes was essential in a context of wider changes in medical education. The disciplines of anatomy and pathology had 'disintegrated into a mosaic of specialities', observed John Edwards, chief technician at the museum of the London Hospital Medical College, in 1959.[19] Sinclair's own surveys of his discipline highlighted the 'process of reduction' that had cut the 'amount of material taught' by one-third since 1900, and was still 'going on fairly rapidly'.[20] The number of hours allocated to dissection in Aberdeen were cut from 690 to 356 between 1945 and 1970, making time for other areas of study such as human genetics, growth and development.[21] As Sinclair explained, 'the professional study of regional topography' in dissecting rooms was being eroded, and this was problematic because this was precisely what

> helps students and doctors find their way confidently round human bodies which daily mangle themselves in roads, cut their wrists on glass doors, and develop acute appendicitis, frozen shoulders, pains in their backs, enlarged lymph-nodes in their necks, and sprained ankles.[22]

Due to institutional decisions to shift curricular teaching time from topography to subjects such as biochemistry and psychology, 'the human body is being squeezed out' to the detriment of medical practice, Sinclair worried.

In this context of curricular change there was perceived need to redesign and repurpose medical collections, as otherwise it was difficult to justify the space, staff and expenditure they required. Many such collections in Britain, therefore, underwent serious modification in the second half of the twentieth century: some were divided into specialist groupings, some were transferred to other medical institutions, some were destroyed or placed in long-term storage.[23] To achieve the effective redesign of Marischal College's Anatomy Museum, a process of separation and transfer was initiated by Sinclair; certain preserved body parts were removed and relocated in order to clear the way for those defined as more useful and instructional. If time dedicated to the human body's topography was diminishing in the dissecting room, Sinclair expanded the space given over to its display in the Anatomy Museum.

SEPARATION AND TRANSFER

By 1969 the major redisplay of the Anatomy Museum had taken place. Glass-fronted and -topped display cabinets had gone, as had most of the animal skeletons used to teach comparative anatomy (see illus. 90).[24] The nineteenth-century architectural structure of the museum, with its gallery and glazed roof, had been stripped of its overlying exhibitionary apparatus to expose a skeletal framework in which anatomy was displayed in a different way. The ground-floor exhibits were now configured as anatomical regions of the human body, a format which persisted until 2009 (see illus. 35, 42). To make way for this installation, parts of the collection accruing since the 1860s were separated and transferred elsewhere in the university, a museum strategy markedly different to those of previous anatomists at Marischal College who had expanded the collection and preserved its accumulations as far as possible. For when Sinclair arrived in the Anatomy Department, he saw the Anatomy Museum as unusable and cluttered with irrelevant items such as the antelope heads, regarded as no more than antiquated game or hunting 'trophies', not specimens that should be in a space for anatomical study.[25]

With assistance from technicians, Sinclair sought to render the displays suitable for the teaching needs of the time to counter the sensation that the Anatomy Museum had somehow remained in the past. Space was cleared by extracting unnecessary animal skeletons so that preserved specimens of human anatomy could be brought to the fore.[26] Criticism of overly packed museum exhibits had also arisen elsewhere. The technician John Edwards advised that 'it is essential to avoid inaccessible, massed regiments of identical preparations, sometimes four lines deep on the shelves'; to ensure its active use by students, a teaching museum must not be a 'storehouse'.[27] Reducing the numbers of displayed specimens displayed was not a new museum principle. In the 1890s William Flower, later applauded by Edwards, had recommended that specimens should be few enough on shelves to be 'perfectly and distinctly seen'.[28] Similar concerns with the profusion of old specimens were expressed during the 1940s when those medical museums seen to offer a 'gleam of light in the darkness' were those that were well preserved, fully catalogued and displaying specimens arranged in ways most useful to students.[29] Between 1965 and 1969 Sinclair began to attend to these issues, dividing the Anatomy Museum into bays with tables so that students could sit and work. In this method of division, museum inscriptions brought specimens, models and images of human anatomy to the 'forefront' of students' 'attention' on open shelves that invited close inspection and interaction with displays.[30]

Zoological haul

In 1966 approximately 250 animal skeletons and skulls were separated from the Anatomy Museum's collection of human body parts and transferred to the university's Zoology Museum (formerly the Natural History Museum) at Marischal College (illus. 157).[31] This substantial 'bequest', as it was termed, from the Anatomy Department to Zoology, embraced the bulk of the comparative anatomy collection, from the earliest dated specimen, a tigress skeleton from Wombwell's menagerie acquired in 1866, to Viscountess Stonehaven's donation of her husband's African 'trophies' in 1945.[32] It included skeletons of reptiles, birds, dogs, cats, deer, anteaters, monkeys, horses, bears, boars, bats, sheep, fish, whales, a fox, kangaroo, camel, hippopotamus and the heads of gazelles, some of the latter in taxidermied form (see illus. 124).[33] By 1966 these preserved animal remains represented antiquated styles of display from the past century that could not be recuperated and made relevant in the study of human anatomy.[34] Within the Zoology Museum, however, they would find new life and a huge removal was coordinated to relocate them.

Not all animals were evacuated, however. Some small dissections of soft tissue were retained on display or in storage. Six articulated skeletons of apes displayed in branches of trees, still considered useful in teaching, were moved to the gallery, as was the crocodile skeleton, whose acquisition history was well known in the Anatomy Department (illus. 158). This placement in the gallery – which was situated above the main ground-floor display space, and was therefore less accessible for students (see illus. 34) –

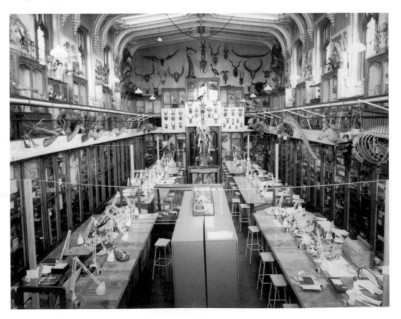

157
Zoology Museum,
Marischal College,
University of
Aberdeen, c. 1967,
photograph.

322

signalled an evaluation of these museum objects as of secondary importance. While these select animals were retained, the large majority of non-human specimens in the Anatomy Museum were removed from display and transported to their next location by technicians. These men were skilled in the construction of anatomical displays; they worked not only on the articulation of skeletons and the continued maintenance of specimens but on the very fabric of the Anatomy Museum and related display spaces, making exhibition supports such as cases, picture frames and specimen jars.[35] During 1966 the task of moving enormous skeletons was especially difficult. An Indian elephant was taken to pieces, its extensive articulations and metal supports undone so that its bony parts could be moved through doorways. Another massive specimen – a 15.25-m (50-ft) sei whale skeleton – was removed from its suspension in the entrance corridor (see illus. 89). Taking down this creature, originally acquired by John Struthers in 1884, was a strenuous event deserving photography on the day (illus. 159).[36] The heavy whale, skull first, was manoeuvred to the floor on ropes and pulleys. The skeleton had been originally articulated with metal rods and wires, and missing vertebrae had been replaced with wooden versions. When it was lowered, as Sinclair later recalled, the removal team could see that insects had made their homes in the skeleton.[37] Over the decades the whale, hung at a height so difficult to clean, had gathered a thick layer of dust. Technicians' white coats and the surrounding floor were covered with it; their shoes walked dusty prints down the corridor and out of the door. To facilitate the reassembly of the skeleton at its destination, the vertebrae were numbered with chalk and the entire bulky frame wheeled away on trolleys.

Anthropological drift

As with animals, so with artefacts: the removal of parts of the anatomical collection continued during the late 1960s and the '70s, when human remains regarded as no longer relevant to anatomical study were transferred to the Anthropological Museum at Marischal College, thereby redefining these objects as ethnographic artefacts (illus. 160). From its foundation in 1907, the Anthropological Museum – open to the public, unlike the Anatomy Museum – had been curated by professors of anatomy, thereby maintaining a connection between anatomy and anthropology for many decades. But when Lockhart retired from his professorship in anatomy he retained his position as curator of the Anthropological Museum until 1979, so from the mid-1960s onwards Sinclair, as professor of anatomy, had no formal institutional responsibilities for anthropological collections and exhibitions.[38] Lockhart expanded the anthropological displays when, in 1970, the Zoology Museum's collection – located in the gallery opposite

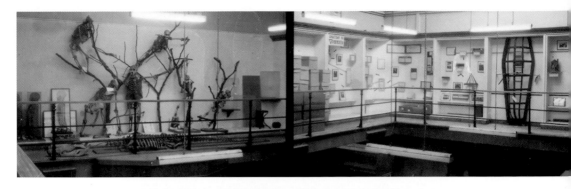

158
Technician's contact
prints showing views
of the gallery in the
Anatomy Museum,
Marischal College,
University of
Aberdeen, c. 1980s.

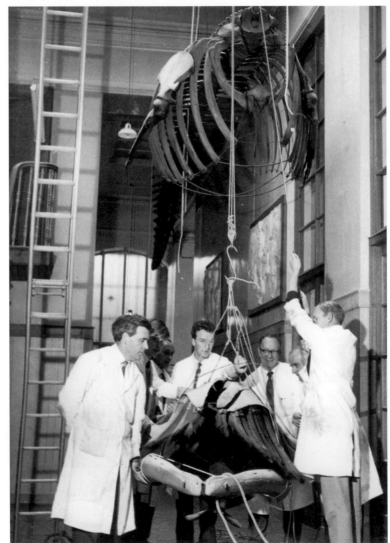

159
Technicians taking
down the whale
skeleton in the
entrance corridor,
Anatomy Department,
Marischal College,
University of
Aberdeen, c. 1966,
photograph.

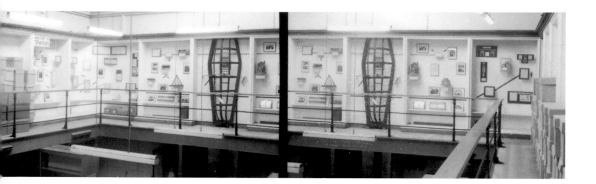

the Anthropological Museum – was moved to a new university building. The wall cases once holding zoology specimens were retained to display, instead, cultural artefacts.

It was into these exhibits that objects from the Anatomy Museum were transferred in the 1970s. Two plaster figures, labelled 'Bush-woman' and 'Bushman', cast from living people in 1880 and displayed in the anthropometric laboratory (see illus. 112) and the Anatomy Museum (see illus. 88), appeared behind glass among other sculptural forms defined as art, and beside cases of artefacts, such as beadwork, from different parts of the world which were grouped together according to their type and function (see illus. 160, back right).[39] Plaster casts of the Parthenon's frieze once displayed in the entrance corridor of the Anatomy Department (see illus. 89) joined framed paintings along the gallery in their new location.[40] These transfers incorporated material objects, previously gathered through the work of anatomists, into a different display scheme which then highlighted their

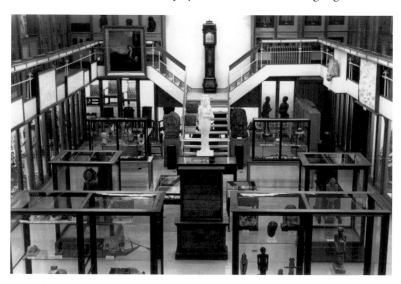

160
Anthropological Museum, Marischal College, University of Aberdeen, 1970s, photograph.

aesthetic qualities: the aim in the Anthropological Museum was to attract visitors by 'showing the arts and crafts of peoples of all nations and times'.[41]

Any object in the Anatomy Museum deemed closer to an anthropological artefact than an anatomical specimen was thus relocated, but unlike the skeletons hauled to the Zoology Museum in one massive consignment, the items redefined as artefacts tended to drift as dispersals at a slower pace. Between 1967 and 1972 approximately twenty carved and embellished skulls from British New Guinea (Papua New Guinea), New Hebrides (Vanuatu) and the Andaman Islands moved from anatomical into anthropological displays (see illus. 110, 113a–d). These human remains had originally been 'decorated' or modified and overlaid with materials and items such as mud, clay, feathers, seeds, shells, bamboo, mother-of-pearl, fibres and beads.[42] By contrast, unadorned skulls, also collected overseas during the late nineteenth and early twentieth century but regarded as free from artificial intervention, were retained in the Anatomy Museum (with their original labels) – although these were displayed in the gallery, rather than the central exhibiting space. When Charles Hunt, newly appointed as curator of the Anthropological Museum, visited the Anatomy Museum in 1979, he saw a 'Maori tattooed head and a New Hebrides overmodelled skull' that he regarded as 'ethnographic specimens', and which he requested as 'important additions' to the anthropological collection. Edward Clegg, Sinclair's successor as professor of anatomy from 1977, duly passed the specimens on.[43]

Transferring objects from spaces of anatomical practice into zoological and anthropological display schemes reclassified those items while also differentiating these three disciplines as distinct fields of knowledge. The composition of collections was significant in defining the subject-matter of anatomy (the human body), anthropology (human culture) and zoology (animal bodies), as was the manner in which material objects were exhibited in particular locations.[44] Inventoried in 1969, the 'furnishings' and 'equipment' in the Anatomy Museum were integral to the complex of interrelated spaces for work and study that composed the Anatomy Department. In addition to the mortuary, workshop and dissecting room, there were photographic and X-ray rooms, and numerous laboratories with microscopes (including an electron microscope), microtomes and collections of microscope slides. So while the Anatomy Museum displayed gross anatomy at the macroscopic level where the body was visible to the naked eye, in the museum's surrounding facilities body parts were magnified.[45] In their learning, then, students moved between spaces in which bodies were displayed at different scales and depths.

Following the removal of outdated materials from the museum and to enable more efficient and effective navigation of its new internal configuration, tailored inscriptions were incorporated into the fabric of anatomical display. Words, as material forms, within the Anatomy Museum were intended to guide students' learning and to increase their capacity to remember the human bodily interior.

REFRAMING AND REWORDING

One visitor, in 1972, was struck by the transformation of the Anatomy Museum. He had known the Anatomy Department in the early 1960s, probably as a medical student, and now he felt 'bewilderment at the structural changes which had been wrought' – so much so that only the technician, William Anderson (appointed in 1945 and about to retire), made the place feel 'more like home'.[46] Despite this visitor's surprise, the museum's new layout was not unusual.[47] It was divided into bays displaying anatomical regions – *Upper Limb, Lower Limb, Thorax, Abdomen, Head and Neck* – as well as *Neuroanatomy*, and *Embryology*, with a further bay for *Demonstrations*. Many anatomy textbooks and manuals for students on how to dissect followed these regional divisions, organizing descriptions and illustrations into chapters headed by these rubrics.[48] And bays were a familiar feature of museums in university medical schools, as in Edinburgh (from 1884) and Glasgow (from 1900; see illus. 74, 36).[49] The latter's ground floor and two galleries were divided into three floors in the 1950s; the contracted museum space located on the top floor, underneath a partly glazed ceiling, retained a bay structure and much of the large comparative anatomy collection was transferred to other museums in Edinburgh (see illus. 37).[50]

Museum as body and library

During the mid-twentieth century detailed practical guidance on how to 'design or modernize' medical museums was readily available in specialist journals and other publications. John Edwards recommended the 'bay system' as the 'best layout of . . . shelving for bottled specimens', and this 'architectural type' was seen to offer the 'most efficient use of floor space in the usual oblong room'.[51] This was adopted in the Anatomy Museum with specimens, three-dimensional models and visual images arranged on open rather than glass-fronted shelves, which were adjustable to accommodate exhibits of various sizes.

The anatomical region displayed in each bay was indicated by a prominent sign, for example *Upper Limb*. In addition, a framed image representing the body region exhibited was hung on the end of each bay which projected into the room (see illus. 42, top left). These images were

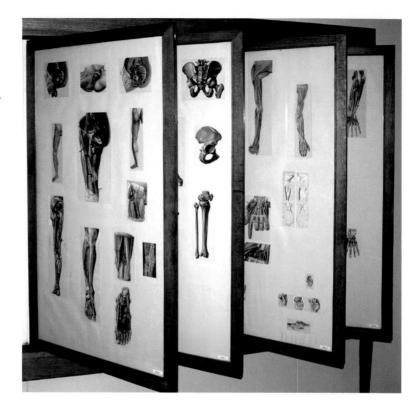

monochrome photographs of 'Anatomy Lesson' paintings originally produced
in the seventeenth and eighteenth centuries. In these compositions
anatomists' hands drew attention to the particular body part they were
dissecting, such as the head, the torso or a limb. In the context of the
Anatomy Museum this gestural framing was used to foreground, in con-
densed and summary form, the area of the body addressed in the bay's
display. This textual and visual signage grounded the Anatomy Museum
in particular forms of authority: it linked the display space to a deep tradition
of anatomical dissection and alluded to another established site of learning,
the library. For the pictures placed at the end of each bay echoed the busts,
such as those of famed writers, that occupied similar positions in libraries
from the Enlightenment onwards.[52] Just as a branch of knowledge was
held in books within each bay of a library, so each bay of the Anatomy
Museum offered knowledge regarding a region of the human body.

In the late 1960s technicians constructed the Anatomy Museum's bays
in oak, and the specimens with related models and images could now be
taken down from the open shelves to be more closely studied on tables, in
parallel with the bodies studied on the dissecting room's tables. Sets of
anatomical illustrations were also displayed in frames with movable hinges

so that they could be turned like the pages of a giant book. Drawings and watercolour illustrations by Alberto Morrocco and others produced for Lockhart's co-authored *Anatomy of the Human Body* had been mounted in over twenty frames and displayed along one wall in the 'bone room', a large study area otherwise known as the general laboratory (see illus. 127). By 1969 this book was split into three smaller segments, one of these mounted in the museum (illus. 161) and the others in two tutorial rooms.[53] Again these frames were made by technicians and fixed to walls on brass hinges so that they could be flipped through and viewed by students with ease and speed.

Erasing, inscribing, remembering

The Anatomy Museum's honed-down collection was effectively reframed in equally spaced bays whose order and purpose could be rapidly discerned by students. With a large part of its nineteenth- and early twentieth-century holdings gone, its new structure was simplified, symmetrical and provided with clear signage to help steer students through it. Now the human body was clearly shown as a unity of anatomical parts with bays/regions to be stepped inside for close study. On the shelves, specimens and models had also been reframed. In 1969 over 160 'wet specimens' preserved in fluid and 90 dry specimens of preserved bone were displayed in Perspex

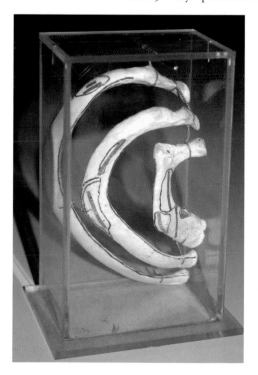

162
Preserved specimens, 'The first three ribs', labelled 'TO 6' c. 1969, in the Anatomy Museum, Marischal College, University of Aberdeen, 2008.

cases.[54] Technicians, in the workshop, had transferred many specimens from older glass jars to purpose-made cases; inside these transparent containers specimens were supported with wire articulations or stitched in place (illus. 162).[55] By the 1950s in many medical museums glass was replaced with Perspex.[56] At the Royal College of Surgeons of England, for instance, technicians also made new cases for exhibits, such as preserved dissections of limbs and casts of airways or tubes in the lungs (illus. 163).

Reframing in this way updated the look of specimens, stripping away many original wooden mounts with their distinctive styles and decorative brass fixtures now seen as unnecessary embellishment inherited from the past. Such adornment was eradicated from many specimens and models (compare the mounting/framing in illus. 27 and 162), often displacing indicators of their provenance, and providing instead cases with clean lines which, according to medical-museum

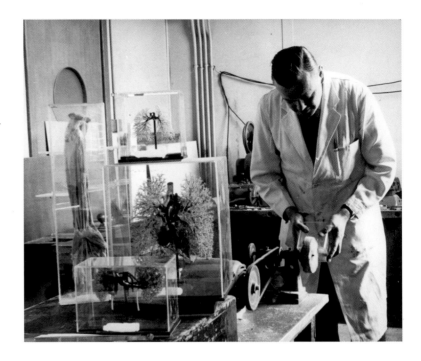

163
Museum technician
Sydney Bartlett
making transparent
Perspex cases for
specimens at the
Royal College of
Surgeons of England,
c. 1960, photograph.

technician John Edwards, became 'almost invisible' with 'careful lighting'.[57]
This reinforced the impression that the viewer had direct and uninterrupted access to the anatomical specimen held inside. Encasing specimens
in Perspex also imparted a certain uniformity to the Anatomy Museum and
created apparently blank surfaces for new labels to be engraved upon.

When signs, labels and a descriptive catalogue were integrated into the
Anatomy Museum in the late 1960s these practices of inscription had a
deep history, despite their role in marking the museum's departure from
past modes of display. Anatomists had long recognized the importance of
labelling in the communication of anatomical knowledge, from the discrete alphabetical and numerical keys of early modern anatomical
illustrations (see illus. 49) to the strategic positioning of image and text
along with the use of colour-coded typefaces in mid-twentieth century
textbooks (see illus. 126, 153).[58] Anatomists have been similarly attentive
to modes of inscription in their museums, from William Hunter's eighteenth-century glass specimen jars engraved with a diamond, to William
Flower's nineteenth-century experiments with inks and printing.[59] Indeed,
Flower was especially alert to the unfortunate fate of specimens lacking
labels: 'dirty, neglected, without label, their identity lost, they are often
finally devoured by insects or cleared away to make room on the crowded
shelves for the new donation.'[60] During the late 1920s at the Wellcome
Museums of Medical Science in London, Sidney Daukes's call for the

'drastic reform' of medical museums emphasized the need for accurate labels and up-to-date catalogues to enhance the educational value of exhibits.[61]

At Marischal College, the Anatomy Museum's new signs placed over bays, such as *Head and Neck*, were constructed in uniform materials and a simple, swiftly legible typeface in capitals. One technician cut out the wooden letters in the workshop and two others sanded down the shapes and applied gold leaf to highlight them.[62] Technicians also carried out the labelling of objects for display within the bays. All objects were categorized according to their location within an anatomical region (directly corresponding with a museum bay) and the surfaces of their transparent cases engraved accordingly. For example three preserved ribs were labelled 'TO 6' (see illus. 162), placing them in the museum's scheme as Thorax Osteology number 6. Students could then find this label in the catalogue, the relevant volume of which was kept in the appropriate bay, for a fuller description of the item.[63]

Objects on display in the museum were thus categorized, and accordingly placed in bays as follows:

UPPER LIMB	= U
LOWER LIMB	= L
THORAX	= T
ABDOMEN	= A
HEAD AND NECK	= H
NEUROANATOMY	= N

Within these regions objects were further categorized according to their method of presentation:

Dissection	= D
Osteology	= O
Cross-section	= X
Model	= M
Radiograph (X-ray)	= R

Lastly, objects were assigned consecutive numerals to produce orderly sequences so that from this system unique identifying codes could be generated for the labelling, locating and study of each object in the museum. This system did not, however, completely erase earlier labels. 'HD 19', for instance, catalogued as a 'Complete set of Deciduous Teeth', remained in its old glass jar with a handwritten label and its newer label on adhesive punch tape, affixed to the surface (illus. 164).[64] Furthermore,

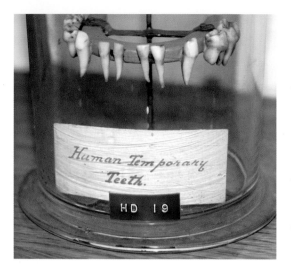

164
Preserved specimen,
'Human Temporary
Teeth', relabelled 'HD
19' c. 1969, in the
Anatomy Museum,
Marischal College,
University of
Aberdeen, 2008.

additional labelling methods were also developed by technicians. The many muscles and blood vessels in a dissected adult arm were identified, for example, with pointers in white thread leading from each anatomical part to an engraved list of labels on a white Perspex panel fixed within the specimen's transparent fluid-filled case. In practice, then, the Anatomy Museum's labelling was flexible to a certain extent, as some previous inscriptions survived and subsequent letterings were incorporated.

The museum's catalogue was specifically designed for use within this display scheme and it promoted efficient learning in this setting, allowing students to rapidly identify specimens and understand their relevance. Efficiency in learning was also a priority in the dissecting room as Sinclair was keenly aware of time slipping away from the study of anatomy in the institutional organization of the medical curriculum.[65] Aligning the Anatomy Museum's structure with the organization of students' dissections, which proceeded through the same anatomical regions, made these two spaces more explicitly mutually reinforcing, potentially speeding up the learning process while boosting its efficacy. Certainly a more rapid identification of specimens was made possible by the museum's new textual apparatus. This closer alignment of the Anatomy Museum with the dissecting room was reinforced with the opening of a doorway in the wall between the two; now staff and students could walk easily from one to the other and back again to work with displays in both.

Organizing the Anatomy Museum so that it could be used by students to augment their work in the dissecting room was especially advantageous given that from the late 1950s medical students in Britain were no longer required to dissect the *entire* body, but instead to gain 'adequate experience of dissection'.[66] Sinclair advised students to 'build' their knowledge of each anatomical region around 'key' structures such as muscles, nerves or arteries, but to avoid studying each region 'in isolation'. He warned: 'you may become seriously confused when you have to make the mental effort of combining the "regions" together . . . into a whole body.'[67] Helping students to understand the anatomy of an integrated whole, then, the Anatomy Museum – which could be surveyed within one space as a (seemingly) complete set of regions – aided in this task of mentally assembling the body parts explored in the dissecting room.

One of the main objectives of practical study through dissection was for students to learn to 'cultivate' their 'visual memory'.[68] This learning required focused embodied activity, as Sinclair recommended:

> when you have finished your dissection, have a good look at it – looking and observing rather than merely looking. Try to impress the picture on your memory. Imagine what a cross-section of the part would look like, draw it, and check your effort against a cross-section in the book or in the museum. Draw a diagram of your dissection on the blackboard from memory; try to visualize it without the book when you are studying at home. Work out the structures you would have to go through in order to reach a given nerve or organ from the intact surface of the body [including your own].[69]

In the dissecting room, Sinclair knew that the main difficulty students had was in 'learning topography in the third dimension': the only way for a student to 'get things straight in his mind', the anatomist advised, was to focus on and handle each body part that the student had themselves 'carved out, like a sculptor, from the material provided' (that is, from the body on the dissecting table).[70] This active engagement with a dissection was extended into the Anatomy Museum where students were expected to remember the bodily anatomy they had sculpted by drawing, imagining and relating that part both to museum specimens and to relevant parts of their own bodies explored anatomically from the surface.

Situated within a region of the museum as body, the active involvement of students in anatomical displays was achieved when they worked through intermedial connections that would develop their visual memory of the bodily interior. This intermediality was promoted through the textual apparatus of the Anatomy Museum. Sinclair advised students to 'work from the body and not the book, but always compare what you actually find with the written description and try to work out the reasons for any discrepancy'.[71] Such an interplay of description and body was set up in the museum catalogue, which explained particular features of specimens and referred students to further related images and sections of anatomical text-books. Thus focused acts of reading were coupled with careful observation to facilitate a deeper and more memorable understanding of anatomy. This was not passive reading of anatomical description to memorize – which was so forcefully rejected in the past – but a questioning and searching mode of reading conducted by students during their comparisons of anatomical parts across a range of media. The Anatomy Museum catalogue was not written simply as a source of information, as it also posed questions and issued tasks with regard to specimens. UD 2, for example, was a preserved dissection of the wrist displaying tendons, nerves and arteries; the catalogue asked students to 'work out for yourself the consequences of injury to any of these structures.'[72]

Anatomy Museum inscriptions were oriented towards the present; their primary purpose was to help students with their current learning. In the catalogue, objects of (then) contemporary anatomical and medical relevance were differentiated from certain museum objects which were described as 'old' or 'of only historic interest'.[73] These temporal distinctions and material divisions were significant. Advice against the 'mixing of historical specimens of little or no teaching value and modern exhibits' had been disseminated in discussions about medical museums since the 1950s.[74] Removing (or relocating) 'old' parts of the collection obscured – or facilitated the forgetting of – aspects of the museum's past, such as its relation to empire, for example, as described in previous chapters. Yet efforts were made to preserve aspects of the museum's local history. On the gallery, a zone peripheral to the main ground-floor space for learning, a display entitled *Anatomy in Aberdeen* provided an historical narrative in texts and photographs (see illus. 34, top). It highlighted some aspects of Aberdeen anatomists' work from around the 1820s to 1939, suggesting continuity in a line of distinguished anatomists during that period. It also displayed late eighteenth- and early nineteenth-century devices placed on graves and built in local cemeteries to prevent grave robbers from taking freshly buried bodies for dissection.[75] Something of the troubled history of anatomy in Scotland's northeast thus manifested in the museum, but this display was consigned to the distanced gallery and presented in such a way as to mark a disjuncture between anatomy as practised in the past and the immediately relevant anatomy of the present (displayed in the museum configured as a 'body'). The effect of this material separation of the past and the present was to display the anatomy of the human body as empirical fact existing outside the historical development of anatomy as a socially and culturally constituted field of knowledge.

Transforming the Anatomy Museum in the late 1960s entailed the use of inscriptions to divide, place and describe the collection in ways that would guide students through anatomical regions of the body to help develop their visual memory of those regions, ideally integrated as a whole body. As we will see below, inscriptions – of a memorial kind dedicated to the anatomized dead – were also significant in the shift from the use of unclaimed bodies for anatomical purposes to donated bodies in Aberdeen from the 1950s to the '70s. When anatomists ceased collecting human remains for the museum in the late 1960s, they became increasingly concerned with how those they anatomized were publicly memorialized.[76]

The unclaimed

The Anatomy Act of 1832 allowed the bodies of those dying in hospitals, poorhouses and other institutions who remained unclaimed for burial by relatives or friends to be acquired for anatomical purposes before their interment. Rather than relying on the limited numbers of executed criminals or obtaining bodies taken from newly filled graves, anatomists were now supposed to have an increased legal supply of cadavers for teaching medical students.[77] In Aberdeen, the funeratory was established in 1833 as the place to temporarily house paupers' bodies until arrangements for burial could be made. It was managed by the Funeratory Committee – composed of city officials and the teachers of anatomy and surgery, overseen by HM Inspector of Anatomy – with a superintendent conducting its daily workings.[78]

The committee saw the funeratory as necessary in order to avoid openly delivering a body directly from the place where the person had died to the place where they were to be dissected, especially following fierce public outrage at the lack of appropriate burial for bodies dissected at a private anatomy theatre in Aberdeen in 1832. Discretion in the conduct of anatomy was therefore of the utmost importance and use of the funeratory allowed a 'supply of bodies' to be 'obtained without the cognisance of any' except those officially involved.[79] Thus the committee aimed to maintain the low public visibility of this method of legal body acquisition to avoid disturbances and protest. It regarded the funeratory as beneficial 'to poor persons who are often compelled to live in the room in which a dead body is lying, and to the public in cases of severe epidemics'.[80] The committee thus saw this institution's workings as a means to deal with the problematic proximity of corpses prior to burial, bodies which they regarded as symbolically polluting if not infectious. These views were not necessarily shared by the poor, many of whom sought to preserve dignity for the dead by preparing them for burial in domestic settings; washing and laying out the corpse for viewing at home remained important aspects of funerary ritual widely observed until the early twentieth century.[81]

At the funeratory the bodies of paupers were laid out for 48 hours after death, during which time they were only 'open to the inspection of friends or relatives, who may claim and bury them thence'.[82] Many were claimed by spouses, parents, siblings, sons, daughters and other relatives. The funeratory also received foetuses, stillborns and unknown infants sometimes found (unburied) in churchyards or on common recreation ground, as well as unidentified people found dead in the sea, canals and harbour. In a register each person was assigned a number alongside a record of their name (unless unknown), age and sex, last place of abode, date and place of death, date of removal from the funeratory, the relative who claimed them or, if they remained unclaimed, the name of the anatomy or surgery teacher who obtained their body, the date the body was sent to the school and, finally, the date of their interment.[83] This documentation thus preserved a written trace of these persons from death to burial, forming a record of either social relatedness after death or of detachment and abandonment with regard to the poorest in the city.

Anatomists selected the suitable unclaimed bodies and any that were overly decomposed were immediately buried. They paid set sums for bodies categorized as 'adult' or 'infant' and as 'opened' or 'entire'; the latter were assigned greater value because the 'great viscera' were 'preserved uninjured'.[84] These payments were funded by students who were charged for each part of a body they dissected (in addition to their class fees), and this money contributed to burial costs of the unclaimed.[85] The Anatomy Act required that each body, after dissection, was 'decently interred in consecrated Ground, or in some public Burial Ground in use for persons of that religious persuasion to which the person whose body was so removed belonged'.[86] In Aberdeen bodies were buried at Footdee near the harbour, and, after 1860, in Nellfield Cemetery in the city centre.[87]

By 1899 a specific section of ground in this cemetery was assigned for these bodies, especially following local newspaper reports of inappropriate burial practices at Nellfield.[88] There was continued emphasis on the 'quiet working' of the Act – on maintaining low public visibility of the body-acquisition process and on making efforts to minimize local opposition to it – which persisted into the early twentieth century when the committee ordered that the transportation of bodies, by this time potentially from outside the city, should be done with the use of a 'proper hearse etc' in 'such a manner that will not wound local feeling'.[89] A professional undertakers' firm was employed, from the 1920s onwards, to transport bodies.[90] From 1921 the anatomized dead were buried in Trinity Cemetery, located between the city and beach; the plot was granted by the cemetery's managers with the requirement that its particular use was not publicly disclosed and that no memorial was erected.[91]

In Aberdeen during the century following the Anatomy Act, then, anatomists and officials maintained a persistent strategy of seclusion combined with attempts to maintain standards of decency when acquiring and burying unclaimed bodies. Furthermore the supply of unclaimed bodies fluctuated, tending to remain low in relation to anatomists' perceived teaching needs. Throughout the nineteenth century bodies were obtained from within the city and then, as numbers became particularly low in the early decades of the twentieth century, they were sought from a wider geographical area in northeast Scotland. In 1914 the Funeratory Committee considered extending its reach further north to Orkney and Shetland, but decided against this due to high cost and logistical difficulties.[92] The scarcity of unclaimed bodies available in Aberdeen, it was suggested, arose from the declining numbers of 'inmates' coming to institutions in the city from 'remote' parts of the region – inmates who, due to geographical distance, would have tended not to have relatives or friends who could claim them when they died.[93] By 1918 the committee observed that war conditions had 'emptied the Poor Houses', thereby further reducing body supply.[94] The decreased death rate was cited in 1928 as a further factor in the continued difficulties in obtaining adequate numbers, and from the mid-1930s to the 1960s some bodies were transferred to Aberdeen from medical schools and hospitals in England in attempts to provide students with enough bodies to dissect.[95] It was not until 1970 that the committee could report that the Anatomy Department did not require bodies from elsewhere as it now had a 'healthy' supply of bodies from its own region.[96] This shift was attained not by increasing the intake of unclaimed bodies but by calling for and receiving bequests.

The bequeathed

The number of people bequeathing their bodies in Britain gradually began to increase in the 1930s, this rising trend becoming most apparent from the mid-1940s onwards. Since the Second World War, as Ruth Richardson suggests, a 'culture of medical donation' has developed in which people willingly donate their blood during life, their bodies for dissection or their organs for transplant after death.[97] The rise in whole-body donation coincided with the growing popularity of cremation: in the early 1930s only 1 per cent of people in Britain were cremated, rising to 50 per cent during the 1960s and to 66.5 per cent in the early 1970s, so that for these people there was a move away from the preference for traditional burial.[98] A further factor identified by Richardson was a 'more benign public view of scientific medicine' developing especially after the National Health Service was formed in 1948 to provide free healthcare for everyone.[99] In Scotland, however, during the 1950s, there was a slower increase in bodies donated for dissection in comparison with England.[100] This shift to bequests, gaining momentum during the 1960s and '70s, was encouraged through the forging of local connections between anatomists, other professionals, potential donors and their relatives.

In Aberdeen the activities of the Funeratory Committee, whose membership continued to include anatomists, were crucial in securing donations. From the mid-1940s onwards the committee's strategy was to boost public awareness of the necessity of bequests to anatomy by cultivating a network of sympathetic local and regional contacts. In Lockhart's view there was 'too much secrecy' about the need for bodies and the 'University's requirements' needed to be publicized.[101] The Funeratory Committee was renamed the Anatomy Act Committee (1955), as members considered the latter more conducive to 'public interest and support'.[102] The local press was used to disseminate information to people on how to donate. One press article in 1960, describing a widow's bequest, included excerpts from an interview with Lockhart in which he pointed out that 'BBC stars' and 'eminent people' had 'given their bodies quite recently'. He explained that body donations to anatomy were

> not by any means confined to people in poorer circumstances. Many people whose lives were in the highest classes decided that it was the sensible thing to do. It is a very desirable bequest to make in a worthwhile cause.[103]

Such publicity carried the message that donors were prominent individuals and from wealthy groups, whose deaths were dignified, prepared for and dealt with sensibly. In this way anatomists attempted to adjust public perceptions of the persons associated with dissection, shifting emphasis from the criminal and the poor to exemplary individuals and affluent groups. This public reporting in Aberdeen also emphasized the orderliness of the bequest procedure and the ease with which an intending donor, relative or executor could contact the professor of anatomy to deal with a bequest: the anatomist was represented as friendly and sympathetic, only a telephone call away.

Cultivating contacts and disseminating media messages generated written correspondence between anatomists and potential donors. Letters from the 1960s and '70s, originally archived in the Anatomy Department, reveal aspects of these unfolding dialogues, and indicate the importance of key intermediaries through whom anatomists extended their call for donations.[104] The Anatomy Act Committee sent information about donation procedures to solicitors in the region and considered a similar approach to churches and the governing boards of hospitals, aiming to recruit authoritative and respected members of communities who would circulate accurate advice to potential donors.[105] These messages yielded responses as doctors, solicitors and ministers replied with indications regarding their patients, clients and parishioners who expressed wishes to bequeath their bodies. Through letters, intending donors discussed with anatomists their views and preferences for the future disposal of their bodies.[106]

Donations were registered by people who had no surviving relatives, and by those with relatives who were in sympathy with the bequest. Some

338

donors wanted to make a bequest together with a relative (such as a mother with her daughter) or a spouse, to ensure a shared future and mode of disposal for their deceased bodies. One requested that his skeleton be preserved to instruct students, but David Sinclair explained that this would not be legally possible as anatomists are required to 'substantially reassemble a body after dissection' in preparation for burial or cremation.[107] Such dialogues were part of the bequest-making process and by 1970 the Anatomy Department had filed bequest forms from 800 people stating their intention to donate.[108] By 1973 all of the bodies received by the department were bequeathed and no unclaimed bodies had been dissected for the past three years.[109]

The 'subjects' dissected by anatomists and their students were no longer bodies necessarily from among the destitute and socially isolated; instead they were deceased persons – many still very much socially connected at death with their surviving families – who had explicitly chosen to give their bodies. Anatomists took a leading part in cultivating the social relations through which bequests were forthcoming and a significant aspect of this was the formation of several interrelated memorials for donors – a service, a book and a cemetery memorial, all of which are, to date, actively maintained. These memorial forms focus on the names of donors through spoken words and manuscript records or through memorial lettering that makes reference to names without literally displaying them. These words have been performed and inscribed within a necro-topography that encompasses sites for the ritualized treatment of the anatomized dead in Aberdeen since the 1950s: from Marischal College's Anatomy Department to a cemetery, chapel, crematorium and, most recently, as anatomists' memorial practices continue into the twenty-first century, a garden of remembrance.

WITNESSING THE NAME

The memorial service to thank and remember those who had donated their bodies to medical science was inaugurated in the Anatomy Department at Marischal College during the early 1950s – the first of its kind in Scotland, and possibly in Britain.[110] Initially referred to as the 'annual funeral service', it was held, prior to the burial or cremation of bodies, in the refurbished dissecting room where dissecting tables were wheeled aside for a minister to conduct the service for staff, students, city officials, HM Inspector of Anatomy and some relatives of donors.[111] The service developed in a context where anatomists were paying increased attention to the attitudes and intentions of donors, especially by observing donors' requirements for their burial. For instance, Robert Lockhart followed donors' instructions regarding their coffins (some supplied their own), where to return their remains for private burial and further requests, such as the burial of one Catholic donor with a rosary according to his wishes.[112]

Lockhart also respected the mourning practices of relatives. When a woman donor of 91 years died in 1958 a wreath was sent to her by mourners, and Lockhart instructed the undertakers to deliver it with her to the Anatomy Department, keeping it with her body until she was dissected. When the woman was buried he arranged for a new wreath to accompany her to the grave. Exchanges between Lockhart and donors' next of kin could involve intensely emotional issues, as in the case of one grieving widow whose husband, a doctor, donated his body. The widow wrote that when her husband died her 'world crashed'. She continued: 'I should like to come to the last ceremony if I survive in June 1958. Then I can scatter my husband's ashes in secret on his parents' grave.'[113] Thus the memorial service developed in this context of increased communication between anatomists, donors and their relatives regarding personal preferences for the ritualized treatment of donors' bodies.

By 1972 the memorial service had relocated from the dissecting room at Marischal College to the Chapel at King's College, where it was led by the chaplain to the university. This encouraged donors' relatives and friends to attend, the chapel being a more publicly accessible and perhaps less daunting venue. The service featured hymns and readings, the details of which were recorded each year in an archive currently kept by the chaplain. She uses this to guide her own present-day addresses as, from her perspective, she has inherited a 'tradition' that she actively maintains.[114] As a minister of the Church of Scotland she conducts the service with 'Judeo-Christian overtones', regarded as broadly consistent with the beliefs of donors. The chaplain is aware that most people attending might not be 'religious', and the intention is to create a service that is 'very open'. From her perspective, the service expresses 'gratitude to God as well as for the huge gift of the body to anatomy', and provides a setting for people to grieve and say goodbye. The service's messages emphasize that the 'value of life continues after death' and suggest, in spiritual terms, that 'death is not an end to life.'[115]

The memorial service is an annual event currently (to date) attended on a weekday in May by about 300 people, including university and city officials, the Anatomy Department's staff and students, and many people who knew the donors in life – whether as close relatives, friends or residential-home nurses. The long-serving anatomy bequest administrator, in the department, takes a leading role in the organization of the service. She manages the process of donation, receiving enquiries from and advising potential donors, coordinating undertakers' deliveries of bodies at the department and arranging their disposal, while also maintaining an archive of donors' bequest forms that began in 1965.[116] The administrator is thus a central figure in the practice and ongoing social relations of donation: she participates in matters personal and legal, emotional and bureaucratic, mundane and ceremonial.

At the time of the memorial service (prior to 2009) donors' coffins were not taken to the chapel, but were laid out in the dissecting room at Marischal College before their delivery by undertakers to Aberdeen Crematorium or Trinity Cemetery. Each donor was placed in a coffin and the number they had been given upon entry into the Anatomy Department was linked back to their name.[117] At the chapel, during the memorial service, an emotive reconnection of each deceased person with family and friends takes place through the witnessing of the donor's name.[118] Hearing and also viewing a person's name in a special book remain the central acts of the memorial service. There are hymns, prayers and readings from scripture, some by medical students, but the chaplain's address is especially emotionally heightened as she reads aloud the full names of the men and women who donated their bodies and the places they were from in northeast Scotland. This is a potent point of recognition and recall for donors' relatives and friends for whom the name can evoke memories of a donor's living actions, expressions, and voice. Students, however, hearing those names for the first time, are unable to retrospectively associate the numbered bodies they encountered in the dissecting room with those persons' actual names – for students, the bodies of donors are remembered primarily as a more generally applicable human anatomy. Nevertheless hearing donors' names in the service is especially moving: it reinforces students' sense of those anatomized bodies as persons to whom relatives and friends are still emotionally attached.[119]

Those attending the service can also read donors' names in the memorial book, opened for the duration of the event on a table at the chapel's entrance. Here, in the antechapel through which visitors pass into the chapel, there is also a temporary convergence of memorials, for anatomy donors and for the war dead – a connection that is also echoed in the cemetery memorial discussed below. Into the oak-panelled walls of the antechapel are carved the names of 524 members of the university who died serving during the First World War and the Second World War, and these names are also recorded in a dedicated book of remembrance. This war memorial's inscription explains that these people 'gave their lives . . . in the sacred cause of justice and freedom' for their survivors, and the memorial service for body donors narrates a comparable gesture of giving as a valuable contribution to collective bodily health and the continuity of spiritual life.[120]

In the entrance corridor of the Anatomy Department at Marischal College, from the late 1960s to 2009, the memorial book was displayed in a locked glass-fronted case built into the wall, lined with dark red velvet and framed in oak. This casing, like that in the Anatomy Museum, was made by technicians (illus. 165).[121] Its accompanying brass plaque was inscribed: *This book records in gratitude the names of those who bequeathed their bodies for the advancement of medical science.* Viewers could see the dark blue and the dark green covers of two volumes embossed with gold lettering: one entitled *In Memoriam*, the other – the oldest – *The Book of Memory*. As memorial objects, the closed books remained on permanent display and their written contents were periodically viewed. Inside the books each right-hand page is assigned to a consecutive year and the names of donors who died in that year inscribed on it. Alongside each person's name is the place that person was associated with, usually the place where they dwelt in later life. The occasions when the memorial book is opened are specifically framed as acts of remembrance: when people related to a donor request to see that person's name and during the annual memorial service. By virtue of its inscriptions the memorial book has become a focus for personal acts of memory-making, and it is also central to collective memorial occasions in the chapel.

The memorial book was established in the 1960s. During the Anatomy Act Committee's discussions about the need for bequests, and ways of publicizing that need, HM Inspector of Anatomy Denis Dooley suggested that 'a book of remembrance' could be 'kept in the Anatomy Department as a form of memorial and to which the public could have access'.[122] David Sinclair obtained the book and the first names were recorded from 1966 onwards.[123] A similar book of remembrance was established at the University of Glasgow in 1974. There donors' names and their dates of death have been decoratively written in ink and the pages embellished with floral motifs by the medical artist at the Laboratory of Human Anatomy. Following the layout of the first entries, over the last decade she has written twelve names on each page which she makes distinctive with the application of varied motifs in the margins. The two volumes of the book are displayed, closed, in Glasgow's

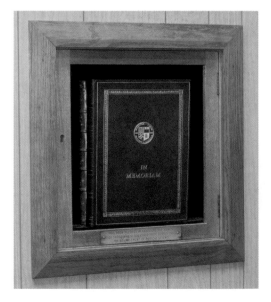

165
In Memoriam, two volumes in display case with brass inscription plate, books inscribed from 1966 onwards. In the entrance corridor, Anatomy Department, Marischal College, University of Aberdeen, 2007.

Museum of Anatomy in a locked glass-topped case containing a red artificial rose.

In Aberdeen the memorial book is currently maintained by the anatomy bequest administrator. She arranges for donors' names to be inscribed by a person with calligraphy skills – an anatomist in the department and a photographic technician have entered the names in the past and from 1999 it was done by an art teacher, now retired, from an local school. As the only formal memorial inscription of a donor's name, these words are significant for relatives: it is through them that a person is memorialized and connections potentially sustained between a donor's relatives and the Anatomy Department.

From anatomists' point of view, the inscription of donors' names expresses gratitude for the bequest. The book is a memorial for individual persons, which also associates those persons with a wider culturally valued process – the 'advancement of medical science'. As the memorial inscription records the name of a person alongside the place where they lived, the person retains a connection with their home while also being memorialized in a place of anatomical learning. On each page of the memorial book, individuals are also memorialized as part of a group of persons whose commonality is the act of donating their own bodies. Each page in the book marks another year that passes and an ever-growing community of donors. Yet for the donor's relatives and friends the inscribed name retains the unique features of the person whom they knew, providing the material from which memories of a particular life can be generated and renewed.

LETTERING ON STONE

These memorial forms – a service and a book – are also related to a further memorial structure at Aberdeen's Trinity Cemetery (illus. 166). Facing into the cemetery, with the beach and sea behind, the memorial's prominent dedication reads: *In memory of those who gave their bodies for the increase of knowledge and the advance of medicine.* A plaque, on its central panel, is inscribed: *'Their name liveth for ever. The people will tell of their wisdom and the congregation will show forth their praise' Ecclesiasticus 44.* The first inscription is legible at a distance; the second has to be approached from shallow steps leading to a paved platform. An impression of austere simplicity is conveyed by the structure with its bold lines in stone and concrete, uninterrupted except for a few flowers and shrubs.[124] In its elevated position, it creates definition for the expanse of ground before it – a third of an acre for the exclusive use of the Anatomy Department. This is where donors' remains are buried in assigned plots but the grass remains

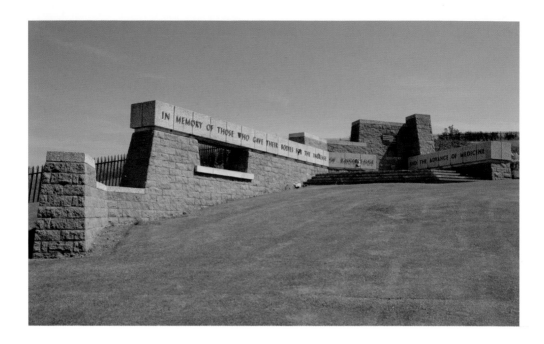

166
Memorial established
by the Anatomy
Department, University
of Aberdeen in 1974,
at Trinity Cemetery,
Aberdeen, 2007.

unmarked by individual headstones. The memorial thus operates as a collective marker that registers the presence of donors, while also maintaining their anonymity. Viewed in relation to nearby headstones that mark individual or family graves, the memorial is clearly devoid of personal names, yet its inscription draws attention to the significance of the name and its remembrance through the quotation from Ecclesiasticus. Like the memorial book, it highlights one central gesture in the lives of those buried, that they gave their bodies, linking this gesture to the powerful narrative of medicine's advancement and claims regarding the growth of knowledge.

The cemetery memorial was built in 1974 – the first in Britain – as part of anatomists' efforts to give aspects of anatomical practice a positive public visibility while expressing gratitude to donors and their relatives.[125] Planning for the memorial had begun six years earlier. With the notable increase in bequests of bodies during the 1960s, David Sinclair raised the issue of a memorial with the Anatomy Act Committee in 1968, pointing out that although many donors were opting for cremation, many still preferred burial.[126] Yet where they were interred, at Trinity Cemetery, the ground 'was not marked in any way as indicative of who lay there' and so Sinclair suggested that 'some form of headstone be instructed and erected'.[127] He explained further that donors' families and friends greatly appreciated the book of remembrance instituted by the department, and argued that the burial plot in Trinity Cemetery 'ought also to carry some visible recognition of its purpose and of our gratitude to those who are buried there'. This issue had become particularly acute at the time of the annual service, when relatives asked where donors were buried and were 'distressed' to hear that there was no 'commemorative stone or memorial' for them.[128] The committee's concern was that 'there was nothing for such people to see except a stretch of grass', and this absence was recognized as troubling for the bereaved.[129] The memorial was thus conceived and designed in relation to the concerns expressed by families and friends of donors as well as anatomists' perceptions of those people's bereavement and memorial needs.

Although the original allocation of ground at Trinity Cemetery in 1921 had stipulated that no memorial be built, 50 years later cemetery managers granted permission, recognizing the value of body donation to medical science.[130] David Sinclair secured this agreement and also raised funds, using finances from the previous sale of the funeratory and contributions from the university, the town council and a private donor whose mother had previously bequeathed her own body.[131] The Anatomy Act Committee maintained control of the memorial's design, deciding not to consult relatives of donors in case of conflicts of opinion.[132] One suggestion from the committee, in 1969, was for a 'boulder', 'in view of the nature of the site' which was sloping and exposed to the sea.[133] Subsequently various motifs, such as hands, eyes and a heart, were sketched as well as memorial forms including crosses, headstones, wreaths and praying hands (illus. 167). Although these traditional Christian images and familiar gestures were initially considered, the cemetery memorial developed as a much more honed and minimal structure.

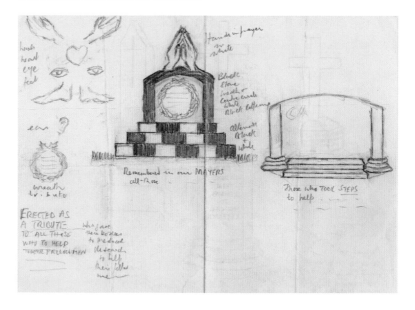

167
Draft sketches of designs for the memorial planned by the Anatomy Department, University of Aberdeen, c. 1970.

Guiding principles for the memorial's design were outlined in 1970: it 'should not be one which should attract particular attention and . . . it should be a simple form' appropriate to its function and achievable with the available funds.[134] Its main feature was to be an inscription which the committee decided should be along the lines of the one displayed beside the memorial book in the Anatomy Department – a 'general inscription' devoid of any 'individual names' to form a collective memorial that also respected donors' privacy.[135] The wording went through many drafts with subtle amendments that adjusted its tone and memorial reach. Many variations on the line 'In grateful memory of those who bequeathed their bodies for the advancement of medical education and research' were discussed. The words 'in Aberdeen' were deleted from an earlier version, enlarging the scope of the inscription so that it became generalized rather than locally specific.[136]

Unlike the memorial book, which was instituted exclusively for donors, the cemetery memorial was to mark a plot where, in addition to donors, unclaimed bodies were buried from 1921 to around 1970. Consequently an important question for the committee was how the memorial might address both categories of bodies, one having actively chosen to donate and the other having been acquired as no one objected. It was recognized that the term 'bequeathed' did not 'cover unclaimed bodies' and the final inscription became a dedication to 'those who gave their bodies'.[137] These shifts indicate an attempt to include the unclaimed but not directly as such, the emphasis of the inscription falling on the act of giving. This highlighted donors rather than the unclaimed, even though the word 'gave' was intended to embrace both intentional and unknowing acts seen to be of benefit to medical practice and hence the health of many. The unclaimed thus remained an invisible category, subsumed by the memorial's narrative in which undifferentiated persons gave their bodies. The graves of the anatomized dead buried prior to 1920 at Footdee and Nellfield cemeteries also remained unmarked. With its selective emphases the memorial is implicated in processes of forgetting where one social category is memorialized while another becomes invisible.[138]

Reference to those who 'gave their bodies', intentionally or not, for a greater good resonates with war memorial inscriptions dedicated to those who 'gave their lives' and thus made sacrifices for others. Indeed, the devising of the cemetery memorial for the anatomized dead was perhaps informed by those memorials for the British war dead which, after the First World War, displayed the quotation from Ecclesiasticus 'Their names liveth evermore' – as does one in Trinity Cemetery dedicated to local men who served in the military.[139] A further possible influence on the memorial's design was the modernist architecture of the 1937 Aberdeen Crematorium (at Kaimhill Road), the majority of crematoria in Britain having been purpose-built between 1950 and 1970.[140]

If the memorial's design was negotiated among a number of participants, and in relation to further memorials and architectures, it was also shaped within its immediate material context. The Anatomy Act Committee obtained assistance, in 1972, from the architect William Coutts Youngson, a member of staff at Aberdeen's Scott Sutherland School of Architecture. Youngson's formal designs for the 'memorial stone' were guided by advice from the cemetery superintendent regarding practicalities of maintenance, and they took advantage of the plot's high ground, positioning the memorial so that visitors would be oriented towards the sea.[141] Youngson proposed a 'simple silhouette', a 'wall designed to present

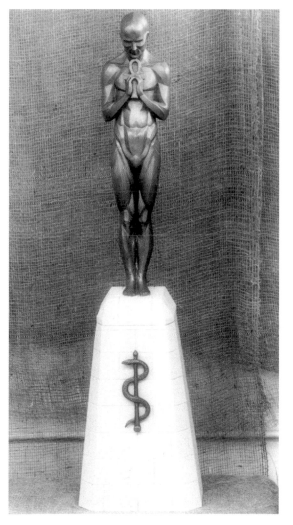

a bold inscription in metal roman capitals, a small bronze plaque and a base or platform for a piece of symbolic sculpture which might be acquired in due course'.[142] An approach path and bollards defining the boundaries of the site were planned but funds were only sufficient to finance the wall, though it was hoped that the memorial would be completed in due course.[143] To date these elements have not been added and with the passage of time the memorial's status as incomplete has dissolved so that its once 'missing' parts have become invisible.

There were plans to install a sculpture, but these did not come to fruition. In 1974 Youngson approached the sculpture department at Gray's School of Art in Aberdeen and arranged for students to produce some designs.[144] They made seven models for possible sculptures and one of these, a human figure standing on a plinth, perhaps in a praying posture, designed by a Mr Alexander, was selected for the memorial (illus. 168). The figure, with angular lines, is accompanied by ancient symbols: an ankh (the Egyptian hieroglyph for life) and the staff of Asclepius the Greek god of medicine. The plan was to construct the figure, at

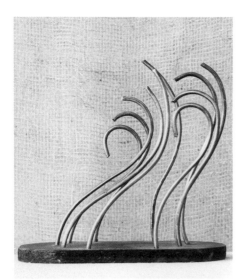

a height of 0.9 m (3 ft), in 'cement fondue' – a highly durable substance which would be applied over an armature and then coated with a material resembling bronze.[145] The rejected designs for the memorial's sculpture included models of an obelisk and of several abstract forms with curved, interlocking or rising shapes. Also declined was a model with ten metal components, separate fluid lines apparently moving in unison (illus. 169). So the art students' models proposed a range of ways in which the memorial could have been further developed. However, the chosen sculpture was never commissioned, for reasons unrecorded in the archive but probably due to lack of finances, despite the efforts of the university's chaplain and Marischal College's anatomy professor Edward Clegg as well as medical students around 1978.[146] With this sculptural omission the memorial's textual inscriptions have remained predominant features.

Visitors to Trinity Cemetery read and respond to these inscriptions in different ways. For instance, the metal letters of the main text have been pressed into service as improvised resting places for small floral tributes. In 2007 visitors had left once fresh daisies lodged in the letter *W* in the word *who*, an artificial rose at the *O* of *bodies*, and a Christmas basket of flowers was also hooked onto the word *knowledge* (illus. 170). These are personal ritualized gestures that make the memorial meaningful for particular persons. For the bereaved, visiting the memorial is an occasion for remembering the deceased, for animating and renewing memories of them. Fresh, or artificial and therefore enduring, flowers brought to the memorial can represent a regeneration of the departed, making them feel alive and in close proximity.[147] In this context the memorial's inscriptions express gratitude for what the anatomist David Sinclair termed 'invaluable gifts' while also operating as foci of intense remembering for those who knew donors when alive.[148]

Relatives also scatter donor's ashes at the cemetery memorial. And as most donors are now cremated, a further memorial was established in 2007, this time at the Aberdeen Crematorium (located at Hazlehead from 1975). Set in the garden of remembrance, a pink granite stone 0.5 metres square (1.5 ft square) has a slanted surface for its inscription, these words taken from Trinity Cemetery's memorial. This was initiated and organized by the Anatomy Department's senior anatomy lecturer and the anatomy bequest administrator, and funded by the university. They wanted to mark a place where relatives and friends of donors could visit, especially on

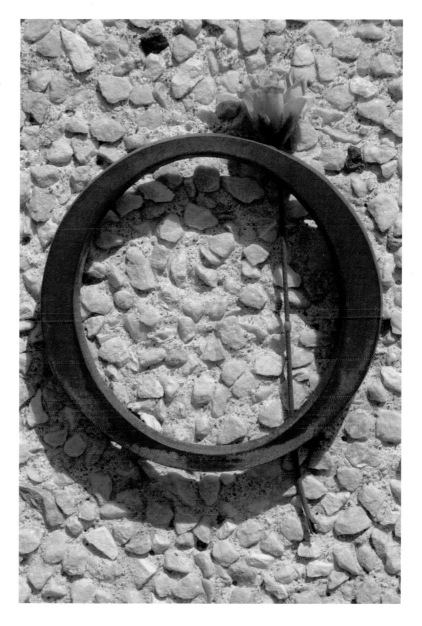

170
'O' in the word
'bodies', on the
memorial established
by the Anatomy
Department, University
of Aberdeen, at Trinity
Cemetery, Aberdeen,
with an artificial
flower placed by
a visitor, 2007.

future anniversaries of deaths, where donors could be remembered and grief expressed. The stone also defined another site where donors' ashes can be scattered. This latest memorial stone, like the memorial at Trinity Cemetery, arose out of anatomists' respect for the mourning practices of donors' relatives. Both memorials shared the inscription, which was itself derived from that displayed with the memorial book in the Anatomy Department. Memorial and anatomical sites were connected through materialized words.

In the late 1960s the Anatomy Museum was transformed into a 'body', with interrelated material and textual displays designed to facilitate students' active, efficient learning. With the reduction in time for dissecting the body's anatomical topography, the Anatomy Museum was configured as that very topography which students could physically enter to develop their visual memory of an integrated bodily interior. Following the separation of the human and animal, the anatomical specimens and the anthropological artefacts, and the historical objects from the current materials for learning, the museum was made spatially and conceptually continuous with the dissecting room; learning practices in both spaces were mutually reinforcing through the active forging of intermedial connections. From *c.* 1965 dissected parts of human bodies were no longer collected for the Anatomy Museum; unreliable supplies of unclaimed bodies for dissection were replaced by a more dependable influx of donors' bodies and with this shift the collecting of dissected parts was seen as less necessary and less appropriate. Within the social relations of body donation, anatomists became increasingly attentive to the perspectives and requests of body donors as well as their relatives. While the topography of the body within the Anatomy Museum was displayed to stimulate students' remembering of anatomized bodies, this museum was related – within the necro-topography of the city – to memorial displays designed to sustain memories of body donors among their kin and friends. Such memorials have become part of the public profile of anatomical practice, displays that perhaps work indirectly to invite further people to donate their bodies after death.

INCOMPLETION

The cemetery memorial remains incomplete in three important respects. First, its sculptural component was not realized, although this has now been mostly forgotten and the omission is not visible as such – it is only evident in archival traces. Second, when this memorial is explored in terms of the ongoing social, cultural and material processes in which it is enmeshed, it appears not as a fixed entity but as emergent in its making and uses. Its initial design was realized differently in practice, its stone becomes weathered and requires cleaning, its plants grow, die and are replanted, its lettering is used to mount floral tributes brought by the bereaved. Third, the memorial as process is connected with other memorials dedicated to anatomy donors – on the one hand it was devised in relation to a memorial book, a book which is integrated into a memorial service, and on the other, its inscription was reiterated when a further stone was installed at another site of mourning, a crematorium's garden of remembrance. Over time interrelated memorials have been generated, directly referring to their immediate predecessors and indirectly evoking further memorial forms such as those of war.

Memorials are processual and relational, rather than fixed and completed, and so are museums as explored throughout this book. Museums of anatomy are made, used, taken apart and composed, just as the bodies they display have been dissected, framed as specimens, preserved, repaired and removed. In their formation such museums have been modelled on and refer to others; when their exhibits are built, destroyed, rebuilt and modified they are caught up in processes of intermuseality. A plethora of visual images and material objects for displaying anatomy are caught up in an unfolding intermediality. Human anatomy has been rendered through such a variety of media that anatomy museums become echo chambers of repeated yet modified body parts. Those involved in designing medical museums in the early twentieth century claimed that in such a museum 'there can be no finality – progress is the essence of its existence.' Displays had to be kept up to date to prevent them fading into the past. From this point of view, the completion of a museum was impossible; as one commentator suggested, 'it is doubtful if . . . completeness can ever be attained in view of the rapid advance of scientific knowledge.'[149] Here was the notion that as knowledge was ever-expanding, museums which were enmeshed in that knowledge creation and communication could consequently never be finished.

In practice, anatomy museums have expanded and contracted in contexts shaped by their social relations as much as the material resources and technologies available to them. During the 1940s and '50s the Anatomy Museum was animated with the use of new visual technologies and methods of display that focused on living anatomy. Changes during the 1960s introduced discontinuities with past modes of display, but these did not entirely eradicate material traces of the museum's historical formation. During the 1980s there was a wave of questioning within the university with regard to the Anatomy Museum's relevance along with concerns that its specimens had been 'inherited unquestioningly from past actions', and with reductions in staff as well as in funds, it was feared that the collection was suffering an 'inevitable process of attrition'.[150] This collection, perceived in some ways as a difficult material inheritance, was, however, maintained and actively used to generate and communicate anatomical knowledge through teaching and learning. In 2009 the Anatomy Museum's collection was removed from its Victorian shell to be relocated and reconfigured in its most recent site in the new medical school building at Aberdeen's hospital complex.[151] Here the again pared-down collection is displayed alongside the dissected deceased so that the human body can come to be known in

intimate anatomical terms, so that the anatomy of the dead can be imagined as that of the living, so that the anatomy of the living can be seen and
felt though the dead.

ABBREVIATIONS

AMCS Aberdeen Medico-Chirurgical Society

AUAAS Aberdeen University Anatomical and Anthropological Society

PAAS University of Aberdeen Proceedings of the Anatomical and Anthropological Society

RCS Royal College of Surgeons of England

RCSEd Royal College of Surgeons of Edinburgh

UAAD University of Aberdeen, Anatomy Department

UAAM University of Aberdeen, Anatomy Museum

UAMM University of Aberdeen, Marischal Museum

UASC University of Aberdeen, Special Collections

UAZM University of Aberdeen, Zoological Museum

REFERENCES

Introduction: Articulating Anatomy

1 'Las Ruinas Circulares' was first published in *Sur 75*, in December 1940. The quotation cited is from Jorge Luis Borges, *Labyrinths: Selected Stories and Other Writings*, ed. Donald A. Yates and James E. Irby (Harmondsworth, 1970), pp. 74–5.

2 Historical distinctions between specimens and preparations are explained in Simon Chaplin, 'John Hunter and the "Museum Oeconomy", 1750–1800', PhD thesis, King's College London (2009), pp. 101–2.

3 See Arjun Appadurai, ed., *The Social Life of Things: Commodities in Cultural Perspective* (Cambridge, 1986); Cara Krmpotich, Joost Fontein and John Harries, 'The Substance of Bones: The Emotive Materiality and Affective Presence of Human Remains', *Journal of Material Culture*, xv (2010), pp. 371–84; Henrik B. Lindskoug and Anne Gustavsson, 'Stories from Below: Human Remains at the Gothenburg Museum of Natural History and the Museum of World Culture', *Journal of the History of Collections*, xxvii (2015), pp. 97–109; Katherine Verdery, *The Political Lives of Dead Bodies: Reburial and Postsocialist Change* (New York, 1999).

4 For studies of anatomy and pathology museums and collections, see Eva Åhrén, *Death, Modernity, and the Body: Sweden 1870–1940*, trans. Daniel W. Olson (Rochester, NY, 2009); Samuel J.M.M. Alberti, *Morbid Curiosities: Medical Museums in Nineteenth-century Britain* (Oxford, 2011); Chaplin, 'John Hunter'; Elizabeth Hallam and Samuel J.M.M. Alberti, 'Bodies in Museums', in *Medical Museums: Past, Present, Future*, ed. Samuel J.M.M. Alberti and Elizabeth Hallam (London, 2013), pp. 1–15; Dawn Kemp with Sara Barnes, *Surgeons' Hall: A Museum Anthology* (Edinburgh, 2009); Jonathan Reinarz, 'The Age of Museum Medicine: The Rise and Fall of the Medical Museum of Birmingham's School of Medicine', *Social History of Medicine*, xviii (2005), pp. 419–37; Steve Sturdy, 'Making Sense in the Pathology Museum', in *Anatomy Acts: How We Come to Know Ourselves*, ed. Andrew Patrizio and Dawn Kemp (Edinburgh, 2006), pp. 107–15. For histories of public anatomical exhibitions, see Richard D. Altick, *The Shows of London: A Panoramic History of Exhibitions, 1600–1862* (Cambridge, MA, 1978); Alan W. Bates, '"Indecent and Demoralising Representations": Public Anatomy Museums in Mid-Victorian England', *Medical History*, lii (2008), pp. 1–22; Maritha Rene Burmeister, 'Popular Anatomical Museums in Nineteenth-century England', PhD thesis, Rutgers University (2000); Elizabeth Stephens, *Anatomy as Spectacle: Public Exhibitions of the Body from 1700 to the Present* (Liverpool, 2011).

5 For histories of medical education, see William F. Bynum and Roy Porter, eds, *Medicine and the Five Senses* (Cambridge, 1993); William F. Bynum et al., *The Western Medical Tradition, 1800–2000* (Cambridge, 2006); Thomas Neville Bonner, *Becoming a Physician:*

Medical Education in Britain, France, Germany, and the United States, 1740–1945 (Oxford, 1995); Elizabeth Hurren, *Dying for Victorian Medicine: English Anatomy and Its Trade in the Dead Poor, c. 1834–1929* (London, 2012); Fiona Hutton, *The Study of Anatomy in Britain, 1700–1900* (London, 2013); Vivian Nutton and Roy Porter, eds, *The History of Medical Education in Britain* (Amsterdam, 1995); Keir Waddington, *Medical Education at St Bartholomew's Hospital, 1123–1995* (Woodbridge, Suffolk, 2003). Mark Weatherall, *Gentlemen, Scientists, and Doctors: Medicine at Cambridge, 1800–1940* (Baltimore, MD, 2000).

6 For analysis of the constitution of knowledge in practice, as discussed in historical studies of science, see for example Lorraine Daston and Peter Galison, *Objectivity* (New York, 2007); Lorraine Daston and Elizabeth Lunbeck, eds, *Histories of Scientific Observation* (Chicago, IL, 2011); Jan Golinski, *Making Natural Knowledge: Constructivism in the History of Science* (Cambridge, 1998); Simon Shapin, *A Social History of Truth: Civility and Science in Seventeenth-century England* (Chicago, IL, 1994), Simon Shapin, *Never Pure: Historical Studies of Science as if It Was Produced by People with Bodies, Situated in Time, Space, Culture, and Society, and Struggling for Credibility* (Baltimore, MD, 2010).

7 There is an extensive literature on the history of anatomy, see for example Andrea Carlino, *Books of the Body: Anatomical Ritual and Renaissance Learning* (Chicago, IL, 1999); Andrew Cunningham, *The Anatomist Anatomis'd: An Experimental Discipline in Enlightenment Europe* (Farnham, 2010); Anita Guerrini, 'Anatomists and Entrepreneurs in Early Eighteenth-century London', *Journal of the History of Medicine and Allied Sciences*, LIX (2004), pp. 219–39; Hurren, *Dying for Victorian Medicine*; Hutton, *Study of Anatomy*; Cynthia Klestinec, *Theatres of Anatomy: Students, Teachers, and Traditions of Dissection in Renaissance Venice* (Baltimore, MD, 2011); Helen MacDonald, *Possessing the Dead: The Artful Science of Anatomy* (Melbourne, 2010); Katherine Park, *Secrets of Women: Gender, Generation and the Origins of Human Dissection* (New York, 2006); Lynda Payne, *With Words and Knives: Learning Medical Dispassion in Early Modern England* (Aldershot, 2007); Ruth Richardson, *Death, Dissection and the Destitute*, 2nd edn (London, 2001); Jonathan Sawday, *The Body Emblazoned: Dissection and the Human Body in Renaissance Culture* (London, 1995); Michael Sappol, *A Traffic of Dead Bodies: Anatomy and Embodied Social Identity in Nineteenth-century America* (Princeton, NJ, 2002).

8 See Elizabeth Hallam and Tim Ingold, eds, *Making and Growing: Anthropological Studies of Organisms and Artefacts* (Farnham, 2014).

9 On embodiment, see for example Thomas J. Csordas, *Embodiment and Experience: The Existential Ground of Culture and Self* (Cambridge, 1994); Christopher Lawrence and Simon Shapin, eds, *Science Incarnate: Historical Embodiments of Natural Knowledge* (Chicago, IL, 1998); Margaret Lock and Judith Farquhar, eds, *Beyond the Body Proper: Reading the Anthropology of Material Life* (Durham, NC, 2007); Rachel Prentice, *Bodies in Formation: An Ethnography of Anatomy and Surgery Education* (Durham, NC, 2013).

10 The University of Aberdeen's Anatomy Department (or Anatomy Facility) is currently (to date) part of the School of Medicine and Dentistry. Acknowledgements regarding my research at this site are given at the end of this book. Elizabeth Hallam, 'Anatomy Museum: Anthropological and Historical Perspectives', in *Museus, discursos e representações*, ed. Alice Semedo and João Teixeira Lopes (Porto, 2005), pp. 111–34; Elizabeth Hallam, 'Disappearing Museums? Medical Collections at the University of Aberdeen', in *Medical Museums*, ed. Alberti and Hallam, pp. 44–59.

11 R. D. Lockhart, G. F. Hamilton and F. W. Fyfe, *Anatomy of the Human Body* (London, 1959), p. 23.

12 Bronwyn Parry and Cathy Gere, 'Contested Bodies: Property Models and the Commodification of Human Biological Artefacts', *Science as Culture*, XV (2006), pp. 139–58, p. 139.

13 On the cultural significance of skin, see Steven Connor, *The Book of Skin* (London, 2004).

14 For studies that trace and identify some of the dead who were dissected and/or preserved in parts as specimens during the eighteenth and nineteenth centuries, see Simon Chaplin, 'The Divine Touch, or Touching Divines: John Hunter, David Hume and the Bishop of

Durham's Rectum', in *Vital Matters: Eighteenth-century Views of Conception, Life and Death*, ed. Helen Deutsch and Mary Terrall (Toronto, 2012), pp. 222–45; Hurren, *Dying for Victorian Medicine*; Karen Ingham and Simon Chaplin, *Narrative Remains* (London, 2009); Helen MacDonald, *Human Remains: Dissection and Its Histories* (Melbourne, 2005); Ruth Richardson, *The Making of Mr Gray's Anatomy: Bodies, Books, Fortune, Fame* (Oxford, 2008).

15 See Richardson, *Death, Dissection*; Sappol, *Traffic of Dead Bodies*.

16 See D. Gareth Jones and Maja I. Whitaker, *Speaking for the Dead: The Human Body in Biology and Medicine*, 2nd edn (Aldershot, 2009); Margaret Lock and Vinh-Kim Nguyen, *An Anthropology of Biomedicine* (Chichester, 2010); Parry and Gere, 'Contested Bodies'.

17 'Report by Museum Committee, University of Aberdeen', 1920–21, archive of University of Aberdeen, Marischal Museum (UAMM).

18 Lockhart, Hamilton and Fyfe, *Anatomy*, pp. 23–4.

19 On visual images in science and medicine, see Nancy Anderson and Michael R. Dietrich, eds, *The Educated Eye: Visual Culture and Pedagogy in the Life Sciences* (Hanover, NH, 2012); Lisa Cartwright, *Screening the Body: Tracing Medicine's Visual Culture* (Minneapolis, MN, 1995); Catelijne Coopmans et al., eds, *Representation in Scientific Practice Revisited* (Cambridge, MA, 2014); Michael Lynch and Steve Woolgar, eds, *Representation in Scientific Practice* (Cambridge, MA, 1990); Roberta McGrath, *Seeing Her Sex: Medical Archives and the Female Body* (Manchester, 2002); Luc Pauwels, ed., *Visual Cultures of Science: Rethinking Representational Practices in Knowledge Building and Science Communication* (Hanover, NH, 2006); Catherine Waldby, *The Visible Human Project: Informatic Bodies and Posthuman Medicine* (London, 2000). The present book seeks to situate visual images of anatomy, and the ways of seeing they help to form, in relation to material processes of anatomical display involving embodied practices.

20 Prentice, *Bodies in Formation*, p. 112.

21 For anthropological studies of embodied practices in the formation of knowledge, see Mark Harris, ed., *Ways of Knowing: Anthropological Approaches to Crafting Experience and Knowledge* (Oxford, 2007); Tim Ingold, *The Perception of the Environment: Essays on Livelihood, Dwelling and Skill* (London, 2000); Trevor H. J. Marchand, 'Making Knowledge: Explorations of the Indissoluble Relation between Minds, Bodies, and Environment', *Journal of the Royal Anthropological Institute*, XVI (2010), S1–S21.

22 Sandra Dudley, 'Museum Materialities: Objects, Sense and Feeling', in *Museum Materialities: Objects, Engagements, Interpretations*, ed. Sandra Dudley (London, 2010), pp. 1–17, p. 11. See also Fiona Candlin, *Art, Museums and Touch* (Manchester, 2010); Nina Levent and Alvaro Pascual-Leone, eds, *The Multisensory Museum: Cross-disciplinary Perspectives on Touch, Sound, Smell, Memory, and Space* (Lanham, MD, 2014). Helen Rees Leahy, *Museum Bodies: The Politics and Practices of Visiting and Viewing* (Farnham, 2012).

23 Lockhart, Hamilton and Fyfe, *Anatomy*, p. 18.

24 See Elizabeth Hallam, 'Articulating Bones: An Epilogue', *Journal of Material Culture*, XV (2010), pp. 465–92; Prentice, *Bodies in Formation*.

25 For general discussion of archives in the analysis of science as practice, see Soraya de Chadarevian, 'Things and the Archives of Recent Sciences', *Studies in the History and Philosophy of Science*, XLIV (2013), pp. 634–8.

26 On the predominant (though not exclusive) London focus of historical studies of anatomy in Britain, see Piers Mitchell, ed., *Anatomical Dissection in Enlightenment England and Beyond: Autopsy, Pathology and Display* (Farnham, 2012). On analysis of knowledge production in localities that are enmeshed in wider developments, and on the circulation of knowledge, see for example Bruno Latour, *Science in Action: How to Follow Scientists and Engineers through Society* (Milton Keynes, 1987); Soraya de Chadarevian, *Designs for Life: Molecular Biology after World War II* (Cambridge, 2002); Peter Galison, *Image and Logic: A Material Culture of Microphysics* (Chicago, IL, 1997); James A. Secord, 'Knowledge in Transit, *Isis*, XCV (2004), pp. 654–72; David N. Livingstone, *Putting Science in Its Place: Geographies of Scientific Knowledge* (Chicago, IL, 2004).

27 For anthropological discussion of the category 'the body' see Lock and Nguyen, *Anthropology of Biomedicine*.

28 On approaches to material objects in museums, see for example Samuel J.M.M. Alberti, 'Objects and the Museum', *Isis*, XCVI (2005), pp. 559–71; Dudley, *Museum Materialities*; Sandra H. Dudley, ed., *Museum Objects: Experiencing the Properties of Things* (London, 2012); Elizabeth Edwards, Chris Gosden and Ruth B. Phillips, eds, *Sensible Objects: Colonialism, Museums and Material Culture* (Oxford, 2006).

29 Nicholas Thomas, *Entangled Objects: Exchange, Material Culture, and Colonialism in the Pacific* (Cambridge, MA, 1991), p. 125, p. 4.

30 See Alberti, *Morbid Curiosities*; Simon Harrison, *Dark Trophies: Hunting the Enemy Body in Modern War* (Oxford, 2012).

31 For discussions of the material dimensions of deceased bodies, see Zoë Crossland, 'Materiality and Embodiment', in *The Oxford Handbook of Material Culture Studies*, ed. Dan Hicks and Mary C. Beaudry (Oxford, 2010), pp. 386–405; Elizabeth Hallam, Jenny Hockey and Glennys Howarth, *Beyond the Body: Death and Social Identity* (London, 1999); Joanna R. Sofaer, *The Body as Material Culture: A Theoretical Osteoarchaeology* (Cambridge, 2006).

32 Sarah Ferber and Sally Wilde, eds, *The Body Divided: Human Beings and Human 'Material' in Modern Medical History* (Farnham, 2011); Lock and Nguyen, *Anthropology of Biomedicine*.

33 See Penny Harvey et al., eds, *Objects and Materials: A Routledge Companion* (London, 2014); Tim Ingold, *Being Alive: Essays on Movement, Knowledge and Description* (London, 2011); Tim Ingold, *Making: Anthropology, Archaeology, Art and Architecture* (London, 2013); Christopher Tilley with Wayne Bennett, *The Materiality of Stone: Explorations in Landscape Phenomenology* (Oxford, 2004).

34 For anthropological and historical studies of making and materials, see for example Christy Anderson, Anne Dunlop and Pamela H. Smith, eds, *The Matter of Art: Materials, Practices, Cultural Logics, c. 1250–1750* (Manchester, 2015); Myrlem Naji and Laurence Douny, 'Editorial: "Making" and "Doing" the Material World', *Journal of Material Culture*, XIV (2009), pp. 411–32; Hallam and Ingold, *Making and Growing*; Pamela H. Smith, Amy R. W. Meyers and Harold J. Cook, eds, *Ways of Making and Knowing: The Material Culture of Empirical Knowledge* (Ann Arbor, MI, 2014).

35 See Samuel J.M.M. Alberti, 'Anatomical Craft: A History of Medical Museum Practice', *The Fate of Anatomical Collections*, ed. Rina Knoeff and Robert Zwijnenberg (Farnham, 2015), pp. 231–46; Stephen Graham and Nigel Thrift, 'Out of Order: Understanding Repair and Maintenance', *Theory, Culture and Society*, XXIV (2007), pp. 1–25.

36 I am very grateful to Caroline Morris for providing information about these models in August 2007.

37 Umberto Eco, *The Open Work*, trans. Anna Cancogni (London, 1989 [1962]).

38 Martin Kemp, *Visualizations: The Nature Book of Art and Science* (Oxford, 2000), p. 4.

39 Chris Gosden and Chantal Knowles, *Collecting Colonialism: Material Culture and Colonial Change* (Oxford, 2001), pp. 17–18. Tim Ingold, 'Making Culture and Weaving the World', in *Matter, Materiality and Modern Culture*, ed. Paul M. Graves-Brown (London: 2000), pp. 50–71.

40 For discussions of material objects in terms of relations, see Alfred Gell, *Art and Agency: An Anthropological Theory* (Oxford, 1998); Penny Harvey and Hannah Knox, 'Objects and Materials: An Introduction', in *Objects and Materials*, ed. Harvey et al., pp. 1–17.

41 On material aspects of photographs, see Elizabeth Edwards and Janice Hart, eds, *Photographs, Objects, Histories: On the Materiality of Images* (London, 2004).

42 Lars Elleström, ed., *Media Borders, Multimodality and Intermediality* (New York, 2010); Mary Simonson, *Body Knowledge: Performance, Intermediality, and American Entertainment at the Turn of the Twentieth Century* (Oxford, 2013); Sarah Bay-Cheng et al., eds, *Mapping Intermediality in Performance* (Amsterdam, 2010).

43 Elizabeth Hallam, 'Anatomy Display: Contemporary Debates and Collections in Scotland', in *Anatomy Acts*, ed. Patrizio and Kemp, pp. 119–35.

44 Interview, with retired member of teaching/research staff (A) from University of Aberdeen, Anatomy Department (UAAD), by Elizabeth Hallam, 11 May 2007.

45 For discussion of the living body as medium, see Simonson, *Body Knowledge*; Lisa Jean Moore and Mary Kosut, eds, *The Body Reader: Essential Social and Cultural Readings* (New York, 2010).

46 Interview, with retired member of teaching/research staff (A) from UAAD, by Elizabeth Hallam, 11 May 2007.

47 See Simon J. Knell, Suzanne MacLeod and Sheila Watson, eds, *Museum Revolutions: How Museums Change and Are Changed* (London, 2007).

48 The University of Edinburgh's Anatomical Museum is used by medical students, and since 2012 (to date) it has also admitted the general public on one Saturday per month.

49 Sharon Macdonald, *Behind the Scenes at the Science Museum* (Oxford, 2002).

50 Chris Gosden and Frances Larson with Alison Petch, *Knowing Things: Exploring the Collections at the Pitt Rivers Museum, 1884–1945* (Oxford, 2007), p. 5. See also Helen Southwood, 'A Cultural History of Marischal Anthropological Museum in the Twentieth Century', PhD thesis, University of Aberdeen (2003).

51 J. Struthers, 'The Progress of the Medical School', in *Aurora Borealis Academica: Aberdeen University Appreciations, 1860–1889*, ed. P. J. Anderson (Aberdeen, 1899), pp. 212–36, p. 216.

52 Hans Ulrich Obrist (in conversation with Vivian Rehberg and Stefano Boeri), 'Moving Interventions: Curating at Large', *Journal of Visual Culture*, II (2003), pp. 147–60, p. 150.

53 Sophie Forgan, 'Building the Museum: Knowledge, Conflict, and the Power of Place', *Isis*, XCVI (2005), pp. 572–85, p. 580; Tony Bennett, *The Birth of the Museum: History, Theory, Politics* (London, 1995), p. 60. See also Aileen Fyfe and Bernard Lightman, eds, *Science in the Marketplace: Nineteenth-century Sites and Experiences* (Chicago, IL, 2007); David N. Livingstone and Charles W. J. Withers, eds, *Geographies of Nineteenth-century Science* (Chicago, IL, 2011).

54 Peter Galison, 'Peter Galison Interviewed', in *Laboratorium*, ed. Hans Ulrich Obrist and Barbara Vanderlinden (Antwerp, 2001), p. 107. See also Galison, *Image and Logic*.

55 Elizabeth Hallam, 'Laboratoire anthropométrique: la fabrication du savoir sur le corps en Ecosse, de 1880 à 1930' ('Anthropometric Laboratory: Making Knowledge of the Body in Scotland, 1880–1930'), *Ethnologie française*, II (2007), pp. 275–84.

56 Tim Barringer, ed., *Colonialism and the Object: Empire, Material Culture and the Museum* (London, 1998); Gosden and Knowles, *Collecting Colonialism*; Amiria Henare, *Museums, Anthropology and Imperial Exchange* (Cambridge, 2005); Nicholas Thomas, *Colonialism's Culture: Anthropology, Travel and Government* (Cambridge, 1994); Sadiah Qureshi, *Peoples on Parade: Exhibitions, Empire, and Anthropology in Nineteenth-century Britain* (Chicago, IL, 2011).

57 Displayed in the exhibition *About Human Beings: About Being Human*, 1985–95, curated by Charles Hunt. Southwood, 'A Cultural History of Marischal'.

58 William Knight, 'Inventory of the Principal Curiosities Natural and Artificial, Preserved in the Museum and Library of the Marischal College and University of Aberdeen', *c.* 1840, archive of UAMM (MS M106); 'Aberdeen University Museums. The Anatomical Collection', *Aberdeen Journal*, 15 April 1899, p. 4. See Neil G. W. Curtis, 'Thinking About the Right Home – Repatriation and the University of Aberdeen', in *Utimut: Past Heritage – Future Partnerships – Discussions on Repatriation in the 21st Century*, ed. Mille Gabriel and Jens Dahl (Copenhagen, 2007), pp. 44–54. Neil Curtis, '"A Welcome and Important Part of Their Role": The Impact of Repatriation on Museums in Scotland', in *Museums and Restitution: New Practices, New Approaches*, eds Louise Tythacott and Kostas Arvanitis (Farnham, 2014), pp. 85–104.

59 See Cressida Fforde, Jane Hubert and Paul Turnbull, eds, *The Dead and Their Possessions: Repatriation in Principle, Policy and Practice* (London, 2004); Myra Giesen, ed., *Curating*

Human Remains: Caring for the Dead in the United Kingdom (Woodbridge, 2013); Tiffany Jenkins, *Contesting Human Remains in Museum Collections: The Crisis of Cultural Authority* (London, 2011); Laura Peers, 'On the Treatment of Dead Enemies: Indigenous Human Remains in Britain in the Early Twenty-first Century', in *Social Bodies*, ed. Helen Lambert and Maryon McDonald (Oxford, 2009), pp. 77–99.

60 For discussions of contemporary medical museums from anatomists' perspectives, see for example Yehia M. A-H. Marreez, Luuk N. A. Willems and Michael R. Wells, 'The Role of Medical Museums in Contemporary Medical Education', *Anatomical Sciences Education*, III (2010), pp. 249–53.

61 See Samuel J.M.M. Alberti et al., 'Should We Display the Dead?', *Museum and Society*, VII (2009), pp. 133–49.

62 Elizabeth Hallam, 'Death and Diamonds, Paper and Plastic: Two London Exhibitions in 2012', *Mortality*, XVII (2013), pp. 98–103.

63 'Gunther von Hagens' Body Worlds. The Original Exhibition of Real Human Bodies: Past Exhibitions', www.bodyworlds.com, accessed 1 October 2014.

64 Ken Arnold, 'Book Review, Dream Anatomy: A Unique Blend of Art and Medical Science from the National Library of Medicine' (by Michael Sappol), *Medical History*, LII (2008), pp. 433–4, p. 433.

65 Analysis of 'Body Worlds' is extensive; see for example T. Christine Jespersen, Alicita Rodríguez and Joseph Starr, eds, *The Anatomy of Body Worlds: Critical Essays on the Plastinated Cadavers of Gunther von Hagens* (Jefferson, NC, 2009); John D. Lantos, ed., *Controversial Bodies: Thoughts on the Public Display of Plastinated Corpses* (Baltimore, MD, 2011); Dirk vom Lehn, 'The Body as Interactive Display: Examining Bodies in a Public Exhibition', *Sociology of Health and Illness*, XXVIII (2006), pp. 223–51; Tony Walter, 'Body Worlds: Clinical Detachment and Anatomical Awe', *Sociology of Health and Illness*, XXVI (2004), pp. 464–88; Tony Walter, 'Plastination for Display: A New Way to Dispose of the Dead', *Journal of the Royal Anthropological Institute*, X (2004), pp. 603–27.

66 Gunther von Hagens, 'Anatomy and Plastination', in *Prof. Gunther von Hagens' Körperwelten: Fascination beneath the Surface*, ed. Gunther von Hagens and Angelina Whalley (Heidelberg, 2001), pp. 9–37, p. 20.

67 Ibid., p. 20.

68 Von Hagens, 'Anatomy', p. 20, p. 34, p. 13, p. 32; 'Gunther von Hagens' Body Worlds: Body Donation for Plastination', www.bodyworlds.com, accessed 1 October 2014.

69 Von Hagens, 'Anatomy', p. 13, p. 32, p. 33.

70 Juan Valverde de Hamusco, *Historia de la composicion del cuerpo humano* (Rome, 1556). See K. B. Roberts and J.D.W. Tomlinson, *The Fabric of the Body: European Traditions of Anatomical Illustration* (Oxford, 1992).

71 Von Hagens and Whalley, *Prof. Gunther von Hagens' Körperwelten*, p. 268, p. 181.

72 See Christophe Degueurce, *Fragonard Museum: The Écorchés: The Anatomical Masterworks of Honoré Fragonard* (New York, 2011).

73 'Gunther von Hagens' Body Worlds: Questions and Answers, What Does Body Worlds Show?', www.bodyworlds.com, accessed 1 October. 2014.

74 Gunther von Hagens, 'Letter from Gunther von Hagens', *Journal of Plastination*, XXIV (2009–12), pp. 2–22.

75 Stefan Hirschauer, 'Animated Corpses: Communicating with Post Mortals in an Anatomical Exhibition', *Body and Society*, XII (2006), pp. 25–52, p. 41.

76 Institute for Plastination, Heidelberg, Germany, 'Donating Your Body for Plastination', p. 13, brochure download at www.koerperspende.de, accessed 1 October 2014.

77 Von Hagens, 'Anatomy', p. 33.

78 D. Gareth Jones and Maja I. Whitaker, 'Engaging with Plastination: A Cultural and Intellectual Challenge for Anatomists', *Clinical Anatomy*, XXII (2009), pp. 770–76.

79 Jo Revill, 'The Lovely Bones', www.theguardian.com, 23 January 2005.

80 Wendy Moore, 'Hunterian Museum Reopens after a Two Year Closure', *British Medical Journal*, CCCXXX/7485 (2005), p. 214.

81 Simon Chaplin, 'Nature Dissected, Or Dissection Naturalized? The Case of John Hunter's Museum', *Museum and Society*, VI (2008), pp. 135–51.

82 Fay Bound Alberti and Samuel J.M.M. Alberti, 'The Hunterian Museum at the Royal College of Surgeons of England, London, opened 12 February 2005', Media Reviews, *Bulletin of the History of Medicine*, LXXX (2006), pp. 571–73, p. 573; Chaplin, 'John Hunter'.

83 Marguerite Dupree, 'Surgeons' Hall: A Museum in Transition', *The Lancet*, 22 September 2012, p. 1048.

84 Anna Crowe, 'From the Hinterland', in *The Hand That Sees: Poems for the Quincentenary of the Royal College of Surgeons of Edinburgh*, ed. Stewart Conn (Edinburgh, 2005), pp. 31–3, p. 31.

85 Kathleen Jamie, 'Surgeons' Hall', in *Findings* (London, 2005), pp. 129–45, p. 135.

86 Ibid., p. 130.

87 Ibid., p. 140.

88 Ibid., p. 140, p. 142.

89 On Henry Wellcome's collection see Ken Arnold and Danielle Olsen, eds, *Medicine Man: The Forgotten Museum of Henry Wellcome* (London, 2003); Frances Larson, *An Infinity of Things: How Sir Henry Wellcome Collected the World* (Oxford, 2009). Aspects of human anatomy were also displayed in the exhibition *Assembling Bodies: Art, Science and Imagination*, Museum of Archaeology and Anthropology, University of Cambridge, 2009–10; see Anita Herle, Mark C. Elliott and Rebecca Empson, *Assembling Bodies: Art, Science and Imagination* (Cambridge, 2009).

90 Martin Kemp and Marina Wallace, *Spectacular Bodies: The Art and Science of the Human Body from Leonardo to Now*, exh. cat., Hayward Gallery, London (2000), p. 165.

91 Adrian Searle, 'From the Cradle to the Grave', www.theguardian.com, 21 October 2000.

92 Fiona Bradley, 'Introduction', in *Christine Borland: Preserves*, ed. Fiona Bradley (Edinburgh, 2006), p. 4.

93 Michael Tarantino, 'Vulnerable', in *Christine Borland: Bullet Proof Breath*, exh. cat., Art Gallery of York University, Toronto (2002), pp. 9–36.

94 Alfred Gell, 'Vogel's Net: Traps as Artworks and Artworks as Traps', *Journal of Material Culture*, I (1996), pp. 15–38, p. 30.

95 Julian Stallabrass, *High Art Lite: British Art in the 1990s* (London, 1999), p. 25.

96 Sean O'Hagan, 'Hirst's Diamond Creation Is Art's Costliest Work Ever', www.theguardian.com, 21 May 2006. See Damien Hirst, Rudi Fuchs and Jason Beard, *For the Love of God: The Making of the Diamond Skull* (London, 2007).

97 *For the Love of God*, exhibited in 'Beyond Belief' at White Cube, London (2007), Tate Modern's Turbine Hall, London (2012). Tom Sutcliffe, 'For the Love of God: A £50m Work of Art', *The Independent*, 2 June 2007.

98 'Works: *In the Eyes of Others*, Towner the Contemporary Art Museum, Eastbourne, 2009', www.jodiecarey.co.uk, accessed 1 October 2014.

99 Paul Koudounaris, *The Empire of Death: A Cultural History of Ossuaries and Charnel Houses* (London, 2011).

100 On contemporary ritualized disposal and memorialization in Britain, see for example Andy Clayden et al., *Natural Burial: Landscape, Practice and Experience* (London, 2014); Doris Francis, Leonie A. Kellaher and Georgina Neophytou, *The Secret Cemetery* (Oxford, 2005); Jenny Hockey, Kate Woodthorpe and Carol Komaromy, eds, *The Matter of Death: Space, Place and Materiality* (Basingstoke, 2010).

101 C. Nadia Seremetakis, *The Last Word: Women, Death and Divination in Inner Mani* (Chicago, IL, 1991), p. 177. See also Elizabeth Hallam and Jenny Hockey, *Death, Memory and Memorial Culture* (Oxford, 2001); Lambert and McDonald, *Social Bodies*; Lock and Farquhar, *Beyond the Body Proper*.

102 Jack Goody and Cesare Poppi, 'Flowers and Bones: Approaches to the Dead in Anglo-American and Italian Cemeteries', *Comparative Studies in Society and History*, XXXVI (1994), pp. 146–75.

103 Koudounaris, *Empire of Death*; Michael Taussig, 'The Language of Flowers', *Critical Inquiry*, xxx (2003), pp. 98–131.

104 Michael Camille, *Master of Death: The Lifeless Art of Pierre Remiet, Illuminator* (New Haven, CT, 1996), p. 177. Yves Le Fur and Jean-Hubert Martin et al., *"la mort n'en saura rien": Reliques d'Europe et d'Océanie*, exh. cat., Musée national des Arts d'Afrique et d'Océanie, Paris (1999).

105 Le Fur and Martin et al., *"la mort n'en saura rien"*.

106 Two anonymous albums, 1882–5, archive of University of Aberdeen, Anatomy Department (UAAD).

107 Goody and Poppi, 'Flowers and Bones', p. 160, note 39.

108 Charles Bell, *A System of Dissections, Explaining the Anatomy of the Human Body*, vol. 1 (Edinburgh, 1798). On natural history collecting see Kate Hill, '"He Knows Me . . . But Not at the Museum": Women, Natural History Collecting and Museums, 1880–1914', in *Narrating Objects, Collecting Stories*, eds Sandra H. Dudley et al. (London, 2012), pp. 184–95; N. Jardine, J. A. Secord and E. C. Spary, eds, *Cultures of Natural History* (Cambridge, 1996).

109 See Andrea Kunard, 'Traditions of Collecting and Remembering: Gender, Class and the Nineteenth-century Sentiment Album and Photographic Album', *Early Popular Visual Culture*, IV (2006), pp. 227–43; Martha Langford, *Suspended Conversations: The Afterlife of Memory in Photographic Albums* (Montreal, 2001).

110 Kunard, 'Traditions of Collecting', p. 231; Susan Tucker, Katherine Ott and Patricia B. Buckler, eds, *The Scrapbook in American Life* (Philadelphia, PA, 2006).

111 See Hallam and Hockey, *Death, Memory*; Ann Louise Luthi, *Sentimental Jewellery: Antique Jewels of Love and Sorrow* (Princes Risborough, Buckinghamshire, 1998); Deborah Lutz, *Relics of Death in Victorian Literature and Culture* (Cambridge, 2015); Marcia Pointon, *Brilliant Effects: A Cultural History of Gems and Jewellery* (New Haven, CT, 2009).

112 Luthi, *Sentimental Jewellery*; Pointon, *Brilliant Effects*.

113 Geoffrey Batchen, 'Ere the Substance Fade: Photography and Hair Jewellery', in Edwards and Hart, *Photographs, Objects, Histories*, pp. 32–46; Jay Ruby, *Secure the Shadow: Death and Photography in America* (Cambridge, MA, 1995).

114 Audrey Linkman, 'Taken from Life: Post-mortem Portraiture in Britain, 1860–1910', *History of Photography*, xxx (2006), pp. 309–47; Ruby, *Secure the Shadow*.

115 Ruby, *Secure the Shadow*.

116 Stanley B. Burns, *Sleeping Beauty: Memorial Photography in America* (Altadena, CA, 1990).

117 Linkman, 'Taken from Life'; Ruby, *Secure the Shadow*.

118 Pat Jalland, *Death in the Victorian Family* (Oxford, 1996); Julie-Marie Strange, *Death, Grief and Poverty in Britain, 1870–1914* (Cambridge, 2005).

119 Glennys Howarth, *Last Rites: The Work of the Modern Funeral Director* (New York, 1996); Pat Jalland, *Death in War and Peace: Loss and Grief in England, 1914–1970* (Oxford, 2010); Linkman, 'Taken from Life'; Ruby, *Secure the Shadow*.

120 Hallam and Hockey, *Death, Memory*; Hallam, Hockey and Howarth, *Beyond the Body*.

121 See Jones and Whitaker, *Speaking for the Dead*; Nuffield Council on Bioethics, *Human Bodies: Donation for Medicine and Research* (London, 2011); Joanne Wilton, 'An Anatomist's Perspective on the Human Tissue Act 2004', in *Death Rites and Rights*, ed. Belinda Brooks-Gordon et al. (Oxford, 2007), pp. 261–78.

122 See for example A. V. Campbell and M. Willis, 'They Stole My Baby's Soul: Narratives of Embodiment and Loss', *Medical Humanities*, xxxI (2005), pp. 101–4.

123 Richardson, *Death, Dissection*.

124 Elizabeth Hallam, 'Anatomical Bodies and Materials of Memory', in *Death Rites*, ed. Brooks-Gordon et al., pp. 279–98.

125 See Douglas Davies and Hannah Rumble, *Natural Burial: Traditional-secular Spiritualities and Funeral Innovation* (London, 2012); Hannah Rumble et al., 'Disposal or Dispersal? Environmentalism and Final Treatment of the British Dead', *Mortality*, xIx (2014),

pp. 243–60; Tony Walter, 'Three Ways to Arrange a Funeral: Mortuary Variation in the Modern West', *Mortality*, x (2005), pp. 173–92.

126 See Hallam and Hockey, *Death, Memory*; Francis, Kellaher and Neophytou, *Secret Garden*.

127 Andrew Clayden and Katie Dixon, 'Woodland Burial: Memorial Arboretum Versus Natural Native Woodland', *Mortality*, xii (2007), pp. 240–60.

128 Leonie Kellaher, David Prendergast and Jenny Hockey, 'In the Shadow of the Traditional Grave', *Mortality*, x (2005), pp. 237–50. David Prendergast, Jenny Hockey and Leonie Kellaher, 'Blowing in the Wind? Identity, Materiality, and the Destinations of Human Ashes', *Journal of the Royal Anthropological Institute*, xii (2006), pp. 881–98.

129 See Adam Mosley, 'Objects, Texts and Images in the History of Science', *Studies in History and Philosophy of Science*, xxxviii (2007), pp. 289–302.

130 See note 7, above.

131 Personal communication, member of teaching/research staff at UAAD, with Elizabeth Hallam, 20 May 2008. See S. W. Waterston and I. J. Stewart, 'Survey of Clinicians' Attitudes to the Anatomical Teaching and Knowledge of Medical Students', *Clinical Anatomy*, xviii (2005), pp. 380–84.

132 J. C. McLachlan et al., 'Teaching Anatomy without Cadavers', *Medical Education*, xxxviii (2004), pp 418–24; J. Older, 'Anatomy: A Must for Teaching the Next Generation', *The Surgeon: Journal of the Royal College of Surgeons of Edinburgh and Ireland*, ii (2004), pp. 79–90; Debra Patten, 'What Lies Beneath: The Use of Three-dimensional Projection in Living Anatomy Teaching', *Clinical Teacher*, iv (2007), pp. 10–14; F. R. Pryde and S. M. Black, 'Scottish Anatomy Departments: Adapting to Change', *Scottish Medical Journal*, li (2006), pp. 16–20. Ongoing debates among medical and education professionals regarding the teaching of anatomy are published in journals such as *Journal of Anatomy*, *Clinical Anatomy*, *Medical Education* and *Anatomical Record*.

133 On the development of MRI since the 1970s, including John Mallard's influential work at the University of Aberdeen, see Kelly A. Joyce, *Magnetic Appeal: MRI and the Myth of Transparency* (Ithaca, NY, 2008).

134 See Chaplin, 'Nature Dissected'; Lorraine Daston and Katherine Park, *Wonders and the Order of Nature, 1150–1750* (New York, 2001); Paula Findlen, *Possessing Nature: Museums, Collecting, and Scientific Culture in Early Modern Italy* (Berkeley, CA, 1996); Arthur MacGregor, *Curiosity and Enlightenment: Collectors and Collections from the Sixteenth to the Nineteenth Century* (New Haven, CT, 2007).

135 Alexander Ogston, 'Stereoscopic Photographs of Collection of Ethnological Objects, Weapons and other Curiosities, collected by Professor Ogston, Aberdeen', vols i–iii, *c.* 1900–28, archive of UAMM. Carolyn Pennington, *The Modernisation of Medical Teaching at Aberdeen in the Nineteenth Century* (Aberdeen, 1994).

136 Ogston, 'Stereoscopic Photographs'; 'Report by Museum Committee, University of Aberdeen', 1912–13, archive of UAMM.

137 See Christopher Lawrence, 'Medical Minds, Surgical Bodies: Corporeality and the Doctors', in *Science Incarnate*, eds Lawrence and Shapin, pp. 156–201; John Harley Warner, 'The Aesthetic Grounding of Modern Medicine', *Bulletin of the History of Medicine*, lxxxviii (2014), pp. 1–47.

138 Henry Lonsdale, *A Sketch of the Life and Writings of Robert Knox, the Anatomist* (London, 1870), p. 126, p. 127, p. 129.

139 R. D. Lockhart, 'The Art of Learning Anatomy, *The Lancet*, 27 August 1927, pp. 460–61, p. 460.

140 See Macdonald, *Behind the Scenes*. On the entanglement of the social lives of objects, persons and museums, see Kate Hill, ed., *Museums and Biographies: Stories, Objects, Identities* (Woodbridge, 2012).

141 Ogston, 'Stereoscopic Photographs'. On the transfer of privately owned collections to institutional settings, see Alberti, *Morbid Curiosities*; Simon Chaplin, 'Dissection and Display in Eighteenth-century London', in *Anatomical Dissection in Enlightenment*

England and Beyond: Autopsy, Pathology and Display*, ed. Piers Mitchell (Farnham, 2012), pp. 95–114.

142 Arthur Keith, *An Autobiography* (London, 1950).

143 Post-mortem portrait of Elizabeth Lockhart, 1947, by Alberto Morrocco, held by the archive of the Aberdeen Medico-chirurgical Society, Medical School, Foresterhill, Aberdeen (identified by Alexander Adam, Honorary Librarian, November 2005).

144 Interview, with retired member of staff (technician) from UAAD, by Elizabeth Hallam, 19 August 2003.

145 Keith, *Autobiography*, p. 305.

146 Ibid., p. 308.

147 Steven Shapin, 'The Invisible Technician', *American Scientist*, LXXVII (1989), pp. 554–63. See also E. M. Tansey, 'Keeping the Culture Alive: The Laboratory Technician in Mid-twentieth-century British Medical Research', *Notes and Records of the Royal Society*, LXII (2008), pp. 77–95.

148 'Twenty-five Years' Service at the College: Sidney Charles Bartlett, Charles George Bush, Edward John Noon', *Annals of the Royal College of Surgeons of England*, XXX (1962), pp. 205–6, p. 205.

149 Fieldnotes, University of Aberdeen, Anatomy Department (UAAD), 22 April 2009. Note that all references to fieldnotes throughout this book refer to Elizabeth Hallam's unpublished notes made during fieldwork at the University of Aberdeen, Anatomy Department during the period 1999–2009 (see Acknowledgements).

150 Interview, with member of staff (cleaner) at UAAD, by Elizabeth Hallam, 27 March 2009.

151 H. S. Harrison, 'Presidential Address: Ethnology under Glass', *Journal of the Royal Anthropological Institute of Great Britain and Ireland*, LXVII (1937), pp. 1–14, p. 14.

152 Hallam, 'Articulating Bones'. On the interrelation of the material and the metaphorical, see Hicks and Beaudry, *Oxford Handbook*; Christopher Tilley, *Metaphor and Material Culture* (Oxford, 1999).

153 Andreas Vesalius, *De humani corporis fabrica* (Basel, 1543).

154 University of Aberdeen, Suttie Centre for Teaching and Learning in Healthcare, Foresterhill, Aberdeen.

155 John S. Smith, *A Visitor's Guide to Marischal College, University of Aberdeen* (Aberdeen, 1993).

156 On social, cultural and material processes of architectural decay and destruction more generally, see Victor Buchli, *An Anthropology of Architecture* (London, 2013); Tim Edensor, *Industrial Ruins: Space, Aesthetics and Materiality* (Oxford, 2005).

157 'Split in Council Over Marischal College Move', *Press and Journal*, 30 June 2005.

158 Jennifer J. Carter and Colin A. McLaren, *Crown and Gown: An Illustrated History of the University of Aberdeen, 1495–1995* (Aberdeen, 1994); Royal Commission, *Evidence, Oral and Documentary Taken and Received by the Commissioners Appointed by His Majesty George IV, July 23d 1826; and Re-appointed by His Majesty William IV, October 12th, 1830; for Visiting the Universities of Scotland*, vol. IV: *The University of Aberdeen* (London, 1837).

159 'Shock Discovery of 15th Century Skeletons in Aberdeen', STV, www.news.stv.tv, 8 April 2009; 'Archaeologists to Discuss Marischal College Excavations', www.aberdeencity.gov.uk, 5 November 2013.

One Hand and Eye: Dynamics of Tactile Display

1 'Learning Guide to Practical Anatomy: Systems 1, Phase I MBCHB', 2006–7, document for students, University of Aberdeen, Anatomy Department (UAAD), p. 4, p. 9.

2 The few, but significant, museums of medical schools and colleges in Britain that are currently open to the public include: the Anatomical Museum, University of Edinburgh; Museum of Anatomy, University of Glasgow; Hunterian Museum, Royal College of Surgeons of England (RCS); Surgeons' Hall Museum, Royal College of Surgeons of Edinburgh (RCSEd, see Introduction).

3 Staff and students in the Anatomy Museum, University of Aberdeen, among whom I conducted my fieldwork have preferred to remain anonymous in my account and to be referred to instead by the titles of their professional posts/positions in the university.

4 On front and back stage in funeral directors' practices, see Glennys Howarth, *Last Rites: The Work of the Modern Funeral Director* (Amityville, NY, 2996); and in museums see Sharon Macdonald, *Behind the Scenes at the Science Museum* (Oxford, 2002). For analysis of the desk and the table in scientific work, see Bruno Latour and Steve Woolgar, *Laboratory Life: The Social Construction of Scientific Facts* (Princeton, NJ, 1986 [1979]); Bruno Latour, *Pandora's Hope: Essays on the Reality of Science Studies* (Cambridge, MA, 1999).

5 'Learning Guide', 2006–7, p. 4.

6 Ibid., pp. 8–12.

7 Ibid., p. 7, p. 11.

8 On the use of the present tense in anatomy teaching, see Simon Sinclair, *Making Doctors: An Institutional Apprenticeship* (Oxford, 1997).

9 Constance Classen and David Howes, 'The Museum as Sensescape: Western Sensibilities and Indigenous Artifacts', in *Sensible Objects: Colonialism, Museums and Material Culture*, eds Elizabeth Edwards, Chris Gosden and Ruth Phillips (Oxford, 2006), pp. 199–222, p. 208. On the senses in museums, see Fiona Candlin, *Art, Museums and Touch* (Manchester, 2010); Helen J. Chatterjee, ed., *Touch in Museums: Policy and Practice in Object Handling* (Oxford, 2008); Sandra H. Dudley, ed., *Museum Materialities: Objects, Engagements, Interpretations* (London, 2010).

10 See T. Kenny Fountain, *Rhetoric in the Flesh: Trained Vision, Technical Expertise, and the Gross Anatomy Lab* (New York, 2014); Byron J. Good, *Medicine, Rationality and Experience: An Anthropological Perspective* (Cambridge, 1994); Maryon McDonald, 'Bodies and Cadavers', in *Objects and Materials: A Routledge Companion*, ed. Penny Harvey et al. (London, 2014), pp. 128–43; Rachel Prentice, *Bodies in Formation: An Ethnography of Anatomy and Surgery Education* (Durham, NC, 2013); Sinclair, *Making Doctors*.

11 Fieldnotes, University of Aberdeen, Anatomy Department (UAAD), 14 March 2003; 17 November 2006.

12 'Learning Guide', p. 4.

13 On conceptions of the mind's eye, see Eugene S. Ferguson, *Engineering and the Mind's Eye* (Cambridge, MA, 1994); Shigehisa Kuriyama, Expressiveness of the Body and the Divergence of Greek and Chinese Medicine (New York, 2002); Mary S. Morgan and Marcel Boumans, 'Secrets Hidden by Two-dimensionality: The Economy as Hydraulic Machine', in *Models: The Third Dimension of Science*, ed. Soraya de Chadarevian and Nick Hopwood (Stanford, 2004), pp. 369–401; Prentice, *Bodies in Formation*.

14 'Learning Guide', p. 4.

15 Ibid., p. 4.

16 'Guide to Anatomy Facility and Anatomy Learning', 2009–10, document for students, UAAD, p. 7, p. 9.

17 On the cultural definition of the 'normal body' see Margaret Lock and Vinh-Kim Nguyen, *An Anthropology of Biomedicine* (Chichester, 2010).

18 'Learning Guide', 2006–7, p. 7, p. 11. X-rays, MRI and CT scans were 'drawn from clinical cases', some displayed in 'radiology live demonstrations' by practising radiologists, so that students could begin to learn how to interpret these diagnostic images ('Learning Guide', 2006–7, p. 13).

19 'Learning Guide', 2006–7, p. 12.

20 Ibid., p. 8, p. 9.

21 Michael Lynch, 'The Production of Scientific Images: Vision and Re-vision in the History, Philosophy and Sociology of Science', in *Visual Cultures of Science: Rethinking Representational Practices in Knowledge Building and Science Communication*, ed. Luc Pauwels (Hanover, 2006), pp. 26–40, p. 27.

22 'Learning Guide', 2006–7, p. 11.

23 On the embodied learning of anatomy in medical schools, see Prentice, *Bodies in Formation*.

24 'Learning Guide', 2006–7, p. 7.

25 Fieldnotes, UAAD, 24 May 2005.

26 On anatomical terminology, see Ian Whitmore, 'Terminologia Anatomica: New Terminology for the New Anatomist', *Anatomical Record*, CCLVII (1999), pp. 50–53.

27 Keith L. Moore and Anne M. R. Agur, *Essential Clinical Anatomy*, 2nd edn (Philadelphia, PA, 2002), p. 6.

28 Ibid., p. 7.

29 'MBChB Phase 1 – Guidelines for Learning Anatomy', November 2006, document for students, UAAD, n.p.

30 Fieldnotes, UAAD, 19 June 2007.

31 Moore and Agur, *Clinical Anatomy*, p. 4.

32 Stefan Hirschauer, 'The Manufacture of Bodies in Surgery', *Social Studies of Science*, XXI (1991), pp. 279–319, p. 309, p. 310, p. 312. See also Prentice, *Bodies in Formation*.

33 Hirschauer, 'The Manufacture of Bodies in Surgery', p. 309.

34 'Learning Guide', 2006–7, p. 12.

35 For commentary on this painting see Martin Kemp and Marina Wallace, *Spectacular Bodies: The Art and Science of the Human Body from Leonardo to Now*, exh. cat., Hayward Gallery, London (2000).

36 Lorraine Daston and H. Otto Sibum, 'Introduction: Scientific Personae and Their Histories', *Science in Context*, XVI (2003), pp. 1–8, p. 4. See David S. Jones et al., 'Making the Case for History in Medical Education', *Journal of the History of Medicine and Allied Sciences*, Advance Access published 13 November 2014, doi:10.1093/jhmas/jru026, pp. 1–30. On the intersection of historical and medical knowledge in early modern contexts see Nancy G. Siraisi, *History, Medicine and the Traditions of Renaissance Learning* (Ann Arbor, MI, 2007).

37 'Learning Guide', 2006–7, p. 7, p. 8. Fieldnotes, UAAD, 23 May 2008.

38 'Learning Guide', 2006 7, p. 8.

39 Photography of the mortuary at Marischal College was not permitted during my research, but this mid-twentieth-century photograph shows the layout of the body storage facility that was still in place 1999–2009.

40 'Bequest of Bodies for Anatomy: Information for Potential Donors and their Next-of-Kin/Executors', information sheet (May 2008), issued by UAAD, stated that reasons for the refusal of a body include 'a recent history of AIDS, CJD or rapidly progressive dementia, jaundice (i.e. infective forms of hepatitis, but not obstructive or toxic), tuberculosis or leprosy; severe peripheral vascular disease and/or gangrene; severe contraction deformities; gross obesity; severe muscle wastage/emaciation; certain forms of cancer and recent major surgery'.

41 'University of Aberdeen, Declaration of Bequest, Common Consent Form – Universities of Scotland, Anatomy Act 1984 (as amended 2006)', issued by UAAD.

42 'Learning Guide', 2006–7, p. 7, p. 9.

43 Fieldnotes, UAAD, 7 July 2003.

44 Howarth, *Last Rites*, p. 147.

45 Ibid., p. 169. Elizabeth Hallam, Jenny Hockey and Glennys Howarth, *Beyond the Body: Death and Social Identity* (London, 1999).

46 'Learning Guide', 2006–7, p. 9.

47 Fieldnotes, UAAD, 15 November 2006. On widespread attitudes of respect expressed towards the deceased in dissecting rooms, see Joanne Wilton, 'An Anatomist's Perspective on the Human Tissue Act 2004', in *Death Rites and Rights*, ed. Belinda Brooks-Gordon et al. (Oxford, 2007), pp. 261–78.

48 Fieldnotes, UAAD, 23 July 2006.

49 Fieldnotes, UAAD, 15 November 2006.

50 Fieldnotes, UAAD, 16 November 2006.

51 On comparable perceptions of the deceased in anatomical practices, see Meryl Levin, *Anatomy of Anatomy: In Images and Words* (Manchester, NH, 2001); and Christine Montross, *Body of Work: Meditations on Mortality from the Anatomy Lab* (London, 2008).

52 The Institute of Anatomical Sciences was founded in 1984 as an organization for promoting these skills among professionals involved in this field of work in the UK and Ireland.

53 Fieldnotes, UAAD, 7 July 2003.

54 Interview, with retired member of staff (C) from University of Aberdeen, Anatomy Department (UAAD), by Elizabeth Hallam, 17 July 2003.

55 These skulls were transferred from the Anatomy Museum to Marischal Museum (formerly the Anthropological Museum) in 2009 when the Anatomy Department moved to its new building, thereby finally separating the anatomical and the anthropological collections.

56 A. Low, 'Description of a Specimen', *Journal of Anatomy and Physiology*, XXXIV (1900), pp. 452–57.

57 Fieldnotes, UAAD, 24 May 2005.

58 On the use of Meccano pieces for model building in science, see Soraya de Chadarevian, *Designs for Life: Molecular Biology after World War II* (Cambridge, 2002); Soraya de Chadarevian, 'Models and the Making of Molecular Biology' in *Models*, ed. de Chadarevian and Hopwood, pp. 339–68.

59 See Ingrid Schaffner and Matthias Winzen, eds, *Deep Storage. Collecting, Storing and Archiving in Art* (Munich, 1998).

60 See Sinclair, *Making Doctors*.

61 For anthropological studies of dissecting rooms in medical schools, see for example Good, *Medicine, Rationality*; Sinclair, *Making Doctors*.

62 See Lawrence J. Rizzolo, 'Human Dissection: An Approach to Interweaving the Traditional and Humanistic Goals of Medical Education', *Anatomical Record*, CCLXIX (2002), pp. 242–8. Martin Johnson, 'Male Medical Students and the Male Body', in *Body Lore and Laws*, ed. Andrew Bainham, Shelley Day Sclater and Martin Richards (Oxford, 2002), pp. 91–103.

63 'Learning Guide', 2006–7, p. 7.

64 Ibid., p. 7.

65 Ibid.

66 Malcolm Baker, 2000, '"A Sort of Corporate Company": Approaching the Portrait Bust in Its Setting', in *Return to Life: A New Look at the Portrait Bust*, exh. cat., Henry Moore Institute, Leeds, National Portrait Gallery, London, and Scottish National Portrait Gallery, Edinburgh (Leeds, 2000), pp. 18–35, p. 20.

67 Photography of the dissecting room was not permitted during my research, but this 1950s photograph provides a general indication of the room's architecture which was in place 1999–2009.

68 See F. R. Pryde and S. M. Black, 'Scottish Anatomy Departments: Adapting to Change', *Scottish Medical Journal*, LI (2006), pp. 16–20; S. W. Waterston and I. J. Stewart, 'Survey of Clinicians' Attitudes to the Anatomical Teaching and Knowledge of Medical Students', *Clinical Anatomy*, XVIII (2005), pp. 380–84.

69 'Learning Guide to Systems 1, Practical Anatomy, Phase 1 MBChB', 1999, document for students, UAAD.

70 On the social significance of naming, see Gabriele vom Bruck and Barbara Bodenhorn, eds, *The Anthropology of Names and Naming* (Cambridge, 2006). On students renaming the bodies they dissect, see Sinclair, *Making Doctors*, Wilton, 'Anatomist's Perspective'.

71 Ruth Richardson, *Death, Dissection and the Destitute*, 2nd edn (London, 2001), p. 418.

72 'Learning Guide', 1999, p. 17.

73 See Wilton, 'Anatomist's Perspective'.

74 Heidi K. Lempp, 'Perceptions of Dissection by Students in One Medical School: Beyond Learning about Anatomy. A Qualitative Study', *Medical Education*, XXXIX (2005), pp. 318–25, p. 322.

75 Levin, *Anatomy of Anatomy*; Delese Wear, 'Cadaver Talk: Medical Students' Accounts of their Year-long Experience', *Death Studies*, XIII (1989), pp. 379–91; Wilton, 'Anatomist's Perspective'.

76 Hans Hadders, 'Dealing with the Dead Patient at the Intensive Care Unit', *Mortality*, XII (2007), pp. 207–22, p. 215. See Sheila Harper, 'The Social Agency of Dead Bodies', *Mortality*, XV (2010), pp. 308–22.

77 D. Gareth Jones and Maja I. Whitaker, *Speaking for the Dead: The Human Body in Biology and Medicine*, 2nd edn (Aldershot, 2009), p. 42.

78 Prentice, *Bodies in Formation*, p. 257.

79 See Levin, *Anatomy of Anatomy*; Good, *Medicine, Rationality*; Sinclair, *Making Doctors*.

80 Written instructions on dissection were given in a learning guide prepared by the senior anatomy lecturer, and students also used a manual – *Grant's Dissector,* which advises that fingers should be used as much as possible to dissect, then probes, next scissors and lastly scalpels, except when removing skin; see Patrick W. Tank, *Grant's Dissector*, 14th edn (Baltimore, MD, 2009).

81 Moore and Agur, *Clinical Anatomy*, pp. xi–xii.

82 See F. Gonzalez-Crussi, *The Day of the Dead: And Other Mortal Reflections* (San Diego, CA, 1993).

83 J. Older, 'Anatomy: A Must for Teaching the Next Generation', *The Surgeon: Journal of the Royal College of Surgeons of Edinburgh and Ireland*, II (2004), pp. 79–90, p. 81.

84 Tank, *Grant's Dissector*, p. 1.

85 'Learning Guide', 1999, p. 28, p. 54. Detached tissues from a body were placed in a designated container, kept separately from all other bodies, so that a body's parts could be placed together in a coffin on completion of the dissection.

86 See Steven Connor, *The Book of Skin* (London, 2004); Good, *Medicine, Rationality*.

87 'Learning Guide', 1999, p. 17–18.

88 Interview, with retired member of staff (A) from UAAD, by Elizabeth Hallam, 11 May 2007.

89 'Learning Guide', 1999 p. 6; 'Learning Guide', 2006–7, p. 9, p. 4, p. 12. The other systems studied included the musculo-skeletal, alimentary, urinary, endocrine, reproductive, and nervous systems.

90 Tank, *Grant's Dissector*, p. 3.

91 'Learning Guide', 1999, p. 10.

92 'Learning Guide', 2006–7, p. 12.

93 Fieldnotes, UAAD, 23 October 2001.

94 Ibid.

95 Fieldnotes, UAAD, 11 August 2003.

96 Fieldnotes, UAAD, 14 March 2003. On mistakes in learning anatomy see Prentice, *Bodies in Formation*. For an historical perspective on this issue see Sally Wilde and Geoffrey Hirst, 'Learning from Mistakes: Early Twentieth-century Surgical Practice', *Journal of the History of Medicine and Allied Sciences*, LXIV (2009), pp. 38–77.

97 Fieldnotes UAAD, 23 October 2001.

98 'Learning Guide', 2006–7, p. 5. Fieldnotes, UAAD, 24 July 2003.

99 Fieldnotes, UAAD, 2 July 2003.

100 'Learning Guide', 2006–7, p. 8, p. 9.

101 Ibid., p. 27.

102 Fieldnotes, UAAD, 2 October 2007. See John C. McLachlan and Sam Regan de Bere, 'How We Teach Anatomy without Cadavers', *Clinical Teacher*, I (2004), pp. 49–52; J. W. Op Den Akker, A. Bohnen, W. J. Oudegeest and B. Hillen, 'Giving Colour to a New Curriculum: Bodypaint as a Tool in Medical Education', *Clinical Anatomy*, XV (2002), pp. 356–62.

103 Fieldnotes, UAAD, 2 July 2003.

104 'Learning Guide', 1999, p. 83. For an anthropological analysis of stethoscopes, see Tom Rice, 'Learning to Listen: Auscultation and the Transmission of Auditory Knowledge', *Journal of the Royal Anthropological Institute*, XVI (2010), pp. s41–s61.

105　R. Aggarwal, H. Brough, H. Ellis, 'Medical Student Participation in Surface Anatomy Classes', *Clinical Anatomy*, XIX (2006), pp. 627–31, p. 630.

106　Levin, *Anatomy of Anatomy*, p. 52.

107　Ronald Ruskin 'The Anatomy Museum', *Canadian Medical Association Journal*, CLXVIII (2003), pp. 203–4.

108　Debra Patten, 'What Lies Beneath: The Use of Three-dimensional Projection in Living Anatomy Teaching, *Clinical Teacher*, IV (2007), pp. 10–14, p. 11.

109　'Learning Guide', 1999, p. 18.

110　'Learning Guide', 2006–7, p. 7. Fieldnotes, UAAD, 20 November 2002, 2 July 2003.

111　Questionnaire, devised by Elizabeth Hallam, issued at UAAD, December 2001, completed (anonymously) by 182 students.

112　Cristina Grasseni, 'Introduction', in *Skilled Visions: Between Apprenticeship and Standards*, ed. Cristina Grasseni (Oxford, 2007), pp. 1–20, p. 4. On embodied action in the formation of knowledge, see Brenda Farnell, *Dynamic Embodiment: 'I Move Therefore I Am'* (London, 2012); Prentice, *Bodies in Formation*; also see Introduction (this volume) note 21.

113　Paul Connerton, *How Societies Remember* (Cambridge, 1989), p. 74. See also Sabine C. Koch et al., eds, *Body Memory, Metaphor and Movement* (Amsterdam, 2012).

114　See Waterston and Stewart, 'Survey of Clinicians' Attitudes'.

115　Fieldnotes, UAAD, 5 March 2003.

116　During the removal of cupboards in the science laboratory at Marischal College a wax model of a dissected newborn by Maison Tramond was discovered, this room having previously been used as an embryology laboratory (see illus. 21, and illus. 93).

117　Fieldnotes, UAAD, 2 July 2003.

118　'Learning Guide', 2006–7, p. 11.

119　Fieldnotes, UAAD, 14 March 2003.

120　On medical students' reluctance to volunteer as living models at the Guy's, King's and St Thomas's Medical School, London, see Aggarwal, Brough and Ellis, 'Medical Student Participation'.

121　Fieldnotes, UAAD, 9 May 2007.

122　See Connerton, *How Societies Remember*.

123　Questionnaire, devised by Elizabeth Hallam, issued at UAAD, November 2006, completed (anonymously) by 74 students.

124　'Learning Guide', 2006–7, p. 14.

125　Computer-based anatomical images used in relation to further materials in the Anatomy Museum are not the focus here. On virtual anatomy, see for example Thomas J. Csordas, *Body/Meaning/Healing* (Basingstoke, 2002); José van Dijck, *The Transparent Body: A Cultural Analysis of Medical Imaging* (Seattle, WA, 2005); Prentice, *Bodies in Formation*; Catherine Waldby, *The Visible Human Project: Informatic Bodies and Posthuman Medicine* (London, 2000).

126　'Anatomy Department, Inventory', 1969, typescript/MS list, archive of UAAD.

127　The earliest extant specimens on display in the Anatomy Museum were prepared in 1863–89 (e.g. 'UM. 2', dried bones and blood vessels of the hand), and the most recent in 1964 (e.g. a preserved dissection of the hand).

128　'Learning Guide', 2006–7, p. 12.

129　F. Gonzalez-Crussi, *Suspended Animation: Six Essays on the Preservation of Bodily Parts* (San Diego, CA, 1995), p. 119.

130　'Learning Guide', 2006–7, p. 12.

131　Ibid., p. 12.

132　'Learning Guide', 2006–7, p. 7.

133　An additional bay under the sign *Demonstrations* was used as shelving for textbooks as anatomical demonstrations no longer took place in this area.

134　For photographs of displays at the University of Edinburgh's Anatomical Museum, *c.* 2004, see Karen Ingham, *Anatomy Lessons* (Stockport, 2004).

135 For example, late nineteenth-century models from Auzoux, Ziegler and Maison Tramond; and current models by Somso from Adam,Rouilly.

136 For discussion of the relation of embodiment and architectural spaces, see Victor Buchli, *An Anthropology of Architecture* (London, 2013); Paul Connerton, *The Spirit of Mourning: History, Memory and the Body* (Cambridge, 2011).

137 All of the main anatomical systems were represented by the new signs by 2003. Anatomists note the difficulty of organizing a museum fully according to systems rather than regions, as every system spreads throughout the entire body.

138 Fieldnotes, UAAD, 6 November 2001.

139 'Anatomy Department, Inventory', 1985, typescript/MS list, archive of UAAD.

140 See Elizabeth Hallam, 'Anatomical Design: Making and Using Three-dimensional Models of the Human Body', in *Design Anthropology: Between Theory and Practice*, ed. Wendy Gunn, Ton Otto and Rachel Smith (London, 2013), pp. 100–116.

141 Students were encouraged to use anatomy software packages such as *McMinn's Interactive Clinical Anatomy* and *Acland's DVD Atlas of Human Anatomy*.

142 'Learning Guide', 2006–7, p. 11.

143 Ibid., p. 11.

144 Fieldnotes, UAAD, 6 August 2003.

145 'MBChB Phase 1 – Guidelines for Learning Anatomy', document for students, November 2006, UAAD, n.p.

146 Lorraine Daston, 'Taking Note(s)', *Isis*, XCV (2004), pp. 443–8, p. 444.

147 Fieldnotes, UAAD, 14 March 2003.

148 M. Norton Wise, 'Making Visible', *Isis*, XCVII (2006), pp. 75–82, p. 81.

149 Personal communication, member of teaching staff at UAAD, with Elizabeth Hallam, 12 October 2007. For analysis of the social and cultural significance of colour more generally, see Diana Young, 'The Colours of Things', in *Handbook of Material Culture*, ed. Chris Tilley et al. (London, 2006), pp. 173–85.

150 'Learning Guide', 2006–7, p. 12.

151 Moore and Agur, *Clinical Anatomy*, p. 3. On textbook illustrations as 'typifications' based on a range of sources rather than on one single body, see Dawn Woodgate, 'Taking Things Apart: Ovario-hysterectomy – Textbook Knowledge and Actual Practice in Veterinary Surgery', *Social Studies of Science*, XXXVI (2006), pp. 367–97, p. 367.

152 Patten, 'What Lies Beneath', p. 11.

153 'Learning Guide', 2006–7, p. 12.

154 Fieldnotes, UAAD, 6 August 2003, 17 December 2007.

155 Fieldnotes, UAAD, 16 November 2006, August 2002.

156 On 'toys' as a derogatory term applied to eighteenth-century wax models see Anna Maerker, *Model Experts: Wax Anatomies and Enlightenment in Florence and Vienna, 1775–1815* (Manchester, 2011).

157 Sophie Harrison, 'Diary', www.lrb.co.uk, 5 February 2004.

158 Fieldnotes, UAAD, 24 July 2003; 'Learning Guide' 2006–7, p. 11.

159 'Learning Guide', 2006–7, p. 4.

160 For studies, by medical education professionals, of contemporary learning with anatomical models see Wojciech Pawlina and Richard L. Drake, 'Anatomical Models: Don't Banish Them from the Anatomy Laboratory Yet', *Anatomical Education Sciences*, VI (2013), pp. 209–10.

161 'Learning Guide', 2006–7, p. 11.

162 'Learning Guide', 2006–7, p. 7–8.

163 On play in contexts of learning and professional practice, see Grasseni, *Skilled Visions*.

164 Fieldnotes, UAAD, 17 December 2007.

165 'Learning Guide', p. 11, p. 4.

166 'Appendix A: University of Aberdeen, Anatomy Museum, Existing Collections', www.abdn.ac.uk, accessed 1 October 2014. 'Anatomy Department, Inventory', 1969, typescript/MS list, archive of UAAD.

Two Animations: Relics, Rarities and Anatomical Preparations

1 On Vesalius' influential publication, see: Sachiko Kusukawa, *Picturing the Book of Nature: Image, Text, and Argument in Sixteenth-century Human Anatomy and Medical Botany* (Chicago, IL, 2012); Katharine Park, *Secrets of Women: Gender, Generation, and the Origins of Human Dissection* (New York, 2006).

2 On the social and cultural dimensions of gestures in the early modern period, see Michael J. Braddick, 'Introduction: The Politics of Gesture', *Past and Present*, CCIII/suppl. 4 (2009), pp. 9–35, and articles in this themed issue; Jan Bremmer and Herman Roodenburg, eds, *A Cultural History of Gesture from Antiquity to the Present Day* (Cambridge, 1991); Barbara Furlotti, 'The Performance of Displaying: Gesture, Behaviour and Art in Early Modern Italy', *Journal of the History of Collections*, XXVII (2015), pp. 1–13.

3 On lace and Ruysch's anatomical preparations see Marieke M. A. Hendriksen, *Elegant Anatomy: The Eighteenth-century Leiden Anatomical Collections* (Leiden, 2015); Gijsbert M. van de Roemer, 'From *Vanitas* to Veneration: The Embellishments in the Anatomical Cabinet of Frederik Ruysch', *Journal of the History of Collections*, XXII (2010) pp. 169–86.

4 See Juile V. Hansen, 'Resurrecting Death: Anatomical Art in the Cabinet of Dr Frederik Ruysch', *Art Bulletin*, LXXVIII (1996), pp. 663–79; Luuc Kooijmans, *Death Defied: The Anatomy Lessons of Frederik Ruysch*, trans. Diane Webb (Leiden, 2011).

5 See Janis McLarren Caldwell, 'The Strange Death of the Animated Cadaver: Changing Conventions in Nineteenth-century British Anatomical Illustration', *Literature and Medicine*, XXV (2006), pp. 325–57; K. B. Roberts and J.D.W. Tomlinson, *The Fabric of the Body: European Traditions of Anatomical Illustration* (Oxford, 1992); Michael Sappol, *Dream Anatomy*, exh. cat., National Library of Medicine, Bethesda (Washington, DC, 2002); Katharine Park, 'The Life of the Corpse: Division and Dissection in Late Medieval Europe', *Journal of the History of Medicine and Allied Sciences*, L (1995), pp. 111–32; Jonathan Sawday, *The Body Emblazoned: Dissection and the Human Body in Renaissance Culture* (London, 1995).

6 Park, *Secrets of Women*, p. 15. See Caroline Walker Bynum, *The Resurrection of the Body in Western Christianity, 200–1336* (New York, 1995); Andrea Carlino, *Books of the Body: Anatomical Ritual and Renaissance Learning*, trans. John Tedeschi and Anne C. Tedeschi (Chicago, IL, 1999); Katharine Park, 'Holy Autopsies: Saintly Bodies and Medical Expertise, 1300–1600', in *The Body in Early Modern Italy*, ed. Julia L. Hairston and Walter Stephens (Baltimore, MD, 2010), pp. 61–73.

7 Park, *Secrets of Women*.

8 For historical studies of relics, see Martina Bagnoli et al., eds, *Treasures of Heaven: Saints, Relics, and Devotion in Medieval Europe*, exh. cat., the Cleveland Museum of Art, the Walters Art Museum, Baltimore, and the British Museum, London (London, 2011); Alexandra Walsham, 'Introduction: Relics and Remains', *Past and Present*, CCVI/suppl. 5 (2010), pp. 9–36, and articles in this themed volume.

9 Bynum, *Resurrection of the Body*, p. 179.

10 Ibid., p. 326. See Caroline Walker Bynum, *Wonderful Blood: Theology and Practice in Late Medieval Northern Germany and Beyond* (Philadelphia, PA, 2007).

11 See Paul Binski, *Medieval Death: Ritual and Representation* (London, 1996); Caroline Walker Bynum, *Christian Materiality: An Essay on Religion in Late Medieval Europe* (New York, 2011); Park, *Secrets of Women*.

12 See Caroline Walker Bynum and Paula Gerson, 'Body-part Reliquaries in the Middle Ages, *Gesta*, XXXVI (1997), pp. 3–7; Patrick Geary, 'Sacred Commodities: The Circulation of Medieval Relics', in *The Social Life of Things: Commodities in Cultural Perspective*, ed. Arjun Appadurai (Cambridge, 1986), pp. 169–91.

13 George Didi-Huberman, *Ex-voto image, organe, temps* (Paris, 2006); Geary, 'Sacred Commodities'; Megan Holmes, 'Ex-votos: Materiality, Memory and Cult', in *The Idol in the Age of Art: Objects, Devotions and the Early Modern World*, ed. Michael Wayne Cole

and Rebecca Zorach (Farnham, 2009), pp. 159–82; Ruth Richardson, 'Human Remains', in *Medicine Man: The Forgotten Museum of Henry Wellcome*, ed. Ken Arnold and Danielle Olsen (London, 2003), pp. 319–45.

14 Binski, *Medieval Death*; Lorraine Daston and Katharine Park, *Wonders and the Order of Nature, 1150–1750* (New York, 2001).

15 Caroline Walker Bynum, *Fragmentation and Redemption: Essays on Gender and the Human Body in Medieval Religion* (New York, 1991); Bynum and Gerson, 'Body-part Reliquaries'; Cynthia Hahn, *Strange Beauty: Issues in the Making and Meaning of Reliquaries, 400–circa 1204* (University Park, PA, 2012).

16 Daston and Park, *Wonders*.

17 See Cynthia Hahn, 'The Voices of the Saints: Speaking Reliquaries', *Gesta*, XXXVI (1997), pp. 20–31; Cynthia Hahn, 'What Do Reliquaries Do for Relics?', *Numen*, LVII (2010), pp. 284–316.

18 Bagnoli et al., *Treasures*; Amy G. Remensnyder, 'Legendary Treasure at Conques: Reliquaries and Imaginative Memory', *Speculum*, LXXI (1996), pp. 884–906; Ellen M. Shortell (1997) 'Dismembering Saint Quentin: Gothic Architecture and the Display of Relics', *Gesta*, XXXVI (1997), pp. 32–47.

19 Hahn, *Strange Beauty*; Remensnyder, 'Legendary Treasure'.

20 On monstrances and display see Bynum, *Christian Materiality*.

21 Pinacoteca Giovanni e Marella Agnelli, ed., *Quilling: Devotional Creations from Cloistered Orders*, exh. cat., Pinacoteca Giovanni e Marella Agnelli, Torino (Mantova, 2012); Georges Viard, *Ateliers de Couvents: Paperoles, icônes, broderies d'art, dentelles, santons, crèches* (Longres, 2007).

22 Pinacoteca Giovanni e Marella Agnelli, *Quilling*.

23 Park, *Secrets of Women*, p. 213.

24 Ibid., p. 213; Bynum, *Resurrection of the Body*; Katharine Park, 'The Criminal and the Saintly Body: Autopsy and Dissection in Renaissance Italy', *Renaissance Quarterly*, XLVII (1994), pp. 1–33.

25 See Andrea Carlino *Books of the Body*; Andrew Cunningham, *The Anatomist Anatomis'd: An Experimental Discipline in Enlightenment Europe* (Farnham, 2010); Giovanna Ferrari, 'Public Anatomy Lessons and the Carnival: The Anatomy Theatre of Bologna', *Past and Present*, CXVII (1987), pp. 50–106; Tim Huisman, *The Finger of God: Anatomical Practice in 17th-century Leiden* (Leiden, 2009); Àlvar Martínez-Vidal and José Pardo-Tomás, 'Anatomical Theatres and the Teaching of Anatomy in Early Modern Spain', *Medical History*, XLIX (2005), pp. 251–80; Bjørn Okholm Skaarup, *Anatomy and Anatomists in Early Modern Spain* (Farnham, 2015).

26 Antonio Favaro, ed. (1595), quoted in Cynthia Klestinec, 'A History of Anatomy Theatres in Sixteenth-century Padua', *Journal of the History of Medicine and Allied Sciences*, LIX (2004), pp. 375–412, p. 401. See also Cynthia Klestinec, *Theatres of Anatomy: Students, Teachers, and Traditions of Dissection in Renaissance Venice* (Baltimore, MD, 2011).

27 Andreas Vesailus (1538), quoted in Martin Kemp, 'Temples of the Body and Temples of the Cosmos: Vision and Visualization in the Vesalian and Copernican Revolutions', in *Picturing Knowledge: Historical and Philosophical Problems Concerning the Use of Art in Science*, ed. Brain S. Baigrie (Toronto, 1996), pp. 40–85, p. 54. See also Cunningham, *Anatomist Anatomis'd*; Ruth Richardson, *Death, Dissection and the Destitute*, 2nd edn (London, 2001); Sawday, *Body Emblazoned*.

28 Martin Kemp and Marina Wallace, *Spectacular Bodies: The Art and Science of the Human Body from Leonardo to Now*, exh. cat., Hayward Gallery, London (2000), p. 13. See Andrea Carlino, *Paper Bodies: A Catalogue of Anatomical Fugitive Sheets, 1538–1687*, trans. Noga Arikha (London, 1999); Thomas Laqueur, *Making Sex: Body and Gender from the Greeks to Freud* (Cambridge, MA, 1990); Roberts and Tomlinson, *Fabric of the Body*.

29 See Klestinec, *Theatres of Anatomy*; Park, *Secrets of Women*.

30 Cunningham, *Anatomist Anatomis'd*; Klestinec, 'History of Anatomy'; R. Allen Shotwell,

'Animals, Pictures, and Skeletons: Andreas Vesalius's Reinvention of the Public Anatomy Lesson', *Journal of the History of Medicine and Allied Sciences*, Advance Access published 2 March 2015, doi: 10.1093/jhmas/jrv001, pp. 1–24.

31 Carlino, *Books of the Body*; Cunningham, *Anatomist Anatomis'd*; Park, *Secrets of Women*.

32 Carlino, *Books of the Body*; Klestinec, 'History of Anatomy'.

33 Park, *Secrets of Women*, p. 170.

34 See Jonathan Goldberg, *Writing Matter: From the Hands of the English Renaissance* (Stanford, CA, 1990).

35 Carlino, *Books of the Body*; Sawday, *Body Emblazoned*; Luke Wilson, 'William Harvey's *Prelectiones*: The Performance of the Body in the Renaissance Theatre of Anatomy', *Representations*, XVII (1987), pp. 62–95.

36 Park, *Secrets of Women*, p. 26.

37 Andreas Vesalius (1543), quoted in Park, *Secrets of Women*, p. 243.

38 Carlino, *Books of the Body*; Kemp, 'Temples of the Body'; Sappol, *Dream Anatomy*.

39 Glenn Harcourt, 'Andreas Vesalius and the Anatomy of Antique Sculpture', *Representations*, XVII (1987), pp. 28–61, p. 40.

40 Martin Kemp, 'Style and Non-style in Anatomical Illustration: From Renaissance Humanism to Henry Gray', *Journal of Anatomy*, CCXVI (2010), pp. 192–208; Sawday, *Body Emblazoned*; Nancy G. Siraisi, 'Vesalius and Human Diversity in *De humani corporis fabrica*', *Journal of the Warburg and Courtauld Institutes*, LVII (1994), pp. 60–88; Juan Valverde de Hamusco, *Historia de la composición del cuerpo humano* (Rome, 1556).

41 Kemp, 'Temples of the Body', p. 54. Kemp, 'Style and Non-style'.

42 Carlino, *Books of the Body*; Monique Kornell (2000) 'Vesalius's Method of Articulating the Skeleton and a Drawing in the Collection of the Wellcome Library', *Medical History*, XLIV (2000), pp. 97–110; Shotwell, 'Animals, Pictures'.

43 William Harvey (1616–26), quoted in Wilson, 'William Harvey's *Prelectiones*', p. 76.

44 See Huisman, *Finger of God*, Arthur MacGregor, *Curiosity and Enlightenment: Collectors and Collections from the Sixteenth to the Nineteenth Century* (New Haven, CT, 2007). On visitors, see Rina Knoeff, 'The Visitor's View: Early Modern Tourism and the Polyvalence of Anatomical Exhibits', in *Centres and Cycles of Accumulation in and around the Netherlands during the Early Modern Period*, ed. Lissa Roberts (Berlin, 2011), pp. 155–75.

45 Sawday, *Body Emblazoned*, p. 72. See also Tim Huisman, 'Resilient Collections: The Long Life of Leiden's Earliest Anatomical Collection', in *The Fate of Anatomical Collections*, ed. Rina Knoeff and Robert Zwijnenberg (Farnham, 2015), pp. 73–91.

46 Anita Guerrini, 'Alexander Monro *Primus* and the Moral Theatre of Anatomy', *The Eighteenth Century: Theory and Interpretation*, XLVII (2006), pp. 1–18, p. 7. On the display of skeletons, see also Anita Guerrini, 'Duverney's Skeletons', *Isis*, XCIV (2003), pp. 577–603; Anita Guerrini, 'Inside the Chanel House: The Display of Skeletons in Europe, 1500–1800', in *Fate of Anatomical*, ed. Knoeff and Zwijnenberg, pp. 93–109.

47 Gerard Blancken, *A Catalogue of All the Cheifest Rarities in the Publick Theatre and Anatomie Hall of the University of Leyden* (Leyden, 1695); Hansen, 'Resurrecting Death'.

48 Huisman, *Finger of God*.

49 Blancken, *Catalogue*, p. 3, p. 4, p. 7, p. 6, p. 10, p. 8, p. 11. Huisman, *Finger of God*.

50 John Evelyn, *The Diary of John Evelyn*, vol. II, ed. E. S. de Beer (Oxford, 1955), p. 53.

51 Ibid., p. 53.

52 MacGregor, *Curiosity and Enlightenment*.

53 Evelyn, *Diary*, p. 108, entry 10 July 1654.

54 Martin Kemp, '"Wrought by No Artist's Hand": The Natural, the Artificial, the Exotic and the Scientific in Some Artifacts from the Renaissance', in *Reframing the Renaissance: Visual Culture in Europe and Latin America, 1450–1650*, ed. Claire Farago (New Haven, CT, 1995), pp. 175–96, p. 179.

55 See Ken Arnold, *Cabinets for the Curious: Looking Back at Early English Museums* (Aldershot, 2006); Daston and Park, *Wonders*; R.J.W. Evans and Alexander Marr, eds, *Curiosity and Wonder from the Renaissance to the Enlightenment* (Aldershot, 2006);

MacGregor, *Curiosity and Enlightenment*; Dániel Margócsy, *Commercial Visions: Science, Trade, and Visual Culture in the Dutch Golden Age* (Chicago, IL, 2014); Marjorie Swann, *Curiosities and Texts: The Culture of Collecting in Early Modern England* (Philadelphia, PA, 2001).

56 Daston and Park, *Wonders*; MacGregor, *Curiosity and Enlightenment*.

57 Paula Findlen, *Possessing Nature: Museums, Collecting and Scientific Culture in Early Modern Italy* (Berkeley, CA, 1996).

58 Daston and Park, *Wonders*.

59 MacGregor, *Curiosity and Enlightenment*.

60 See Ole Peter Grell, 'In Search of True Knowledge: Ole Worm (1588–1654) and the New Philosophy', in *Making Knowledge in Early Modern Europe: Practices, Objects and Texts, 1400–1800*, ed. Pamela H. Smith and Benjamin Schmidt (Chicago, IL, 2007), pp. 214–32; Valdimar Tr. Hafstein, 'Bodies of Knowledge: Ole Worm and Collecting in Late Renaissance Scandinavia', *Ethnologia Europaea: Journal of European Ethnology*, XXXIII/1 (2003), pp. 5–20; MacGregor, *Curiosity and Enlightenment*.

61 Ole Worm (1639), quoted in Hafstein, 'Bodies of Knowledge', p. 9. See Harold J. Cook, 'Time's Bodies: Crafting the Preparation and Preservation of Naturalia', in *Merchants and Marvels: Commerce, Science, and Art in Early Modern Europe*, ed. Pamela H. Smith and Paula Findlen (London, 2002), pp. 223–47.

62 On early modern automata, see Jonathan Sawday, *Engines of the Imagination: Renaissance Culture and the Rise of the Machine* (London, 2007).

63 MacGregor, *Curiosity and Enlightenment*.

64 Sawday, *Body Emblazoned*, p. 73.

65 Findlen, *Possessing Nature*.

66 Elizabeth Hallam and Jenny Hockey, *Death, Memory and Material Culture* (Oxford, 2001).

67 On transi tombs, see Binski, *Medieval Death*; Kathleen Cohen, *Metamorphosis of a Death Symbol: The Transi Tomb in the Late Middle Ages and the Renaissance* (Berkeley, CA, 1973); Ashby Kinch, *Imago Mortis: Mediating Images of Death in Late Medieval Culture* (Leiden, 2013).

68 Binski, *Medieval Death*.

69 Michael Camille, *Master of Death: The Lifeless Art of Pierre Remiet Illuminator* (New Haven, CT, 1996), p. 172.

70 Michael Camille, 'The Image and the Self: Unwriting Late Medieval Bodies', in *Framing Medieval Bodies*, ed. Sarah Kay and Miri Rubin (Manchester, 1994), pp. 62–99.

71 See Elina Gertsman, *The Dance of Death in the Middle Ages: Image, Text, Performance* (Turnhout, 2010); Sophie Oosterwijk and Stefanie A. Knöll, eds, *Mixed Metaphors: The Danse Macabre in Medieval and Early Modern Europe* (Newcastle upon Tyne, 2011); Tessa Watt, *Cheap Print and Popular Piety, 1550–1640* (Cambridge, 1991).

72 'Memento mori. Remember to die', c. 1640, woodcut reproduced in Watt, *Cheap Print*, p. 252.

73 'The Map of Mortalitie', 1604, broadside reproduced Watt, *Cheap Print*, p. 245.

74 Hallam and Hockey, *Death, Memory*; Nigel Llewellyn, *The Art of Death: Visual Culture in the English Death Ritual, c. 1500–c. 1800* (London, 1991).

75 Carlino, *Books of the Body*; Sappol, *Dream Anatomy*.

76 See Binski, *Medieval Death*; Camille, *Master of Death*.

77 The term 'arborescent skeleton' was used by Charles Baudelaire (1859), quoted in Ellen Holtzman, 'Félicien Rops and Baudelaire: Evolution of a Frontispiece', *Art Journal*, XXXVIII (1978–79), pp. 102–6, p. 103.

78 See Svetlana Alpers, *The Art of Describing: Dutch Art in the Seventeenth Century* (London, 1983); Fred G. Meijer, *Dutch and Flemish Still-life Paintings* (Zwolle, 2003).

79 Huisman, *Finger of God*.

80 Cook 'Time's Bodies'; Cunningham, *Anatomist Anatomis'd*.

81 See Anthony Anemone, 'The Monsters of Peter the Great: The Culture of the St

Petersburg Kunstkamera in the Eighteenth Century', *Slavic and East European Journal*, XLIV (2000) pp. 583–602; Dániel Margócsy, 'Advertising Cadavers in the Republic of Letters: Anatomical Publications in Early Modern Netherlands', *British Journal for the History of Science,* XLII (2009), pp. 187–210; Dániel Margócsy, 'A Museum of Wonders or a Cemetery of Corpses? The Commercial Exchange of Anatomical Collections in Early Modern Netherlands', in *Silent Messengers: The Circulation of Material Objects of Knowledge in the Early Modern Low Countries*, ed. Sven Dupré and Christoph Lüthy (Berlin, 2010), pp. 185–215.

82　Harold J. Cook, *Matters of Exchange: Commerce, Medicine, and Science in the Dutch Golden Age* (New Haven, CT, 2007).

83　On Ruysch's techniques, see F. J. Cole, *A History of Comparative Anatomy: From Aristotle to the Eighteenth Century* (London, 1949); Cunningham, *Anatomist Anatomis'd*; Margócsy, *Commercial Visions.*

84　Roberts and Tomlinson, *Fabric of the Body*, p. 290; Charles Nicholas Jenty (1757), quoted in Cunningham, *Anatomist Anatomis'd*, p. 238. On the cultural meanings of mercury, see Marieke A. Hendriksen, 'Anatomical Mercury: Changing Understandings of Quicksilver, Blood and the Lymphatic System, 1650–1800', *Journal of the History of Medicine and Allied Sciences*, Advance Access published 16 October 2014, doi:10.1093/jhmas/jru030, pp. 1–33. See also Ursula Klein and E. C. Spary, eds, *Materials and Expertise in Early Modern Europe: Between Market and Laboratory* (Chicago, IL, 2010).

85　F. Gonzalez-Crussi, *Suspended Animation: Six Essays on the Preservation of Bodily Parts* (San Diego, CA, 1995), p. 80. See Cole, *History of Comparative Anatomy*; Kooijmans, *Death Defied.*

86　Frederik Ruysch (1701–7), quoted in Margócsy, 'Advertising Cadavers', p. 198. Gijsbert M. van de Roemer, 'From *Vanitas* to Veneration: The Embellishments in the Anatomical Cabinet of Frederik Ruysch', *Journal of the History of Collections*, XXII (2010) pp. 169–86.

87　Charles Nicholas Jenty (1757), quoted in Cunningham, *Anatomist Anatomis'd*, p. 239.

88　Joseph Gaertner, 'An Account of the Urtica Marina', *Philosophical Transactions (1683–1775)*, LII (1761–62), pp. 75–85, p. 76, p. 75. Rina Knoeff, 'Animals Inside: Anatomy, Interiority and Virtue in the Early Modern Dutch Republic', in *The Body Within: Art, Medicine and Visualization*, ed. Renée van de Vall and Robert Zwijnenberg (Leiden, 2009), pp. 31–50. On Rusch's publications relating to his collection, see Margócsy, *Commercial Visions.*

89　For photographs of Ruysch's preparations currently extant in museum collections, see 'The Anatomical Preparations of Frederik Ruysch', website created by the University of Amsterdam (International Ruysch-researchgroup), www.ruysch.dpc.uba.uva.nl, accessed 10 March 2015; Rosamond Wolff Purcell and Stephen Jay Gould, *Finders Keepers: Eight Collectors* (London, 1992).

90　Van de Roemer, '*Vanitas* to Veneration'.

91　Marsha Meskimmon, *Women Making Art: History, Subjectivity, Aesthetics* (London, 2003); Gonzalez-Crussi, *Suspended Animation*; Roberts and Tomlinson, *Fabric of the Body.*

92　Van de Roemer, '*Vanitas* to Veneration'.

93　Cole, *History of Comparative Anatomy.*

94　See Meijer, *Dutch and Flemish Still-life.*

95　On eighteenth-century developments in colour printing and ceroplastics, see Barbara Maria Stafford, *Body Criticism: Imaging the Unseen in Enlightenment Art and Medicine* (Cambridge, MA, 1991). Colour printing in relation to anatomical practices is also discussed in Cunningham, *Anatomist Anatomis'd*; Margócsy, *Commercial Visions.* For historical studies of the cultural significance and value of colour, see Andrea Feeser, Maureen Daly Goggin and Beth Fowkes Tobin, eds, *The Materiality of Colour: The Production, Circulation, and Application of Dyes and Pigments, 1400–1800* (Farnham, 2012).

96　See Cunningham, *Anatomist Anatomis'd.*

97　Stafford, *Body Criticism.*

98 Simon Chaplin, 'John Hunter and the "Museum Oeconomy", 1750–1800', PhD thesis, King's College London (2009); Ferrari, 'Public Anatomy Lessons'; Anita Guerrini, 'Anatomists and Entrepreneurs in Early Eighteenth-century London', *Journal of the History of Medicine and Allied Sciences*, LIX (2004), pp. 219–39; Huisman, *Finger of God*; Klestinec, *Theatres of Anatomy*; Jonathan Reinarz 'The Transformation of Medical Education in Eighteenth-century England: International Developments and the West Midlands', *History of Education*, XXXVII (2008), pp. 549–66.

99 Guerrini, 'Alexander Monro'.

100 Rina Knoeff, 'Moral Lessons of Perfection: A Comparison of the Mennonite and Calvinist Motives in the Anatomical Atlases of Bidloo and Albinus', in *Medicine and Religion in Enlightenment Europe*, ed. Ole Peter Grell and Andrew Cunningham (Aldershot, 2007), pp. 121–43; Van de Roemer, '*Vanitas* to Veneration'; Sappol, *Dream Anatomy*.

101 Govard Bidloo (1685), quoted in Knoeff, 'Moral Lessons', p. 123. See also Margócsy, 'Museum of Wonders'.

102 Sappol, *Dream Anatomy*, p. 28, p. 33.

103 Ludmilla Jordanova, *Sexual Visions: Images of Gender in Science and Medicine between the Eighteenth and Twentieth Centuries* (New York, 1989), p. 48. Jordanova and Sappol advise caution in the use of the term realism with reference to visual images and practices prior to the nineteenth century.

104 Jordanova, *Sexual Visions*, p. 45, p. 65.

105 Fragonard's preparations (produced 1765–1771) were displayed at the veterinary school in Alfort, currently Le Musée Fragonard at l'École nationale vétérinaire d'Alfort. See Jonathan Simon, 'The Theatre of Anatomy: The Anatomical Preparations of Honoré Fragonard', *Eighteenth-century Studies*, XXXVI (2002), pp. 63–79; Jonathan Simon, 'Honoré Fragonard, Anatomical Virtuoso', in *Science and Spectacle in the European Enlightenment*, ed. Bernadette Bensaude-Vincent and Christine Blondel (Aldershot, 2008), pp. 142–58.

106 Marta Poggesi, 'The Wax Figure Collection in "La Specola" in Florence', in *Encyclopaedia Anatomica: Museo Las Specola Florence*, ed. Monika von Düring, George Didi-Huberman and Marta Poggesi (Cologne, 1999), pp. 6–25.

107 Guillaume Desnoues (1705), quoted in R. W. Lightbrown, 'Gaetano Giulio Zumbo – II: Genoa and France', *Burlington Magazine*, CVI (1964), pp. 563–69, p. 565.

108 Lightbrown, 'Gaetano Giulio Zumbo'. On Zumbo's works see Von Düring, Didi-Huberman and Poggesi, eds, *Encyclopaedia Anatomica*.

109 'A Descriptive Catalogue of Rackstrow's Museum' 1782, n.p., Wellcome Library, London (M0013924). Richard D. Altick, *The Shows of London: A Panoramic History of Exhibitions, 1600–1862* (Cambridge, MA, 1978); Maritha Rene Burmeister, 'Popular Anatomical Museums in Nineteenth-century England', PhD thesis, Rutgers University (2000); Matthew Craske, '"Unwholesome" and "Pornographic": A Reassessment of the Place of Rackstrow's Museum in the Story of Eighteenth-century Anatomical Collection and Exhibition', *Journal of the History of Collections*, XXXIII (2011), pp. 75–99; Thomas N. Haviland and Lawrence Charles Paris, 'A Brief Account of the Use of Wax Models in the Study of Medicine', *Journal of the History of Medicine and Allied Sciences*, XXV (1970), pp. 52–75.

110 Advert, *Daily Advertiser* (25 December 1742), quoted in Craske, '"Unwholesome" and "Pornographic"', p. 2.

111 Harvey Cushing, 'Ercole Lelli and His Écorché', *Yale Journal of Biology and Medicine*, IX (1937), pp. 199–213; Rebecca Messbarger, *The Lady Anatomist: The Life and Work of Anna Morandi Manzolini* (Chicago, IL, 2010).

112 Lucia Dacome, 'Waxworks and the Performance of Anatomy in Mid-18th-century Italy', *Endeavour*, XXX (2006), pp. 29–35; Von Düring, Didi-Huberman and Poggesi, eds, *Encyclopaedia Anatomica*; Messbarger, *Lady Anatomist*.

113 Messbarger, *Lady Anatomist*.

114 Lucia Dacome, 'Women, Wax and Anatomy in the "Century of Things"', *Renaissance*

Studies, XXI (2007), pp. 522–50; Rebecca Messbarger, 'As Who Dare Gaze the Sun: Anna Morandi Manzolini's Wax Anatomies of the Male Reproductive System and Genitalia', in *Italy's Eighteenth Century: Gender and Culture in the Age of the Grand Tour*, ed. Paula Findlen, Wendy Wassyng Roworth and Catherine M. Sama (Stanford, CA, 2009), pp. 251–71.

115 Rebecca Messbarger, 'Re-membering a Body of Work: Anatomist and Anatomical Designer Anna Morandi Manzolini', *Studies in Eighteenth-century Culture*, XXXII (2003), pp. 123–54.

116 See George Didi-Huberman, 'Wax Flesh, Vicious Circles', in *Encyclopaedia Anatomica*, ed. Von Düring, Didi-Huberman and Poggesi, pp. 64–74.

117 Dacome, 'Women, Wax and Anatomy', p. 536; Julie V. Hansen and Suzanne Porter, eds, *The Physician's Art: Representations of Art and Medicine*, exh. cat., Duke University Museum of Art, Durham, NC (1999).

118 See M. Lemire (1992) 'Representation of the Human Body: The Coloured Wax Anatomic Models of the 18th and 19th Centuries in the Revival of Medical Instruction', *Surgical and Radiologic Anatomy*, XIV (1992), pp. 283–91; Anna Maerker, *Model Experts: Wax Anatomies and Enlightenment in Florence and Vienna, 1775–1815* (Manchester, 2011); Alessandro Riva et al., 'The Evolution of Anatomical Illustration and Wax Modelling in Italy from the 16th to the Early 19th Centuries', *Journal of Anatomy*, CCXVI (2010), pp. 209–22.

119 Von Düring, Didi-Huberman and Poggesi, eds, *Encyclopaedia Anatomica*; Anna Maerker, '"Turpentine Hides Everything": Autonomy and Organization in Anatomical Model Production for the State in Late Eighteenth-century Florence', *History of Science*, XLV (2007), pp. 257–86; Maerker, *Model Experts*; Renato G. Mazzolini, 'Plastic Anatomies and Artificial Dissections', in *Models: The Third Dimension of Science*, ed. Soraya de Chadarevian and Nick Hopwood (Stanford, CA, 2004), pp. 43–70; Messbarger, *Lady Anatomist*.

120 Nicolas-René Desgenettes (1793), quoted in Mazzolini, 'Plastic Anatomies', p. 48; Maerker, *Model Experts*.

121 For photographs of this model, see Von Düring, Didi-Huberman and Poggesi, eds, *Encyclopaedia Anatomica*, pp. 582–3, detail p. 335. Kemp and Wallace, *Spectacular Bodies*; Rebecca Messbarger, 'The Re-birth of Venus in Florence's Royal Museum of Physics and Natural History', *Journal of the History of Collections*, XXV (2013), pp. 195–215.

122 See Messbarger, 'The Re-birth of Venus'.

123 The model's maker is identified as Clemente Susini, Florence, 1771–1800, by the Science Museum, London (object number: A627043); see the entry 'Clemente Susini (1754–1814)' on the 'Brought to Life: Exploring the History of Medicine' website, www.sciencemuseum.org.uk, accessed 20 January 2015. The undated photograph in illus. 57 shows the model with damage that has since been repaired, see for example Wellcome Images, www.wellcomeimages.org (record number: L0058207), for a more recent photograph of the model showing the restored torso.

124 On Calenzuoli, see Maerker, *Model Experts*.

125 Kemp and Wallace, *Spectacular Bodies*, p. 50.

126 William Hunter, *Two Introductory Lectures, Delivered by Dr William Hunter to His Last Course of Anatomical Lectures* (London, 1784), p. 56. On Hunter's lectures, see Anita Guerrini, 'The Value of a Dead Body', in *Vital Matters: Eighteenth-century Views of Conception, Life, and Death*, ed. Helen Deutsch and Mary Terrall (Toronto, 2012), pp. 246–64.

127 Hunter, *Introductory Lectures*.

128 Craske, '"Unwholesome" and "Pornographic"'.

129 Martin Kemp, '"The Mark of Truth": Looking and Learning in Some Anatomical Illustrations from the Renaissance and Eighteenth Century', in *Medicine and the Five Senses*, ed. W. F. Bynum and Roy Porter (Cambridge, 1993), pp. 85–121, p. 117.

130 Hunter, *Introductory Lectures*, p. 64, p. 65.

131 On this atlas, see Roberta McGrath, *Seeing Her Sex: Medical Archives and the Female Body* (Manchester, 2002); Deanna Petherbridge and Ludmilla Jordanova, *The Quick and the Dead: Artists and Anatomy*, exh. cat., Hayward Gallery, London (1997).

132 William Hunter (1774), quoted in Kemp and Wallace, *Spectacular Bodies*, p. 44.

133 William Hunter (1774), quoted in Ludmilla J. Jordanova, 'Gender, Generation and Science: William Hunter's Obstetrical Atlas', *William Hunter and the Eighteenth-century Medical World*, ed. W. F. Bynum and Roy Porter (Cambridge, 2002), pp. 385–413, p. 394.

134 Kemp, '"The Mark of Truth"', pp. 113–14.

135 John Bell, *Engravings of the Bones, Muscles, and Joints, Illustrating the First Volume of The Anatomy of the Human Body*, 2nd edn (London, 1804), p. vi. See Sappol, *Dream Anatomy*.

136 Charles Bell, *Engravings of the Arteries; Illustrating the Second Volume of The Anatomy of the Human Body* (Philadelphia, PA, 1812), p. v.

137 Table VI, in William Hunter, *Anatomia Uteri Humani Gravidi Tabulis Illustrata [The Anatomy of the Human Gravid Uterus Exhibited in Figures]* (Birmingham, 1774). See Jordanova, 'Gender, Generation and Science'.

138 Lorraine Daston and Peter Galison, *Objectivity* (New York, 2007).

139 William Hunter, *An Anatomical Description of the Human Gravid Uterus and Its Contents. By the Late William Hunter MD* (London, 1794), p. 45. See Daston and Galison, *Objectivity*.

140 Hunter, *Introductory Lectures*, p. 56. See N. A. McCulloch, D. Russell and S. W. McDonald, 'William Hunter's Casts of the Gravid Uterus at the University of Glasgow', *Clinical Anatomy*, XIV (2001), pp. 210–17.

141 Hunter, *Introductory Lectures*, p. 56.

142 William Hunter (undated), quoted in Alice J. Marshall, *Catalogue of the Anatomical Preparations of Dr William Hunter in the Museum of the Anatomy Department* (Glasgow, 1970), p. 661.

143 On connections between anatomists' practices of dissecting and casting, see Chaplin, 'John Hunter'.

144 Hunter, *Introductory Lectures*, p. 56

145 See McCulloch, Russell, and McDonald, 'William Hunter's Casts'.

146 Hunter, *Introductory Lectures*, p. 87.

147 On connections anatomists made between models, preparations and live patients, see Chaplin, 'John Hunter'.

148 William Hunter (1775), quoted in McCulloch, Russell and McDonald, 'William Hunter's Casts', p. 216. Hunter showed students 'real preparations' of the gravid uterus along with cast plaster of Paris versions, see McCulloch, Russell and McDonald, 'William Hunter's Casts', p. 210.

149 Lawrence Keppie, *William Hunter and the Hunterian Museum in Glasgow, 1807–2007* (Edinburgh, 2007). On Hunter's currently extant casts that correspond with plates in the *Gravid Uterus*, see McCulloch, Russell and McDonald, 'William Hunter's Casts'.

150 Jordanova, 'Gender, Generation and Science', p. 406.

151 Preserved foetus, catalogued as: '48. 117. The Amnion', Hunterian Collection, University of Glasgow, Museum of Anatomy. Photographs of William Hunter's collection can be viewed at 'Hunterian Online Photo Library', www.hopl.gla.ac.uk, accessed 2 March 2015.

152 Hunter, *Anatomical Description*, p. 54, p. 42. On eighteenth-century interests in organic layering, see Jordanova, *Sexual Visions*.

153 Hunter, *Introductory Lectures*, p. 55.

154 Ibid., p. 89, p. 57.

155 Hunter, *Introductory Lectures*, p. 57. On changing collecting practices and definitions of 'rarities' see Chaplin, 'John Hunter'.

156 Marshall, *Catalogue of the Anatomical Preparations*, p. 694.

157 Hunter, *Introductory Lectures*, p. 56.

158 Hunter, *Anatomical Description*, p. 17.

159 Ibid., p. 41.

160 Ibid., p. 17.

161 See Chaplin, 'John Hunter'.

162 Ibid.; Richardson, *Death, Dissection*.

163 Chaplin, 'John Hunter'; Keppie, *William Hunter*.

164 Hunter, *Introductory Lectures*, p. 112, p. 113. For analysis of the cultural meanings of curiosity, see Nicholas Thomas, *Entangled Objects: Exchange, Material Culture, and Colonialism in the Pacific* (Cambridge, MA, 1991).

165 'Rackstrow's Museum', *Morning Chronicle and London Advertiser*, 15 May 1775, p. 3. See Altick, *Shows of London*; Craske, '"Unwholesome" and "Pornographic"'.

166 Johann Christian Fabricius (1782), quoted in Keppie, *William Hunter*, p. 25. Chaplin, 'John Hunter'.

167 Hunter, *Introductory Lectures*, p. 90.

168 Ibid.; Susan C. Lawrence, *Charitable Knowledge: Hospital Pupils and Practitioners in Eighteenth-century London* (Cambridge, 1996); Piers D. Mitchell et al., 'The Study of Anatomy in England from 1700 to the early 20th Century', *Journal of Anatomy*, CCXIX (2011), pp. 91–9; Lynda Payne, *With Words and Knives: Learning Medical Dispassion in Early Modern England* (Aldershot, 2007).

169 Hunter, *Introductory Lectures*, p. 90, p. 88, p. 89; John Fothergill (1768), quoted in Keppie, *William Hunter*, p. 22. Chaplin, 'John Hunter'; Guerrini, 'Value of a Dead Body'; Lawrence, *Charitable Knowledge*; Richardson, *Death, Dissection*.

170 Hunter, *Two Introductory Lectures*, p. 57. See Simon Chaplin, 'Dissection and Display in Eighteenth-century London', in *Anatomical Dissection in Enlightenment England and Beyond: Autopsy, Pathology and Display*, ed., Piers Mitchell (Farnham, 2012), pp. 95–114.

171 For example, illustrations in Francis Sibson, *Medical Anatomy: Or, Illustrations of the Relative Position and Movements of the Internal Organs* (London, 1869), and anatomical models by Joseph Towne. For analysis of Towne's models 1826–79, see Samuel J.M.M. Alberti, 'Wax Bodies: Art and Anatomy in Victorian Medical Museums', *Museum History Journal*, II (2009), pp. 7–36; R. Ballestriero, 'Anatomical Models and Wax Venuses: Art Masterpieces or Scientific Craft Works?', *Journal of Anatomy*, CCXVI (2010), pp. 223–34; Kemp and Wallace, *Spectacular Bodies*.

Three Nerve Centre: Museum Formation I

1 William Hunter, *Two Introductory Lectures, Delivered by Dr William Hunter to His Last Course of Anatomical Lectures* (London, 1784), p. 57.

2 See Samuel J.M.M. Alberti, *Morbid Curiosities: Medical Museums in Nineteenth-century Britain* (Oxford, 2011); Samuel J.M.M. Alberti and Elizabeth Hallam, eds, *Medical Museums: Past, Present, Future* (London, 2013); Tony Bennett, *The Birth of the Museum: History, Theory, Politics* (London, 1995); Sharon Macdonald, ed., *The Politics of Display: Museums, Science, Culture* (London, 1998); Carla Yanni, *Nature's Museums: Victorian Science and the Architecture of Display* (London, 1999).

3 See Simon Chaplin, 'John Hunter and the "Museum Oeconomy", 1750–1800', PhD thesis, King's College London (2009); Elizabeth Hurren, *Dying for Victorian Medicine: English Anatomy and Its Trade in the Dead Poor, c. 1834–1929* (London, 2012); Fiona Hutton, *The Study of Anatomy in Britain, 1700–1900* (London, 2013); Piers D. Mitchell et al., 'The Study of Anatomy in England from 1700 to the early 20th Century', *Journal of Anatomy*, CCXIX (2011), pp. 91–9; Ruth Richardson, *Death, Dissection and the Destitute*, 2nd edn (London, 2001); Keir Waddington, *Medical Education at St Bartholomew's Hospital, 1123–1995* (Woodbridge, Suffolk, 2003).

4 Alberti, *Morbid Curiosities*; Jonathan Reinarz, 'The Age of Museum Medicine: The Rise and Fall of the Medical Museum of Birmingham's School of Medicine', *Social History of*

Medicine, XVIII (2005), pp. 419–37; Michael Sappol, *A Traffic of Dead Bodies: Anatomy and Embodied Social Identity in Nineteenth-century America* (Princeton, NJ, 2002); also see Introduction (this volume) note 4.

5 Tony Bennett, *Pasts beyond Memory: Evolution, Museums, Colonialism* (London, 2004); Pratik Chakrabarti, *Medicine and Empire, 1600–1960* (Basingstoke, 2014); Annie E. Coombes, *Reinventing Africa: Museums, Material Culture and the Popular Imagination in Late Victorian and Edwardian England*; Amiria Henare, *Museums, Anthropology and Imperial Exchange* (Cambridge, 2005); John M. MacKenzie, *Museums and Empire: Natural History, Human Cultures and Colonial Identities* (Manchester, 2010).

6 Marjory Harper, *Adventurers and Exiles: The Great Scottish Exodus* (London, 2003); John D. Hargreaves, *Academe and Empire: Some Overseas Connections of Aberdeen University, 1860–1970* (Aberdeen, 1994); Lawrence Keppie, *William Hunter and the Hunterian Museum in Glasgow, 1807–2007* (Edinburgh, 2007).

7 Chris Gosden and Chantal Knowles, *Collecting Colonialism: Material Culture and Colonial Change* (Oxford, 2001), p. 4, p. 23.

8 Nicholas Thomas, *Entangled Objects: Exchange, Material Culture and Colonialism in the Pacific* (Cambridge, MA, 1991).

9 Ian Hodder, 'Human-thing Entanglement: Towards an Integrated Archaeological Perspective', *Journal of the Royal Anthropological Institute*, XVII (2011), pp. 154–77.

10 Arthur Keith, *An Autobiography* (London, 1950), pp. 299–300.

11 J. Arthur Thomson, 'The Evolution of Museums', in *The North-east: The Land and Its People*, ed. J. Arthur Thomson et al. (Aberdeen, 1930), pp. 13–16, p. 16. See Helen Southwood, 'A Cultural History of Marischal Anthropological Museum in the Twentieth Century', PhD thesis, University of Aberdeen (2003).

12 W. H. Flower, *Diagrams of the Nerves of the Human Body, Exhibiting Their Origin, Divisions and Connections, with Their Distributions to the Various Regions of the Cutaneous Surface and to All the Muscles*, 2nd edn (London, 1872). The copy held by the University of Aberdeen, Anatomy Museum is stamped on title page: 'Anatomy Class, Aberdeen University, J. Struthers, Professor'.

13 J. Arthur Thomson, *Introduction to Science* (London, 1911), p. 30, p. 178.

14 On nineteenth-century metaphors used to describe nerves, see Laura Otis, *Networking: Communicating with Bodies and Machines in the Nineteenth Century* (Ann Arbor, MI, 2001).

15 'Catalogue of Miscellaneous Articles, as Arranged in Old Museum, 1847–48' (Banchory House), MS list, archive of University of Aberdeen, Marischal Museum (UAMM).

16 Ibid.; 'General Catalogue of Banchory House Museum', 1862, n. pag., MS list, archive of UAMM.

17 Keppie, *William Hunter*; Arthur MacGregor, *Curiosity and Enlightenment: Collectors and Collections from the Sixteenth to the Nineteenth Century* (New Haven, CT, 2007); Susan Pearce, 'Bodies in Exile: Egyptian Mummies in the Early Nineteenth Century and Their Cultural Implications', in *Displaced Persons: Conditions of Exile in European Culture*, ed. Sharon Ouditt (Aldershot, 2002), pp. 54–72; Christina Riggs, *Unwrapping Ancient Egypt* (London, 2014).

18 Minute Book, 1816–55, p. 77, records of Aberdeen Medico-Chirurgical Society (AMCS) (AMCS/1/1/1/18), catalogued by University of Aberdeen, Special Collections; Human skulls, collection of University of Aberdeen, Anatomy Museum (UAAM), museum labels undated.

19 *Catalogue of the Exhibition of Objects Illustrative of the Fine Arts, Natural History, Philosophy, Machinery, Manufactures, Antiquities, Curiosities, &c. in connection with The Aberdeen Mechanics' Institution, 1840*, 4th edn (Aberdeen, 1840).

20 *Catalogue of the Exhibition*, title page.

21 Sydney Wood, 'Education', in *Aberdeen, 1800–2000: A New History*, ed. W. Hamish Fraser and Clive H. Lee (East Linton, 2000), pp. 323–47.

22 'Aberdeen Mechanics' Institution . . ., Exhibition of Articles in The Fine Arts, Natural History, Experimental Philosophy, Antiquities, &c.', *Aberdeen Journal*, 2 September 1840, p. 2.

23 *Catalogue of the Exhibition*, title page, p. 36. For analysis of 'curiosities' as a cultural category, see Macgregor, *Curiosity and Enlightenment*; Thomas, *Entangled Objects*.

24 *Catalogue of the Exhibition*, p. 36, p. 37, p. 38. On the collection and display of material objects from New Zealand, see Henare, *Museums, Anthropology and Imperial Exchange*; Steven Hooper, *Pacific Encounters: Art and Divinity in Polynesia, 1760–1860* (London, 2006); Conal McCarthy, *Exhibiting Maori: A History of Colonial Cultures of Display* (Oxford, 2007).

25 Pennington, *The Modernisation of Medical Teaching at Aberdeen in the Nineteenth Century* (Aberdeen, 1994).

26 On university collections see Marta C. Lourenço, 'Between Two Worlds: The Distinct Nature and Contemporary Significance of University Museums and Collections in Europe', PhD thesis, Conservatoire National des Arts et Métiers, Paris (2005); Macgregor, *Curiosity and Enlightenment*.

27 Macgregor, *Curiosity and Enlightenment*.

28 King's College was founded in 1495, Marischal College in 1593, and the 1860 fusion formed the united University of Aberdeen; see Jennifer J. Carter and Colin A. McLaren, *Crown and Gown: An Illustrated History of Aberdeen* (Aberdeen, 1994); Fraser and Lee, eds, *Aberdeen, 1800–2000*.

29 'Appendix, Part 1' (1754), in Royal Commission, *Evidence, Oral and Documentary Taken and Received by the Commissioners Appointed by His Majesty George IV, July 23d, 1826; and Re-appointed by His Majesty William IV, October 12th, 1830; for Visiting the Universities of Scotland*, vol. IV: *The University of Aberdeen* (London, 1837), p. 178. See also Carter and McLaren, *Crown and Gown*; Neil Curtis, 'A History of the University of Aberdeen and Its Museums', *A Handbook for Academic Museums: Exhibitions and Education*, ed. Stephanie S. Jandl and Mark S. Gold (Edinburgh, 2012), pp. 62–86.

30 Paul B. Wood, *The Aberdeen Enlightenment: The Arts Curriculum in the Eighteenth Century* (Aberdeen, 1993).

31 John Stuart, *Essays, Chiefly on Scottish Antiquities* (Aberdeen, 1846 [1798]), p. 29. Wood, *Aberdeen Enlightenment*.

32 John S. Reid, 'Scientific Apparatus of Professor Patrick Copland of Marischal College, Aberdeen' (2004), University of Aberdeen, Natural Philosophy Collection website, www.abdn.ac.uk, accessed 4 November 2014. On Copland's teaching, see Wood, *Aberdeen Enlightenment*.

33 John S. Reid, 'Head of Despair', *Viewpoint: Newsletter of the British Society for the History of Science*, XCII (2010), p. 6.

34 Stuart, *Essays*, p. 31. William Knight, 'The Marischal College and University of Aberdeen', in *The New Statistical Account of Scotland by the Ministers of the Respective Parishes*, vol. XII: *Aberdeen* (Edinburgh, 1845), pp. 1163–92; 'Order LXI', in *Evidence, Oral and Documentary*, pp. 303–4.

35 William Knight, evidence given 19 September 1827, in *Evidence, Oral and Documentary*.

36 Knight, 'The Marischal College and University of Aberdeen', p. 1185; 'List of Some of the Curiosities in the Museum of Marischal College', 26 April 1833, n. pag., MS list, archive of UAMM. 'Order LXI', in *Evidence, Oral and Documentary*, pp. 303–04.

37 William Knight, 'Inventory of the Principal Curiosities Natural and Artificial, Preserved in the Museum and Library of the Marischal College and University of Aberdeen', *c.* 1840, archive of UAMM (MS M106).

38 Donated 1823, see Knight, 'Inventory of the Principal Curiosities', n. pag.

39 On footbinding, see Dorothy Ko, *Cinderella's Sisters: A Revisionist History of Footbinding* (Berkeley, CA, 2005).

40 Knight, 'Inventory of the Principal Curiosities', n. pag. See Charles Hunt, *Shark Tooth and Stone Blade: Pacific Island Art from the University of Aberdeen*, exh. cat., Anthropological Museum, Marischal College, University of Aberdeen (Aberdeen, *c.* 1982).

41 Knight, 'Inventory of the Principal Curiosities', n. pag.

42 Ibid., n. pag.

43 David M. Walker, 'The Rebuilding of King's and Marischal Colleges, 1723–1889', *Aberdeen University Review*, LV (1993), pp. 123–45. At the fusion of King's College and Marischal College in 1860 items of natural history at King's were transferred to the Natural History Museum at Marischal, and some artefacts in the latter were probably moved to King's College's Archaeological Museum. See Charles Michie, *Catalogue of Antiquities in the Archaeological Museum of King's College, University of Aberdeen* (Aberdeen, 1887); Southwood, 'Cultural History of Marischal'.

44 Hugh McPherson, evidence given 17 September 1827, in *Evidence, Oral and Documentary*, p. 29.

45 Charles Skene, evidence given 19 September 1827, in *Evidence, Oral and Documentary*. See Pennington, *Modernisation of Medical Teaching*.

46 Alexander Ewing, evidence given 20 September 1827, in *Evidence, Oral and Documentary*, p. 113.

47 Ibid., p. 112.

48 Skene, ibid., p. 70

49 Ewing, ibid., p. 114.

50 J. Struthers, *Historical Sketch of the Edinburgh Anatomical School* (Edinburgh, 1867), p. 50. See also Dawn Kemp with Sara Barnes, *Surgeons' Hall: A Museum Anthology* (Edinburgh, 2009). Violet Tansey and D.E.C. Mekie, *The Museum of the Royal College of Surgeons of Edinburgh* (Edinburgh, 1982).

51 Keppie, *William Hunter*.

52 J. Laskey, *A General Account of the Hunterian Museum, Glasgow: Including Historical and Scientific Notices of the Various Objects of Art, Literature, Natural History, Anatomical Preparations, Antiquities, &c. in that Celebrated Collection* (Glasgow, 1813), p. v.

53 Keppie, *William Hunter*.

54 On the wider 'cartography' of anatomical and pathological collecting in Britain, see Alberti, *Morbid Curiosities*.

55 Thomas Hodgkin, *Catalogue of the Preparations in the Anatomical Museum of Guy's Hospital* (London, 1829), p. iii.

56 *Brookesian Museum. The Museum of Joshua Brookes, Esq. FRS, FLS, Blenheim Street, Great Marlborough Street. Consists of a Collection of Anatomical & Zoological Preparations* (London, 1828). On the auction of anatomical collections see Alberti, *Morbid Curiosities*; Chaplin, 'John Hunter'.

57 Dissection was legally permitted in Britain from the early sixteenth century onwards (from 1506 in Scotland, and from 1540 in England), and the 1752 Murder Act made provision for bodies of executed murderers to be dissected without subsequent burial, see Richardson, *Death, Dissection*. On the 1832 Anatomy Act and its effects, see also Elizabeth T. Hurren, *Dying for Victorian Medicine*; Hutton, *Study of Anatomy*.

58 Privy Council (*c.* 1636), quoted in G.A.G. Mitchell, 'Anatomical and Resurrectionist Activities in Northern Scotland', *Journal of the History of Medicine and Allied Sciences*, IV (1949), pp. 417–30, p. 418.

59 John Scott Riddell, *The Records of the Aberdeen Medico-chirurgical Society from 1789 to 1922* (Aberdeen, 1922); Mitchell cites evidence of resurrectionist activity in the Aberdeen Medico-Chirurgical Society's records from 1800 to 1832, see Mitchell, 'Anatomical and Resurrectionist Activities'. On resurrectionism in Britain see Chaplin, 'John Hunter'; Hutton, *Study of Anatomy*; Helen MacDonald, *Human Remains: Dissection and its Histories* (New Haven, CT, 2006); Richardson, *Death, Dissection*.

60 Minute Book, 1816–55, p. 45, records of AMCS (AMCS/1/1/1/18).

61 Martyn L. Gorman, 'Scottish Echoes of the Resurrection Men', M.Litt. thesis, University of Aberdeen (2010).

62 See A. W. Bates, *The Anatomy of Robert Knox: Murder, Mad Science and Medical Regulation in Nineteenth-century Edinburgh* (Brighton, 2010); Helen MacDonald, *Possessing the Dead: The Artful Science of Anatomy* (Melbourne, 2010); Richardson, *Death, Dissection*.

63 'Destruction of the Theatre of Anatomy, St Andrew's Street', *Aberdeen Journal*, 21 December 1831, p. 3. See Pennington, *Modernisation of Medical Teaching*.

64 Alberti, *Morbid Curiosities*; Sean Burrell and Geoffrey Gill, 'The Liverpool Cholera Epidemic of 1832 and Anatomical Dissection: Medical Mistrust and Civil Unrest', *Journal of the History of Medicine and Allied Sciences*, LX (2005), pp. 478–98; Richardson, *Death, Dissection*; Mark Weatherall, *Gentlemen, Scientists and Doctors: Medicine at Cambridge, 1800–1940* (Woodbridge, 2000).

65 Caroline Walker Bynum, *Fragmentation and Redemption: Essays on Gender and the Human Body in Medieval Religion* (New York, 1991); Lucia Dacome, 'Resurrecting by Numbers in Eighteenth-century England', *Past and Present*, CXCIII (2006), pp. 73–110; Richardson, *Death, Dissection*.

66 'An Act for Regulating Schools of Anatomy', 1 August 1832 (2&3 Gul. IV c.75); Hurren, *Dying for Victorian Medicine*; Helen MacDonald, 'Procuring Corpses: The English Anatomy Inspectorate, 1842 to 1858', *Medical History*, LIII (2009), pp. 379–96; Richardson, *Death, Dissection*.

67 Anatomy Act Committee Minutes, Aberdeen, vol. I, 1856–1959, p. 19, University of Aberdeen, Special Collections (UASC) (MSU 1332/4/1/1). See Elizabeth Hallam, 'Anatomical Bodies and Materials of Memory', in *Death Rites and Rights*, ed. Belinda Brooks-Gordon et al. (Oxford, 2007), pp. 279–98.

68 In the 1850s the majority of medical students in Aberdeen attended Marischal College, which had the advantage of being located near to the Aberdeen Royal Infirmary, see Anatomy Act Committee Minutes, vol. I, p. 42, p. 57; Pennington, *Modernisation of Medical Teaching*.

69 Anatomy Act Committee Minutes, vol. I, p. 80; Anatomy Act Committee cash book, Aberdeen, 1833–53, UASC (MSU 1332/4/2/1); Register of Bodies Brought to the Parochial Burying House, Aberdeen, 1843–1921, UASC (MSU 1332/4/3/1). See Hallam, 'Anatomical Bodies'. On Footdee Cemetery (Churchyard), see Robert Wilson, *An Historical Account and Delineation of Aberdeen* (Aberdeen, 1822).

70 'An Act for Regulating Schools of Anatomy', section XIII.

71 Richardson, *Death, Dissection*.

72 Anatomy Act Committee Minutes, vol. I, p. 48, p. 41.

73 Human skulls, collection of UAAM, museum labels dated 1835 and 1857.

74 Londa Schiebinger, 'The Anatomy of Difference: Race and Sex in Eighteenth-century Science', *Eighteenth-century Studies*, XXIII (1990), p. 390; Human skulls, collection of UAAM, museum labels undated. See also George W. Stocking, 'Bones, Bodies, Behaviour', in *Bones, Bodies and Behaviour: Essays on Biological Anthropology*, ed. George W. Stocking (Madison, WI, 1988) pp. 3–17. On the collecting of human skulls during the late eighteenth century and the first half of the nineteenth, see for example Ann Fabian, *The Skull Collectors: Race, Science, and America's Unburied Dead* (Chicago, IL, 2010); Paul Turnbull, 'British Anatomists, Phrenologists and the Construction of the Aboriginal Race, c. 1790–1830', *History Compass*, V (2007), pp. 26–50.

75 Human skulls, collection of UAAM, museum label dated 1838. On MacGillivray and Audubon see Kemp and Barnes, *Surgeons' Hall*; R. Ralph (1999) *William MacGillivray: Creatures of Air, Land and Sea* (London, 1999).

76 Human skull, collection of UAAM, museum label undated; *Catalogue of the Collections in Natural History Which Belonged to the Deceased William Macgillivray, LLD Professor of Natural History, in Marischal College and University, Aberdeen* (n.p., 1853).

77 Allen Thomson (1839), quoted in L. S. Jacyna, *Philosophic Whigs: Medicine, Science and Citizenship in Edinburgh, 1789–1848* (London, 1994), p. 165.

78 W. Aitken, 'Obituary of Allen Thomson', in 'Obituary Notices of Fellows Deceased', *Proceedings of the Royal Society of London*, XLII (1887), pp. xi–xxviii; Arthur Keith, 'Anatomy in Scotland during the Lifetime of Sir John Struthers (1823–1899)', *Edinburgh Medical Journal*, VIII (1912), pp. 7–33.

79 Aitken, 'Obituary of Allen Thomson', p. xx, see also p. xxvi.

80 'The Late Professor John Lizars', *The Lancet*, 9 June 1860, p. 582. John Lizars's additional surgical and pathological collection was sold to Dr Peter David Handyside when Lizars retired from teaching in 1839; see Matthew H. Kaufman, *Medical Teaching in Edinburgh During the 18th and 19th Centuries* (Edinburgh, 2003).

81 Knight, 'The Marischal College and University of Aberdeen'. See also Walker, 'Rebuilding of King's and Marischal Colleges'.

82 See Struthers, *Historical Sketch*.

83 '*Text Book of Anatomy for Students*. By Alexander Jardine Lizars, MD, Professor of Anatomy in the Marischal College and University of Aberdeen. Parts 2 and 3. 1844', *The Medico-chirurgical Review, and Journal of Practical Medicine*, 1 (1 October 1844–31 March 1845), pp. 484–9, p. 485, p. 487. On the use of microscopes in early nineteenth-century anatomical practices, see Andrew Cunningham, *The Anatomist Anatomis'd: An Experimental Discipline in Enlightenment Europe* (Farnham, 2010).

84 John Lizars, *A System of Anatomical Plates of the Human Body; Accompanied with Descriptions, and Physiological, Pathological and Surgical Observations* (Edinburgh, 1822–6), Part II, p. xii; Part I, Preface, p. vii. For discussion of Lizars's work, see Roberta McGrath, *Seeing Her Sex: Medical Archives and the Female Body* (Manchester, 2002).

85 Ibid., Part II, p. xii; Part IV, p. viii.

86 '*System of Anatomical Plates, with Descriptive Letter Press, &c.* By John Lizars, FRSE, &c. Part VII . . ., Edinburgh . . . 1825', *The Lancet*, 26 March 1825, p. 370.

87 Angus Fraser, 'Notes on Lectures on Anatomy. By Dr Lizars, Marischal College, Aberdeen', 1856, archive of the Aberdeen Medico-chirurgical Society.

88 See Elizabeth Hallam, 'Anatomists' Ways of Seeing and Knowing', in *Fieldnotes and Sketchbooks: Challenging the Boundaries Between Descriptions and Processes of Describing*, ed. Wendy Gunn (Frankfurt, 2009), pp. 69–107.

89 The Aberdeen Phrenological Society (1836–*c.* 1840s) also formed a museum of skulls and casts thereof, see Jacqueline Jenkinson, *Scottish Medical Societies, 1731–1939: Their History and Records* (Edinburgh, 1993); 'Proceedings of the Phrenological Society of Aberdeen', *Phrenological Journal*, X (June 1836–September 1837), pp. 616–18; 'Intelligence: Aberdeen', *Phrenological Journal*, XIX (1846), pp. 197–8. The museum of this society was possibly subsequently transferred to Marischal College's Anatomy Department, as 32 casts of the heads of individuals (in miniature form) were recorded in the collection, see 'Museum Material', 1959–69, MS/typescript list, *c.* 17 pages, archive of University of Aberdeen, Anatomy Department.

90 Minute Book, 1816–55, p. 68, p. 72, p. 73, records of AMCS (AMCS/1/1/1/18).

91 Ibid., p. 74, p. 94, p. 98, p. 109.

92 Ibid., p. 64.

93 Ibid., p. 376.

94 Ibid., p. 58.

95 Ibid., p. 218, p. 396.

96 Ibid., p. 106, p. 107, p. 111.

97 Ibid., p. 111, p. 112. The crocodile skeleton was originally recorded, when received in 1822, as that of an alligator, see Riddell, *Records of the Aberdeen Medical-chirurgical Society*.

98 Minute Book, 1816–55, p. 119, records of AMCS (AMCS/1/1/1/18).

99 Ibid., p. 266, p. 271, p. 300, p. 302, p. 352.

100 Ibid., p. 403. On methods used to preserve body parts in museums see Samuel J.M.M. Alberti, 'Anatomical Craft: A History of Medical Museum Practice', in *The Fate of Anatomical Collections*, ed. Rina Knoeff and Robert Zwijnenberg (Farnham, 2015), pp. 231–46.

101 Minute Book, 1816–55, p. 519, p. 537, records of AMCS (AMCS/1/1/1/18).

102 Minute Book, 1854–86, p. 72, p. 70, records of AMCS (AMCS/1/1/1/19).

103 Ibid., p. 74, p. 26.

104 Ibid., p. 74, p. 75.

105 Ibid., pp. 70–7, p. 117, p. 141; Riddell, *Records of the Aberdeen Medical-chirurgical*

Society, p. 111. Surviving AMCS records do not state the number of preparations in spirits that were transferred from the AMCS's Museum to Marischal College. They were removed from the AMCS's Museum by the end of 1859, see Minute Book, 1854–86, pp. 70–141, records of AMCS (AMCS/1/1/1/19).

Four Skeletal Growth: Museum Formation II

1 William Leslie Mackenzie, 'The Professor of Anatomy, 1863–1889: John Struthers', in *Aurora Borealis Academica: Aberdeen University Appreciations, 1860–1889*, ed. P. J. Anderson (Aberdeen, 1899), pp. 237–48, p. 244.

2 See Elizabeth Hallam, 'Articulating Bones: An Epilogue', *Journal of Material Culture*, xv (2010), pp. 465–92.

3 Caroline Pennington, *The Modernisation of Medical Teaching at Aberdeen in the Nineteenth Century* (Aberdeen, 1994), p. 19.

4 Mackenzie, 'Professor of Anatomy', p. 241. On Struthers, see Matthew H. Kaufman, 'Sir John Struthers (1823–1899), Professor of Anatomy in the University of Aberdeen (1863–1889), President of the Royal College of Surgeons of Edinburgh (1895–1897)', *Journal of Medical Biography*, Advance Access published 30 January 2014, doi: 10.1177/0967772013506808, pp. 1–8; Pennington, *Modernisation of Medical Teaching*. On the influence of Darwin, see Jane R. Goodall, *Performance and Evolution in the Age of Darwin: Out of the Natural Order* (London, 2002); Arthur MacGregor, 'Exhibiting Evolutionism: Darwin and Pseudo-Darwinism in Museum Practice after 1859', *Journal of the History of Collections*, xxi (2009), pp. 77–94.

5 Charles Darwin, *On the Origin of Species by Means of Natural Selection, Or the Preservation of Favoured Races in the Struggle for Life*, 1st edn (London, 1859), pp. 129–30.

6 Mackenzie, 'Professor of Anatomy', p. 244, p. 243. See Carla Yanni, 'Development and Display: Progressive Evolution in British Victorian Architecture and Architectural Theory', in *Evolution and Victorian Culture*, ed. Bernard Lightman and Bennett Zon (Cambridge, 2014).

7 J. Struthers, in *Report of the Committee on Professional Education* (1869), General Medical Council (London, 1869), pp. 85–6; J. Struthers, 'Progress of the Medical School', in *Aurora Borealis*, ed. Anderson, pp. 212–36.

8 J. Struthers 'Medical Education', *Aberdeen Journal*, 8 November 1865, p. 8; Struthers, 'Progress of the Medical School', p. 216.

9 See Samuel J.M.M. Alberti, *Morbid Curiosities: Medical Museums in Nineteenth-century Britain* (Oxford, 2011); Rina Knoeff and Robert Zwijnenberg, eds, *The Fate of Anatomical Collections* (Farnham, 2015); Jonathan Reinarz, 'The Age of Museum Medicine: The Rise and Fall of the Medical Museum of Birmingham's School of Medicine', *Social History of Medicine*, xviii (2005), pp. 419–37.

10 See, for example Alberti, *Morbid Curiosities*; Tony Bennett, *Pasts beyond Memory: Evolution, Museums, Colonialism* (London, 2004); John M. MacKenzie, *Museums and Empire: Natural History, Human Cultures and Colonial Identities* (Manchester, 2010); Susan Sheets-Pyenson, *Cathedrals of Science: The Development of Colonial Natural History Museums during the Late Nineteenth Century* (Kingston, Ont., 1988).

11 Sheets-Pyenson, *Cathedrals of Science*, p. 5.

12 J. Struthers, Evidence, 1 December 1876, in *Report of the Royal Commissioners Appointed to Inquire into the Universities of Scotland, with Evidence and Appendix*, vol. iii, *Evidence – Part II* (Edinburgh, 1878), pp. 5–48, p. 46. See Pennington, *Modernisation of Medical Teaching*.

13 Struthers, 'Progress of the Medical School'.

14 J. Struthers, *Osteological Memoirs, No. 1: The Clavicle* (Edinburgh, 1855), p. iii.

15 Struthers, Evidence, 1 December 1876, p. 45, p. 47.

16 Mackenzie, 'Professor of Anatomy', p. 238; Struthers, 'Progress of the Medical School', p. 226.

17 Sophie Forgan, 'Bricks and Bones: Architecture and Science in Victorian Britain', in *The*

Architecture of Science, ed. Peter Galison and Emily Thompson (Cambridge, MA, 1999), pp. 181–208; David N. Livingstone, *Putting Science in Its Place: Geographies of Scientific Knowledge* (Chicago, IL, 2003).

18 'Progress of the Medical School', p. 226.

19 'Opening of New Anatomical Buildings', *Aberdeen Journal*, 27 October 1881, p. 3; J. Struthers, *References to Papers in Anatomy: Human and Comparative* (Edinburgh, 1889), p. 38. 'On the Preservation of Subjects for Dissection', *The Lancet*, 20 October 1877, p. 585; J. Struthers, 'Account of Methods for Preparing and Preserving the Brain, Museum Specimens, and Dissections', in 'Proceedings of the Anatomical Society of Great Britain and Ireland', *Journal of Anatomy and Physiology*, XXII (1888), pp. ix–xi.

20 'Opening of New Anatomical Buildings'; Struthers, Evidence, 1 December 1876, p. 46.

21 Struthers, 'Progress of the Medical School', p. 226, p. 244. See Ludmilla Jordanova, *Defining Features: Scientific and Medical Portraits, 1660–2000* (London, 2000).

22 Plaster casts of blocks of Parthenon frieze, dated *c.* 1881, slip catalogue, 3 and 10 July 1975, archive of University of Aberdeen, Marischal Museum.

23 See Martin Kemp and Marina Wallace, *Spectacular Bodies: The Art and Science of the Human Body from Leonardo to Now*, exh. cat., Hayward Gallery, London (2000); Ann L. Poulet et al., *Jean-Antoine Houdon: Sculptor of the Enlightenment* (Chicago, IL, 2003).

24 Francis Haskell and Nicholas Penny, *Taste and the Antique: The Lure of Classical Sculpture, 1500–1900* (New Haven, CT, 1981); Cinzia Sicca and Alison Yarrington, eds, *The Lustrous Trade: Material Culture and the History of Sculpture in England and Italy, c. 1700–1860* (London, 2000).

25 Malcolm Baker, 'Bodies of Enlightenment: Sculpture and the Eighteenth-century Museum', in *Enlightening the British: Knowledge, Discovery and the Museum in the Eighteenth Century*, ed. R.G.W. Anderson et al. (London, 2003), pp. 142–8; Thorsten Opper, 'Ancient Glory and Modern Learning: The Sculpture-decorated Library', in *Enlightenment: Discovering the World in the Eighteenth Century*, ed. Kim Sloan and Andrew Burnett (London, 2003), pp. 58–67; Rune Frederiksen and Eckart Marchand, eds, *Plaster Casts: Making, Collecting and Displaying from Classical Antiquity to the Present* (Berlin, 2010).

26 Kemp and Wallace, *Spectacular Bodies*, p. 85, p. 78.

27 See Pennington, *Modernisation of Medical Teaching*.

28 Struthers, 'Progress of the Medical School', p. 232.

29 Mackenzie, 'Professor of Anatomy', p. 240.

30 Struthers, 'Progress of the Medical School', p. 226.

31 Mackenzie, 'Professor of Anatomy', p. 241.

32 'VII. The Provision of Assistance and Apparatus', in *Report of the Royal Commissioners Appointed to Inquire into the Universities of Scotland, with Evidence and Appendix*, vol. I: *Report with Index of Evidence* (Edinburgh, 1878), p. 70.

33 'V. Entrance Examinations', in *Report of the Royal Commissioners*, vol. I, p. 50.

34 J. Matthews Duncan, Evidence, 18 November 1876, in *Report of the Royal Commissioners*, vol. III, pp. 885–90, p. 888.

35 Struthers, *Osteological Memoirs*, p. iv.

36 Struthers, 'Modern Improvements in Medical Education', reported in *Aberdeen Journal*, 8 November 1865, p. 8.

37 Struthers, Evidence, 1 December 1876, p. 12. See K. Waddington, 'Mayhem and Medical Students'.

38 See Elizabeth T. Hurren, *Dying for Victorian Medicine: English Anatomy and Its Trade in the Dead Poor, c. 1834–1929* (Basingstoke, 2012); Keir Waddington, 'Mayhem and Medical Students: Image, Conduct and Control in the Victorian and Edwardian London Teaching Hospital', *Social History of Medicine*, XV (2002), pp. 45–64.

39 'Obituary, Sir John Struthers', *The Lancet*, 4 March 1899, pp. 612–15, p. 612; Struthers, in *Report of the Committee on Professional Education*, p. 89; Struthers, 'Progress of the Medical School', p. 227; G. Ellis, in *Report of the Committee on Professional Education*, p. 64.

40 Struthers, in *Report of the Committee on Professional Education*, p. 89.

41 See Lorriane Daston and Peter Galison, *Objectivity* (New York, 2007).

42 Struthers, Evidence, 1 December 1876, p. 45.

43 On the procurement of bodies for medical education, see Hurren, *Dying for Victorian Medicine*; Fiona Hutton, *The Study of Anatomy in Britain, 1700–1900* (London, 2013); Ruth Richardson, *Death, Dissection and the Destitute*, 2nd edn (London, 2001).

44 Joseph Lister, Evidence, 26 June 1876, in *Report of the Royal Commissioners*, vol. III, pp. 231–40, p. 235.

45 Anatomy Act Committee Minutes, Aberdeen, vol. I, 1856–1959, p. 48–9, p. 60, University of Aberdeen, Special Collections (UASC) (MSU 1332/4/1/1).

46 Ibid., pp. 65–132.

47 William Turner, Evidence, 3 July 1876, in *Report of the Royal Commissioners*, vol. III, pp. 303–11, p. 304. See Hurren, *Dying for Victorian Medicine*.

48 William Turner, in *Report of the Committee on Professional Education*, p. 94.

49 'Obituary, Sir John Struthers', *The Lancet*, p. 612. 'Will of the Late Sir John Struthers', *The Scotsman*, 20 April 1899, p.7.

50 Francis Sibson, *Medical Anatomy: Or, Illustrations of the Relative Position and Movements of the Internal Organs* (London, 1869).

51 Ibid., Preface, n. pag., Explanation of Plate I, Explanation of Plate XVI.

52 J. Osborne-Walker, *The Descriptive Atlas of Anatomy. A Representation of the Anatomy of the Human Body* (London, 1880), Preface, pp. v–vi.

53 On *Gray's Anatomy*, see Martin Kemp, 'Gray's Greyness', in *Visualizations: The Nature Book of Art and Science*, Martin Kemp (Oxford: 2000), pp. 70–71; Ruth Richardson, *The Making of Mr Gray's Anatomy: Bodies, Books, Fortune, Fame* (Oxford, 2008).

54 On mechanical objectivity, and the machine as a 'positive ideal of the observer', Daston and Galison, *Objectivity*, p. 139.

55 Struthers, in *Report of the Committee on Professional Education*, p. 92. On activity and passivity within the mid-nineteenth-century scientific self, see Daston and Galison, *Objectivity*.

56 W. H. Flower, 'Note on the Construction and Arrangement of Anatomical Museums', *Journal of Anatomy and Physiology*, IX (1875), pp. 259–62, p. 262.

57 Turner, Evidence, 3 July 1876, p. 307.

58 Struthers, Evidence, 1 December 1876, p. 45.

59 Ibid., p. 45.

60 Matthew H. Kaufman, Medical Teaching in Edinburgh during the 18th and 19th Centuries (Edinburgh, 2003); Pennington, *Modernisation of Medical Teaching*.

61 J. Struthers, *Historical Sketch of the Edinburgh Anatomy School* (Edinburgh, 1867).

62 Turner, Evidence, 3 July 1876, p. 305, p. 306.

63 'Edinburgh University Anatomical Museum', *The Scotsman*, 8 August 1885, p. 7.

64 Struthers, 1878, Evidence, 1 December 1876, p. 45.

65 Simon Chaplin, 'John Hunter and the "Museum Oeconomy", 1750–1800', PhD thesis, King's College London (2009).

66 Royal College of Surgeons of England, *Synopsis of the Arrangement of the Preparations in the Museum of the Royal College of Surgeons of England* (London, 1850), p. 37; J. Dobson, 'The Architectural History of the Hunterian Museum', *Annals of the Royal College of Surgeons*, XXIX (1961), pp. 113–26.

67 Dobson, 'Architectural History'.

68 J. Beveridge to W. H. Flower, MS letters: 23 March 1868, 13 April 1868, Museum Letter Book, vol. I (1862–8), RCS Archives (RCS-MUS/5/2/1).

69 W. H. Flower, 'The Museum of the Royal College of Surgeons of England', in W. H. Flower, *Essays on Museums and Other Subjects Connected with Natural History* (London, 1898 [1881]), pp. 74–94, p. 82. W. H. Flower, 'Note on the Construction'.

70 Struthers, Evidence, 1 December 1876, p. 45, p. 46; 'Obituary, Sir John Struthers', *British Medical Journal*, 4 March 1899, pp. 561–3, p. 563. On pathology museums

see Alberti, *Morbid Curiosities*.

71 'Obituary, Sir John Struthers', *British Medical Journal*, p. 561.

72 Mackenzie, 'Professor of Anatomy', p. 241. See T. H. Huxley, *Evidence as to Man's Place in Nature* (London, 1863) with a drawing by Waterhouse Hawkins from specimens in the Museum of the Royal College of Surgeons of England; and Bennett, *Pasts beyond Memory*; Pennington, *Modernisation of Medical Teaching*.

73 Struthers, 'Progress of the Medical School', p. 227.

74 'Dr John Struthers', *Aberdeen Weekly Journal*, 2 May 1885. Caricature of John Struthers, *Bon-Accord*, 13 November 1886.

75 The image could also have referred to 'grinders' in anatomy teaching. These were instructors who 'beat into the heads of negligent students that information which they had failed to learn during the proper period of their studies, and when thus ground, polished, or wound up to the proper point, they select their day for examination, and very often succeed. Information thus acquired is evanescent', 'Westminster Hospital. Mr Guthrie's Introductory Address', *The Lancet*, 8 October 1853, pp. 336–8, p. 337. Struthers was openly critical of grinding as a method of learning, see J. Struthers 'Medical Education', *Aberdeen Journal*, 8 November 1865, p. 8.

76 Pennington, *Modernisation of Medical Teaching*.

77 Struthers, Evidence, 1 December 1876, p. 46.

78 J. Struthers (n.d.), quoted in Mackenzie, 'Professor of Anatomy', p. 244. J. Struthers to the Museum Committee of the RCSEd, 16 October 1896, copy of letter, RCSEd Library and Special Collections (GD4/420).

79 In 1897 Struthers estimated the number of specimens in his collection: 1304 in Human Anatomy, 300 in Comparative Anatomy. See List of specimens presented by Struthers to the RCSEd museum, 19 December 1897, MS list, RCSEd Library and Special Collections (GD4/421).

80 Samuel J.M.M. Alberti, 'Owning and Collecting Natural Objects in Nineteenth-century Britain', in *From Private to Public: Natural Collections and Museums*, ed. Marco Beretta (Sagamore Beach, MA, 2005), p. 145.

81 J. Struthers, *Anatomical and Physiological Observations*, Part 1 (Edinburgh, 1854); Struthers, *References to Papers in Anatomy*.

82 J. Struthers, 'On Variations of the Vertebrae and Ribs in Man', *Journal of Anatomy and Physiology*, IX (1874), pp. 17–96, p. 17.

83 J. Struthers, 'Case of Additional Bone in the Human Carpus', *Journal of Anatomy and Physiology*, III (1869), pp. 354–6.

84 Anatomy Act Committee Minutes, vol. 1, p. 3, p. 68.

85 List of specimens presented by Struthers to the RCSEd museum, 19 December 1897. See Pennington, *Modernisation of Medical Teaching*.

86 'Development of the Human Skeleton. Paris. 1873', collection of the University of Aberdeen, Anatomy Museum (UAAM).

87 Struthers, *Historical Sketch*, p. 81, p. 82.

88 Kaufman, *Medical Teaching in Edinburgh*.

89 Frederick John Knox, *The Anatomist's Instructor, and Museum Companion. Being Practical Directions for the Formation and Subsequent Management of Anatomical Museums*, (Edinburgh, 1836), p. vii. See Matthew H. Kaufman, 'Frederick Knox, Younger Brother and Assistant of Dr Robert Knox: His Contribution to "Knox's Catalogues"', *Journal of the Royal College of Surgeons of Edinburgh*, XLVI/1 (2001), pp. 44–56.

90 A. W. Bates, *The Anatomy of Robert Knox: Murder, Mad Science and Medical Regulation in Nineteenth-century Edinburgh* (Brighton, 2010); Henry Lonsdale, *A Sketch of the Life and Writings of Robert Knox the Anatomist* (London, 1870). Robert Knox, *Great Artists and Great Anatomists: A Biographical and Philosophical Study* (London, 1852); Isobel Rae, *Knox: The Anatomist* (Edinburgh, 1964).

91 See Kaufman, 'Frederick Knox'. On the contents of Knox's collection see also J. A. Ross and H.W.Y. Taylor, 'Robert Knox's Catalogue', *Journal of the History of Medicine and*

Allied Sciences, x (1955), pp. 269–76.

92   Struthers, Evidence, 1 December 1876, p. 46.

93   John Scott Riddell, *The Records of the Aberdeen Medico-chirurgical Society from 1789 to 1922* (Aberdeen, 1922).

94   Struthers, 'On Variations of the Vertebrae and Ribs in Man', p. 39.

95   Struthers, 'Progress of the Medical School'; J. Struthers, 'On the Cervical Vertebrae and their Articulations in Fin-whales', *Journal of Anatomy and Physiology*, VII (1872), pp. 1–55.

96   J. Struthers, 'On the Bones, Articulations, and Muscles of the Rudimentary Hind-limb of the Greenland Right-whale (*Balaena mysticetus*)', *Journal of Anatomy and Physiology*, XV (1881), pp. 141–76. Struthers, *References to Papers in Anatomy*.

97   J. Struthers, 'On Some Points in the Anatomy of a Great Fin-whale (*Balaenoptera musculus*)', *Journal of Anatomy and Physiology*, VI (1871), pp. 107–25; Struthers, *Aurora*; J. Struthers, 'The Whale at Aberdeen', *Aberdeen Weekly Journal*, 28 October 1888.

98   Struthers, 1872, 'On the Cervical Vertebrae and their Articulations in Fin-whales', p. 1. J. Struthers, 'The Whale at Aberdeen'.

99   J. Struthers, 'On the External Characters and Some Parts of the Anatomy of a Beluga (*Delphinapterus leucas*)', *Journal of Anatomy and Physiology*, XXX (1895), pp. 124–56.

100   See Irene Maver, 'Leisure and Culture: The Nineteenth Century', in *Aberdeen, 1800–2000: A New History*, ed. W. Hamish Fraser and Clive H. Lee (East Linton, 2000), pp. 398–421.

101   J. Struthers, 'On the Rudimentary Hind-limb of a Great Fin-whale (*Balaenoptera musculus*) in Comparison with those of the Humpback Whale and the Greenland Right-whale', *Journal of Anatomy and Physiology*, XXVII (1893), pp. 291–33.

102   Ibid., p. 291. On Robert Gibb, see Arthur Keith, 'Anatomy in Scotland during the Lifetime of Sir John Struthers (1823–1899)', *Edinburgh Medical Journal*, VIII (1912), pp. 7–33.

103   'Aberdeen University Museums', *Aberdeen Weekly Journal*, 15 April 1899.

104   J. Struthers, *Memoir on the Anatomy of the Humpback Whale Megaptera Longimana* (Edinburgh, 1889).

105   'Whale at Peterhead', *Aberdeen Journal*, 5 July 1871, p. 8. 'The Tay Whale', *Aberdeen Weekly Journal*, 22 January 1884; 'The Tay Whale on Exhibition', *Aberdeen Weekly Journal*, 26 January 1884; M. J. Williams, 'Professor Struthers and the Tay Whale', *Scottish Medical Journal*, XLI (1996), pp. 92–4.

106   Struthers, *Memoir on the Anatomy*.

107   Ibid., p. 3.

108   'Dundee – Dissection of the Tay Whale', *Dundee Courier*, 26 January 1884, p. 2.

109   Struthers, *Memoir on the Anatomy*, p. 3.

110   'Come and See the Great Tay Whale', *Aberdeen Weekly Journal*, 5 February 1884; 'The Whale', *Aberdeen Weekly Journal*, 1 February 1884.

111   'The Tay Whale', 1 Jan 1884, *Aberdeen Weekly Journal*; 'The Tay Whale', Liverpool Mercury, 5 March 1884, p 6.

112   Struthers, *Memoir on the Anatomy*, p. 2.

113   'The Tay Whale: Lecture by Professor Struthers', *Aberdeen Weekly Journal*, 5 February 1884.

114   J. Struthers, 'On the Rudimentary Hind Limb of Megaptera Longimana', *The American Naturalist*, XIX (1885), pp. 124–5, p. 125.

115   Mackenzie, 'Professor of Anatomy', p. 243.

116   'The Tay Whale', *Aberdeen Weekly Journal*, 6 August 1886; 'The Skeleton of the Tay Whale', *Aberdeen Weekly Journal*, 6 September, 1887; 'The Tay Whale', *Aberdeen Weekly Journal*, 6 February 1888.

117   R. Sinclair Black (1899), quoted in Pennington, *Modernisation of Medical Teaching*, p. 21.

118   The skeleton was installed at Dundee Museum by Robert Gibb, see 'Removal of the Tay Whale to Dundee', *Aberdeen Weekly Journal*, 31 December 1889.

119   'The Tay Whale', *Dundee Courier*, 15 January 1891, p. 4.

120 Struthers, 'On the Cervical Vertebrae and Their Articulations in Fin-whales'; Struthers, 'On Some Points in the Anatomy of a Great Fin-whale (*Balaenoptera Musculus*)'; Struthers, *References to Papers in Anatomy*.

121 Struthers, *Memoir on the Anatomy*, p. 16. See Gavin Sutherland, *The Whaling Years: Peterhead, 1788–1893* (Aberdeen, 1993).

122 J. Struthers, 'On the Carpus of the Greenland Right Whale (*Balaena mysticetus*) and of Fin-Whales', *Journal of Anatomy and Physiology*, xxix (1895), pp. 146–87, p. 187.

123 Sutherland, *The Whaling Years*.

124 Struthers, 'On the Carpus of the Greenland Right Whale (*Balaena mysticetus*) and of Fin-whales'.

125 George Sim, ms Diary/notebook, vol. i: 1862–70, p. 34, Aberdeen City Library.

126 Struthers, 'Progress of the Medical School', p. 229.

127 Struthers, 'On the Rudimentary Hind-limb of a Great Fin-whale'; Struthers, *Memoir on the Anatomy*.

128 Sim, ms Diary/notebook, vol. i, p. 41; vol. iii, 1874–7, p. 59.

129 Sim, ms Diary/notebook vol. iii, p. 114.

130 Sim, ms Diary/notebook, vol. i, p. 33.

131 J.W.H. Trail, 'Obituary – George Sim, als', *The Annals of Scottish Natural History*, ed. J. A. Harvie-Brown, James W. H. Trail and William Eagle Clarke (Edinburgh, 1909), pp. 129–33 (with Plate ii).

132 Sim, ms Diary/notebook, vol. ii, p. 3; vol. iii, p. 55; Book of ms letters to George Sim from: W. F. Forbes, 22 March 1875; Lady Sydney, 6 March 1876; Alexander Gray, 9 January 1877, Aberdeen City Library.

133 Sim, ms Diary/notebook, vol. i, p. 82.

134 Struthers, 'Progress of the Medical School', p. 229.

135 Flower, 'Museum Organisation', in Flower, *Essays on Museums*, pp. 1–29, p. 17. On techniques used to preserve animals, Samuel J.M.M. Alberti, 'Constructing Nature behind Glass', *Museum and Society*, VI (2008), pp. 73–97, and articles in this themed issue; Ann C. Colley, *Wild Animal Skins in Victorian Britain: Zoos, Collections, Portraits, and Maps* (Farnham, 2014); Pat Morris, *Rowland Ward: Taxidermist to the World* (Ascot, 2003); Rachel Poliquin, *The Breathless Zoo: Taxidermy and the Cultures of Longing* (Philadelphia, pa, 2012).

136 William Turner differentiated between 'skins and stuffed specimens' and 'preparations displaying internal structure', see Turner, Evidence, 3 July 1876, p. 305. Some taxidermists also prepared and articulated animal skeletons, see P. A. Morris, *Edward Gerrard & Sons: A Taxidermy Memoir* (Ascot, 2004).

137 Sim, ms Diary/notebook, vol. vii, 1885–90, p. 51; vol. iii, p. 2; volume of ms letters to George Sim from: Charles O. Waterhouse (British Museum), 15 May 1868.

138 See Diarmid A. Finnegan, *Natural History Societies and Civic Culture in Victorian Scotland* (London, 2009).

139 'Natural History Society', 16 December 1868, *Aberdeen Journal*, p. 4.

140 'Aberdeen Natural History Society: Proposed Public Museum', *Aberdeen Weekly Journal*, 30 June 1885; 'East of Scotland Naturalist's Union, *Aberdeen Weekly Journal*, 9 August 1886.

141 Sim, ms Diary/notebook, vol. vi, 1882–84/5, p. 70; vol. viii, 1890–91, p. 53.

142 'Aberdeen Natural History Society', *Aberdeen Weekly Journal*, 20 February 1889.

143 Sim, ms Diary/notebook, vol. iii, p. 67, p. 105; vol. viii, p. 109.

144 Book of ms letters to George Sim: Sim to Charles Darwin, 18 October 1879; Darwin to Sim, 22 October 1879.

145 J. Struthers to Charles Darwin, 31 December 1864, letter, University of Cambridge, Darwin Correspondence Database.

146 Struthers, 'Progress of the Medical School'; Richard Perren, 'The Nineteenth-century Economy', *Aberdeen 1800–2000*, ed. Fraser and Lee, pp. 75–98.

147 Struthers, 'Progress of the Medical School'; 'Miscellaneous Business of the Meeting on February 4, 1873', *Journal of the Anthropological Institute*, iii (1874), pp. 1–2.

148 Struthers, 'Progress of the Medical School';

149 J. Struthers to W. H. Flower, MS letters: 22 July 1868, Museum Letter Book, vol. I (1857–68); 7 November 1871, 18 November 1871, Museum Letter Book, vol. II (1868–73); 26 January 1875, Museum Letter Book, vol. III (1874–78), RCS Archives (RCS-MUS/5/2/1, RCS-MUS/5/2/2, RCS-MUS/5/2/3).

150 Struthers, 'Progress of the Medical School'.

151 John D. Hargreaves, *Academe and Empire: Some Overseas Connections of Aberdeen University, 1860–1970* (Aberdeen, 1994).

152 File of MS Letters, late 19th–early 20th century, archive of University of Aberdeen Anatomy Department (UAAD).

153 Struthers, *Anatomical and Physiological Observations*, p. 105.

154 Megan J. Highet, 'Body Snatching and Grave Robbing: Bodies for Science', *History and Anthropology*, XVI (2005), pp. 415–40; Elise Juzda, 'Skulls, Science, and the Spoils of War: Craniological Studies at the United States Army Medical Museum, 1868–1900', *Studies in History and Philosophy of Biological and Biomedical Sciences*, XL (2009), pp. 156–67; Helen MacDonald, *Human Remains: Dissection and Its Histories* (New Haven, CT, and London, 2006); Christine Quigley, *Skulls and Skeletons: Human Bone Collections and Accumulations* (London, 2001); Ricardo Roque, *Headhunting and Colonialism: Anthropology and the Circulation of Human Skulls in the Portuguese Empire, 1870–1930* (Basingstoke, 2010); Paul Turnbull, 'Australian Museums, Aboriginal Skeletal Remains, and the Imagining of Human Evolutionary History, c. 1860–1914', *Museum and Society*, XIII (2015), pp. 72–87.

155 Correspondent to J. Struthers, 26 June 1867, MS letter, archive of UAAD.

156 H. Wheeler to J. Struthers, 16 November 1870, MS letter, archive of UAAD.

157 See Paul Turnbull, 'Indigenous Australian People, their Defence of the Dead and Native Title', in *The Dead and Their Possessions: Repatriation in Principle, Policy and Practice*, ed. Cressia Fforde, Jane Hubert and Paul Turnbull (London, 2002), pp. 63–86; Paul Turnbull, 'British Anthropological Thought in Colonial Practice: The Appropriation of Indigenous Australian bodies, 1860–1880', in *Foreign Bodies: Oceania and the Science of Race, 1750–1940*, ed. Bronwen Douglas and Chris Ballard (Canberra, 2008), pp. 205–28.

158 Struthers, 'On Variations of the Vertebrae and Ribs in Man', p. 17; Struthers, 'On a New Craniometer', *Edinburgh Medical Journal*, IX (1863), p. 368. The craniometer was a glass cube in a brass frame with panes etched with lines from which to take measurements. It was designed by Struthers and made by Peter Stevenson, an Edinburgh philosophical instrument maker.

159 J. Struthers, MS note, 1873; Dr Vandersmaght to J. Struthers, 9 November 1887, MS letter, archive of UAAD.

160 Marshall Lamb to J. Struthers, 24 June 1889, MS letter, archive of UAAD.

161 W. J. Simpson to J. Struthers, 21 July 1888, MS letter, archive of UAAD. See R. A. Baker and R. A. Bayliss, 'William John Ritchie Simpson (1855–1931): Public Health and Tropical Medicine', *Medical History*, XXXI (1987), pp. 450–65; Hargreaves, *Academe and Empire*.

162 John Robb to J. Struthers, 14 May 1888, MS letter, archive of UAAD; Struthers, 'Progress of the Medical School'.

163 Flower, 'Modern Museums', in Flower, *Essays on Museums*, pp. 30–53, p. 32.

164 John S. Billings, 'Medical Museums', *Science*, XII (1888), pp. 134–6, p. 135.

165 Flower, 'Museum Organisation', p. 13.

166 Flower, 'Local Museums', in Flower, *Essays on Museums*, p. 57. Flower was quoting George Brown Goode, director of the United States National Museum of the Smithsonian Institution in Washington.

167 Flower, 'Museum Organisation', p. 12, p. 13.

168 Flower, 'Local Museums', p. 55; Flower, 'Modern Museums', p. 35, p. 36.

169 'Aberdeen University Court', *Aberdeen Weekly Journal*, 3 September 1889.

170 Struthers, 'Progress of the Medical School', p. 226, p. 227; F. J. Shepherd, 'Notes of a

Visit to Some of the Anatomical Schools and Surgical Clinics of Europe in 1887',
Canadian Medical Association Journal, XIV (1924), pp. 59–65, p. 62.

171 Mackenzie, 'Professor of Anatomy', p. 242. See Nélia Dias, 'The Visibility of Difference:
Nineteenth-century French Anthropological Collections', in *The Politics of Display:
Museums, Science, Culture*, ed. Sharon Macdonald (London, 1998).

172 Struthers, 'Progress of the Medical School', p. 227.

173 Struthers, Evidence, 1 December 1876, p. 46.

174 Ibid., p. 46.

175 Struthers, account of methods, in 'Proceedings of the Anatomical Society of Great Britain
and Ireland', p. x, p. ix.

176 Allen Thomson, Evidence, 8 July 1876, in *Report of the Royal Commissioners*, vol. III,
pp. 353–81, p. 377.

177 Struthers, *References to Papers in Anatomy*.

178 William Turner, Minutes of Evidence, 1878, p. 304, p. 305.

179 Struthers, Evidence, 1 December 1876, p. 46.

180 Ibid., p. 25.

181 Struthers, Evidence, 1 December 1876, pp. 46–7. An account of an Edinburgh dissecting-room servant, whose sister and mother washed the students' dissecting clothes, is
given in 'David Paterson', *Aberdeen Journal*, 4 February 1829, p. 4.

182 Struthers, 'Progress of the Medical School', p. 229.

183 Keith, 'Anatomy in Scotland', p. 24. 'The Tay Whale', *Dundee Courier*, 15 January 1891,
p. 4.

184 J. Struthers to W. H. Flower, MS letter: 22 July 1868, Museum Letter Book, vol. 1
(1857–68), RCS Archives (RCS-MUS/5/2/1).

185 For example, 'Three Preparations of Foetal Blood Vessels', with wax-injected blood vessels, dissected by John Struthers, 1842, RCSEd Collections (GC 14141). See Dawn Kemp
with Sara Barnes, *Surgeons' Hall: A Museum Anthology* (Edinburgh, 2009).

186 Flower, 'Modern Museums', p. 32.

187 Keith, 'Anatomy in Scotland'; 'Obituary, Sir John Struthers', *British Medical Journal*.

188 Daston and Galison, *Objectivity*, p. 229.

189 Struthers, 'Progress of the Medical School'; J. Struthers, 'On a Method of Promoting
Maceration for Anatomical Museums by Artificial Summer Temperature', *Journal of
Anatomy and Physiology*, XVIII (1883), pp. 49–53.

190 Struthers, 'On Variations of the Vertebrae and Ribs in Man'; Struthers, 'On the Bones,
Articulations, and Muscles of the Rudimentary Hind-limb of the Greenland Right-whale'.

191 Anatomy Act Committee Minutes, vol. 1, p. 92, p. 96.

192 For example, a case of 'Models of the Red Corpuscles of the Blood in Various Animals',
presented to Struthers by Hermann Welcker, professor of anatomy at the University of
Halle in 1871, RCSEd Collections (N12 M19).

193 See Tricia Close-Koenig, 'Betwixt and Between: Production and Commodification of
Knowledge in a Medical School Pathological Anatomy Laboratory in Strasbourg (mid-
19th Century to 1939)', PhD thesis, Université de Strasbourg (2011); Nick Hopwood,
Embryos in Wax: Models from the Ziegler Studio (Cambridge and Bern, 2002); Ross L.
Jones, Humanity's Mirror: 150 Years of Anatomy in Melbourne (Melbourne, 2007);
Michael Sappol, *A Traffic of Dead Bodies: Anatomy and Embodied Social Identity in
Nineteenth-century America* (Princeton, NJ, 2002).

194 On Rudolf Weisker, see Sabine Hackethal, 'The Blachka Models of the Humboldt
University of Berlin and their Historical Context', *Historical Biology*, XX (2008), pp. 19–28.

195 On Franz Josef Steger, see Jon Cornwall and Chris Smith, 'Anatomical Models by F. J.
Steger (1845–1938): The University of Otago Collection', *European Journal of Anatomy*,
XVIII/3 (2014), pp. 209–11.

196 See Aileen Fyfe and Bernard Lightman, eds, *Science in the Marketplace: Nineteenth-century
Sites and Experiences* (Chicago, IL, 2007); Jane R. Goodall, *Performance and Evolution
in the Age of Darwin: Out of the Natural Order* (London, 2002); Bernard Lightman,

Victorian Popularizers of Science: Designing Nature for New Audiences (Chicago, IL, 2007).

197 'Professor Struthers on the Higher Education of Women', *Aberdeen Weekly Journal*, 6 November 1879.

198 Ibid.; 'Evening Lectures on Science in Aberdeen, *Aberdeen Journal*, 14 February 1872, p. 5.

199 Advert for 'Wombwell's Royal No. 1' visiting Aberdeen, *Aberdeen Journal*, 27 October 1869, p. 4. On animal displays, see Helen Cowie, *Exhibiting Animals in Nineteenth-century Britain: Empathy, Education, Entertainment* (Basingstoke, 2014); Robert J. Hoage and William A. Deiss, eds, *New Worlds, New Animals: From Menagerie to Zoological Park in the Nineteenth Century* (London, 1996).

200 Struthers, 'Progress of the Medical School'; 'The Aquarium at Berlin', *The American Journal of Education*, V (1870), pp. 285–6.

201 Struthers, 'Progress of the Medical School'; 'Anatomy Department, University of Aberdeen, Bequest to Zoology Department, February 1966, Preliminary Catalogue Nos'. MS notebook, archive of University of Aberdeen, Zoology Museum.

202 Richard D. Altick, *The Shows of London: A Panoramic History of Exhibitions, 1600–1862* (Cambridge, MA, 1978); Sujit Sivasundaram, 'Trading Knowledge: The East India Company's Elephants in India and Britain', *Historical Journal*, XLVIII (2005), pp. 27–63.

203 'Wombwell's Menagerie', *Aberdeen Journal*, 25 August 1869, p. 1; 'The Queen's Menagerie, Wombwell's Royal No. 1.', *Aberdeen Journal*, 1 September 1869, p. 4.

204 'Messrs Bostock and Wombwell's Menagerie in Aberdeen', *Aberdeen Weekly Journal*, 23 May 1896; 'Bostock and Wombwell's Menagerie', *Aberdeen Weekly Journal*, 26 May 1898.

205 Elizabeth Edwards, 'Evolving Images: Photography, Race and Popular Darwinism', in *Endless Forms: Charles Darwin, Natural Science and the Visual Arts*, ed. Diana Donald and Jane Munro, exh. cat., Fitzwilliam Museum, Cambridge (New Haven, CT, 2009), pp. 167–92; Roslyn Poignant, *Professional Savages: Captive Lives and Western Spectacle* (New Haven, CT, 2004); Pippa Skotnes, 'The Politics of Bushman Representations', in *Images and Empires: Visuality in Colonial and Postcolonial Africa*, ed. Paul S. Landau and Deborah D. Kaspin (Berkeley, CA, 2002), pp. 253–4.

206 See Pascal Blanchard et al., eds, *Human Zoos: Science and Spectacle in the Age of Colonial Empires* (Liverpool, 2008); Pascal Blanchard et al., eds, *Human Zoos: The Invention of the Savage* (Arles, 2011); Poignant, *Professional Savages*; Sadiah Qureshi, *Peoples on Parade: Exhibitions, Empire, and Anthropology in Nineteenth-Century Britain* (Chicago, IL, 2011).

207 Struthers, 'Progress of the Medical School'. For a discussion of how similar casts, at London's Crystal Palace in Sydenham, 1854–66, were used to display human difference see Qureshi, *Peoples on Parade*.

208 William Turner, 'On Variability in Human Structure as Displayed in Different Races of Men, with Especial Reference to the Skeleton', *Journal of Anatomy and Physiology*, XXI (1887), pp. 473–95, p. 482; Struthers, 'On Variations of the Vertebrae and Ribs in Man', p. 17. On the construction of the category 'Bushman', see Pippa Skotnes, ed., *Miscast: Negotiating the Presence of the Bushmen* (Cape Town, 1996); Skotnes, 'Politics of Bushman Representations'.

209 Turner, 'On Variability in Human Structure', p. 482.

210 W. H. Flower and J. Murie, 'Account of the Dissection of a Bushwoman', *Journal of Anatomy and Physiology*, I (1867), pp. 189–208, p. 190.

211 W. H. Flower, 'On the Aims and Prospects of the Study of Anthropology', *Journal of the Anthropological Institute of Great Britain and Ireland*, XIII (1884), pp. 488–501. Struthers, 'On Variations of the Vertebrae and Ribs in Man'; William Turner, 'Notes on the Dissection of a Negro', *Journal of Anatomy and Physiology*, XIII (1879), pp. 382–6.

212 See Sadiah Qureshi, 'Robert Gordon Latham, Displayed Peoples, and the Natural History of Race, 1854–1866', *Historical Journal*, LIV (2011), pp. 143–66.

213 'Liverpool Museum of Anatomy', *Liverpool Mercury*, 12 July 1877, p. 1.

214 Alberti, *Morbid Curiosities*; A. W. Bates, '"Indecent and Demoralising Representations": Public Anatomy Museums in Mid-Victorian England', *Medical History*, LII (2008),

pp. 1–22; Maritha Rene Burmeister, 'Popular Anatomical Museums in Nineteenth-century England', PhD thesis, Rutgers University (2000).

215 'Information against an Anatomical Museum', *Morning Post*, 13 September 1852, p. 7. See Bates, '"Indecent and Demoralising Representations"'.

216 'Reimer's Anatomical Museum', *Bradford Observer*, 3 February 1853, p. 4; 'Reimer's Anatomical Museum', *Huddersfield Chronicle*, 25 August 1855, p. 5.

217 'Signor Sarti's Anatomical Figures', *The Scotsman*, 21 September 1844, p. 3; 'Arrival of Signor Sarti', *The Scotsman*, 18 September 1847, p. 1; 'Venetian Figures', *Dundee Courier*, 12 April 1848, p. 2; '76 Overgate', *Dundee Courier*, 12 February 1883, p. 1.

218 'Dr Kahn's Grand Anatomical Museum', *Glasgow Herald*, 20 September 1852, p. 1. See A. W. Bates, 'Dr Kahn's Museum: Obscene Anatomy in Victorian London', *Journal of the Royal Society of Medicine*, XCIX (2006), pp. 618–24.

219 'Signor Sarti's Florentine Museum of Anatomy', *Aberdeen Journal*, 29 December 1847, p. 4.

220 'Herr Reimers', *Aberdeen Journal*, 1 July 1857, p. 4.

221 'Dr Adair's Anatomical Museum', *Aberdeen Journal*, 3 July 1867, p. 4. Admission tokens were issued for 'Dr Adair's Museum of Science and Anatomy' at the same address, dated *c.* 1867. Following Adair's death his 'medical business and museum' was offered for sale, see *The Scotsman*, 24 April 1876, p. 2. A later owner advertised 'The Museum of Anatomy and Science', *Aberdeen Weekly Journal*, 24 July 1885.

222 'Dr Adair's Anatomical Museum', *Aberdeen Journal*, 3 July 1867, p. 4. 'Dr Adair's Anatomical Museum', *Orcadian*, 24 September 1870, p. 1.

223 See Samuel J.M.M. Alberti, 'The Museum Affect: Visiting Collections of Anatomy and Natural History', in *Science in the Marketplace*, ed. Fyfe and Lightman, pp. 371–403; A. W. Bates, '"Indecent and Demoralising Representations": Public Anatomy Museums in Mid-Victorian England', *Medical History*, LII (2008), pp. 1–22.

224 See Alberti, *Museum Affect*; Sappol, *Traffic of Dead Bodies*.

225 Mackenzie, 'Professor of Anatomy', p. 239. 'Professor Struthers on the Higher Education of Women', *Aberdeen Weekly Journal*, 6 November 1879; 'Death of Sir John Struthers', *Aberdeen Weekly Journal*, 25 February 1899; 'Presentation to Professor Struthers', *Aberdeen Journal*, 2 June 1875, p. 3; 'Lectures on the Human Body', *Aberdeen Journal*, 22 January 1868, p. 5.

226 'Evening Lectures on Science in Aberdeen', *Aberdeen Journal*, 14 February 1872, p. 5. He also invited the women of the Aberdeen Ladies' Educational Association, and their friends, to study in the Anatomical Museum in the 1880s: 'Aberdeen Ladies Educational Association', *Aberdeen Weekly Journal*, 15 April 1882. See Carol Dyhouse, *Students: A Gendered History* (London, 2006).

227 Universities (Scotland) Act 1889, allowing admission of women as students or staff, came into effect 1892, see Jennifer J. Carter and Colin A. McLaren, *Crown and Gown: An Illustrated History of Aberdeen* (Aberdeen, 1994); Lindy Moore, *Bajanellas and Semilinas: Aberdeen University and the Education of Women, 1860–1920* (Aberdeen, 1991).

228 'Professor Struthers on the Higher Education of Women', *Aberdeen Weekly Journal*, 6 November 1879; 'Professor Struthers' Saturday Evening Lectures', *Aberdeen Weekly Journal*, 28 January 1878.

229 'Presentation to Professor Struthers', *Aberdeen Journal*, 2 June 1875, p. 3.

230 'Lecture on Evolution', *Aberdeen Journal*, 25 February 1874, p. 5; 'Saturday Evening Lectures on Anatomy', *Aberdeen Journal*, 3 March 1875, p. 6.

231 *Aberdeen Weekly Journal* ('Dr John Struthers', 2 May 1885) reported that his talents were 'not inferior to that of a good comic actor, who could thus entertain a Saturday night audience of artizans'. On performance in science, see Michael Sappol, 'The Odd Case of Charles Knowlton: Anatomical Performance, Medical Narrative, and Identity in Antebellum America', *Bulletin of the History of Medicine*, LXXXIII (2009), pp. 460–98; Iwan Rhys Morus, 'Worlds of Wonder: Sensation and the Victorian Scientific Performance', *Isis*, CI (2010), pp. 806–16.

232 J. Struthers, 'Evening Lectures on Science', *Aberdeen Journal*, 14 February 1872, p. 5.

233 'Dr John Struthers', *Aberdeen Weekly Journal*, 2 May 1885; 'The British Association', *Aberdeen Weekly Journal*, 9 September 1885.

234 'The Anatomical Museum at Marischal College', *Aberdeen Weekly Journal*, 21 October 1889.

235 Ibid.

Five Visualizing the Interior

1 R. W. Reid, 'Presidential Address to the Aberdeen Anatomical and Anthropological Society', *University of Aberdeen Proceedings of the Anatomical and Anthropological Society* (*PAAS*, 1899–1900), pp. 6–15, p. 10.

2 See Samuel J.M.M. Alberti, *Morbid Curiosities: Medical Museums in Nineteenth-century Britain* (Oxford, 2011); George S. Huntington, 'The Morphological Museum as an Educational Factor in the University System', *Science*, New Series, XIII (1901), pp. 601–11; A. Low, 'University of Aberdeen, Department of Anatomy', *Methods and Problems of Medical Education*, 17th series (1930), pp. 207–12; Jonathan Reinarz, 'The Age of Museum Medicine: The Rise and Fall of the Medical Museum of Birmingham's School of Medicine', *Social History of Medicine*, XVIII (2005), pp. 419–37.

3 George. S. Huntington, 'Anatomy', *Science*, New Series, IX (1899), pp. 85–7, p. 86.

4 On the anthropometric laboratory at Marischal College, see Elizabeth Hallam, 'Laboratoire anthropométrique: La fabrication du savoir sur le corps en Ecosse, de 1880 à 1930' (Anthropometric Laboratory: Making Knowledge of the Body in Scotland, 1880–1930), *Ethnologie française*, XXXVII/2 (2007), pp. 275–84.

5 The arrangement of apes in branches was attributed to Robert Reid, see F. W. Fyfe, 'In Memoriam, R. D. Lockhart', *Journal of Anatomy*, CLV (1987), pp. 203–8, p. 204.

6 'Aberdeen University Museums: The Anatomical Collection', *Aberdeen Journal*, 15 April 1899, p. 4.

7 Low, 'University of Aberdeen'.

8 W. H. Flower, 'Museum Organisation', in W. H. Flower, *Essays on Museums and Other Subjects Connected with Natural History* (London, 1898 [1889]), pp. 1–29, p. 11.

9 Low, 'University of Aberdeen', p. 207.

10 M. V. Portman to R. W. Reid, 25 May 1895, MS letter, archive of University of Aberdeen, Anatomy Department (UAAD); F.H.B. Norrie to A. Low, 4 October 1929, MS letter, archive of UAAD. On M. V. Portman and the context in which he worked, see Satadru Sen, *Savagery and Colonialism in the Indian Ocean: Power, Pleasure and the Andaman Islands* (London, 2010); Claire Wintle, *Colonial Collecting and Display: Encounters with Material Culture from the Andaman and Nicobar Islands* (New York, 2013).

11 'Report by Museum Committee, University of Aberdeen', 1918–19, archive of University of Aberdeen, Marischal Museum (UAMM), n. pag.; R. W. Reid, 'Motor Points in Relation to the Surface of the Body', *Journal of Anatomy*, LIV (1920), pp. 271–5 (with Plates XXVI–XXXI), p. 271. Reid was assisted, when making the original cast, by sculptor William Banbury, from Gray's School of Art, Aberdeen.

12 'Report by Museum Committee, University of Aberdeen', 1920–21, archive of UAMM.

13 J. Struthers, 'The Progress of the Medical School', in *Aurora Borealis Academica: Aberdeen University Appreciations, 1860–1889*, ed. P. J. Anderson (Aberdeen, 1899), pp. 212–36. On Ziegler models, see Nick Hopwood, *Embryos in Wax: Models from the Ziegler Studio* (Cambridge and Bern, 2002).

14 For example, approximately five models were made by Alexander Low during and following a visit to the Anatomical Institute in Freiburg, see A. Low, 'Description of a Human Embryo of 13–14 Mesodermic Somites', *Journal of Anatomy and Physiology*, XLII (1908), pp. 237–51.

15 John S. Billings, 'Medical Museums', *Science*, XII (1888), pp. 134–6, p. 134.

16 E. L. Judah, 'Mounting Moist Specimens', *Canadian Medical Association Journal*, I (1911), pp. 335–6, p. 335. Low, 'Description of a Human Embryo'; J. T. Wilson,

'On a Method of Mounting and Exhibiting Frozen Sections of the Cadaver in the Anatomical Museum', *Journal of Anatomy and Physiology*, XLV (1910), pp. 3–6. On the uses of formaldehyde in medical museums, see Alberti, *Morbid Curiosities*; J. J. Edwards and M. J. Edwards, *Medical Museum Technology* (London, 1959).

17 R. W. Reid, 'Sagittal and Coronal Sections of the Human Head', PAAS (1902–4), pp. 99–100 (with plates XV–XXVIII).

18 Anatomy Act Committee Minutes, Aberdeen, vol. I: 1856–1959, p. 19, University of Aberdeen, Special Collections (UASC), (MSU 1332/4/1/1).

19 'Report by Museum Committee, University of Aberdeen', 1906–7, 1912–13, 1922–3, 1926–31, archive of UAMM.

20 A. Low, 'Obituary: Robert William Reid, MD, LLD, Aberd., FRCS: 1851–1939', *Man*, XXXIX (1939), pp. 179–80; Carolyn Pennington, *The Modernisation of Medical Teaching at Aberdeen in the Nineteenth Century* (Aberdeen, 1994).

21 Low, 'University of Aberdeen', p. 212. Arthur Keith, 'Anatomy in Scotland during the Lifetime of Sir John Struthers (1823–1899)', *Edinburgh Medical Journal*, VIII (1912), pp. 7–33; R. D. Lockhart, 'The Medical School', in *The Fusion of 1860: A Record of the Centenary Celebrations and a History of the United University of Aberdeen, 1860–1960*, ed. W. Douglas Simpson (Edinburgh, 1963), pp. 242–8.

22 'Aberdeen University Celebrations: Description of the Buildings', *Aberdeen Journal*, 22 October 1895, p. 5.

23 Robert Walker and A. M. Munro, *University of Aberdeen Quatercentenary Celebrations, September, 1906: Handbook to City and University* (Aberdeen, 1906).

24 A. Low, 'In Memoriam: Robert William Reid', *Journal of Anatomy*, LXXIV (1940), pp. 409–10 (With 1 Plate), p. 409. 'Report by Museum Committee, University of Aberdeen', 1907–8, archive of UAMM.

25 'Aberdeen University Celebrations: Description of the Buildings', p. 5. Walker and Munro, *University of Aberdeen*.

26 Low, 'University of Aberdeen'; David Wilson, 'Smoking in the Dissecting Room', *The Lancet*, 29 May 2004, p. 1836.

27 The 'anatomical attendant's house' at Marischal College is noted in 'Course of Lectures by Professor Reid', *Aberdeen Journal*, 18 January 1896, p. 6.

28 Low, 'University of Aberdeen'. On X-ray images see, Bernike Pasveer, 'Knowledge of Shadows: The Introduction of X-ray Images in Medicine', *Sociology of Health and Illness*, XI (1989), pp. 360–81; Bernike Pasveer, 'Representing or Mediating: A History and Philosophy of X-ray Images in Medicine', in *Visual Cultures of Science: Rethinking Representational Practices in Knowledge Building and Science Communication*, ed. Luc Pauwels (Hanover, NH, 2006), pp. 41–62; Daniel S. Goldberg, 'Suffering and Death among Early American Roentgenologists: The Power of Remotely Anatomizing the Living Body in Fin de Siècle America', *Bulletin for the History of Medicine*, LXXXV (2011), pp. 1–28.

29 Thomas Cooke and F. G. Hamilton Cooke, *Tablets of Anatomy, Dissectional and Scientific. Part II: Limbs, Abdomen, Pelvis*, 11th edn (London, 1898), p. vii, p. 132ff, p. 132ee. In addition to his Westminster Hospital position, Thomas Cooke founded a private school of anatomy, physiology and surgery in London, c. 1875, where he taught until his death in 1899, assisted by his son F. G. Hamilton Cooke. On his teaching, which was respected among his peers, see 'Obituary: Thomas Cooke, FRCS Eng., MD Paris', *The Lancet*, 18 February 1899, p. 482.

30 Alexander Macalister (n. d.), quoted in Cooke and Cooke, *Tablets of Anatomy*, epigraph, n. pag.

31 Cooke and Cooke, *Tablets of Anatomy*, pp. xxviii–xxix.

32 See Elizabeth Hallam, 'Anatomists Ways of Seeing and Knowing', in *Fieldnotes and Sketchbooks: Challenging the Boundaries between Descriptions and Processes of Describing*, ed. Wendy Gunn (Frankfurt, 2009), pp. 69–107.

33 Reid, 'Presidential Address', p. 11.

34 'Additions to Anatomy Museum and Laboratories', 1908–38, n. pag., MS notebook, archive of UAAD; 'Report by Museum Committee, University of Aberdeen', 1911–12, archive of UAMM; Walker and Munro, *University of Aberdeen*.

35 Anatomy Act Committee Minutes, vol. I, p. 194. On the acquisition of bodies for dissection in the early twentieth century, see Neville M. Goodman, 'The Supply of Bodies for Dissection: A Historical Review', *British Medical Journal*, 23 December 1944, pp. 807–11; Elizabeth T. Hurren, *Dying for Victorian Medicine: English Anatomy and its Trade in the Dead Poor, c. 1834–1929* (Basingstoke, 2012).

36 Low, 'University of Aberdeen, p. 210; Reid, 'Presidential Address, p. 11. James Fowler Fraser, *Doctor Jimmy: Some Reminiscences by Dr James Fowler Fraser, 1893–1979* (Aberdeen, 1980).

37 Reid, 'Presidential Address', p. 11.

38 Ibid., p. 10, p. 11. On practices that define the 'pathological', see Lorraine Daston and Peter Galison, *Objectivity* (New York, 2007) p. 309.

39 R. W. Reid, Anatomical variations occurring in dissections at St Thomas's Hospital, 1874–78, MS book of sketches and notes, UASC (MS 3753/1/1).

40 Anatomical Variations, 1891–1945, drawings and notes made on pre-printed forms by medical students at Marischal College, UASC (MSU 1442/3).

41 For example, Margaret Duncan, see 'Record of Anatomical Variations', *PAAS*, 1899–1900, pp. 45–54 (with plates VII, VIII); Anatomy Act Committee Minutes, vol. I, p. 217; Lindy Moore, *Bajanellas and Semilinas: Aberdeen University and the Education of Women, 1860–1920* (Aberdeen, 1991). On women medical students, see Carol Dyhouse, *Students: A Gendered History* (London, 2006); Ruth Watts, *Women in Science: A Social and Cultural History* (London, 2007); Susan Wells, *Out of the Dead House: Nineteenth-century Women Physicians and the Writing of Medicine* (Madison, 2001).

42 Reid, 'Presidential Address', p. 11.

43 See Jonathan Crary, *Suspensions of Perception: Attention, Spectacle, and Modern Culture* (Cambridge, MA, 2001).

44 F. G. Parsons and William Wright, *Practical Anatomy: The Student's Dissecting Manual, Vol. I, The Head and Neck: The Lower Extremity* (London, 1912), p. xiii.

45 See Lianne McTavish, *Defining the Modern Museum: A Case Study of the Challenges of Exchange* (Toronto, 2013); M. Norton Wise, 'Making Visible', *Isis*, XCVII (2006), pp. 75–82.

46 Reid, 'Presidential Address'.

47 Reid, 'Sagittal and Coronal Sections'.

48 Wilhelm Braune, *An Atlas of Topographical Anatomy After Plane Sections of Frozen Bodies*, trans. Edward Bellamy (London, 1877).

49 The images are signed A. Don and A. H. Lister. Alexander Don graduated MB CM in 1894, and Arthur Hugh Lister graduated MB CM in 1895, see William Johnston, *Roll of the Graduates of the University of Aberdeen, 1860–1900* (Aberdeen, 1906), p. 134, p. 289–90.

50 Huntington, 'Morphological Museum', p.606.

51 See Catelijne Coopmans et al., eds, *Representation in Scientific Practice Revisited* (Cambridge, MA, 2014); Michael Lynch, 'Discipline and the Material Form of Images: An Analysis of Scientific Visibility', *Social Studies of Science*, XV (1985), pp. 37–66; Michael Lynch and Steve Woolgar, eds, *Representation in Scientific Practice* (Cambridge, MA, 1990).

52 W. H. Flower, 'Note on the Construction and Arrangement of Anatomical Museums', *Journal of Anatomy and Physiology*, IX (1875), p. 259–62, p. 260.

53 Dawn Kemp with Sara Barnes, *Surgeons' Hall: A Museum Anthology* (Edinburgh, 2009). On anatomical display see Eva Åhrén, *Death, Modernity, and the Body: Sweden, 1870–1940* (Rochester, NY, 2009).

54 'Report by Museum Committee, University of Aberdeen', 1905–6, archive of UAMM.

55 A. Low, 'The Aberdeen University Anatomical and Anthropological Society', *Aberdeen University Review*, 1944, pp. 333–4.

56 R. W. Reid, 'Notes upon a Mesial Sagittal Section of a Female Subject', *PAAS* (1904–6), pp. 122–3, p. 122.

57 Ibid.

58 Cooke and Cooke, *Tablets of Anatomy*, p. xxviii, p. xxix.

59 Ibid.

60 Low, 'University of Aberdeen', p. 207. 'Report by Museum Committee, University of Aberdeen', 1922–3, 1926–7, archive of UAMM.

61 Massimiano Bucchi, 'Images of Science in the Classroom: Wall Charts and Science Education, 1850–1920', in *Visual Cultures of Science*, ed. Pauwels, pp. 90–119.

62 Wall chart: 'Schematic Representation of the Perilymphatic and Endolymphatic Spaces, the Former Appear in Black and the Latter in Blue (Testut)', labelled by Robert Reid, 1899. The diagram is after Fig. 483 in L. Testut, *Traité d'anatomie humaine, tome troisième, système nerveux périphérique – organes des sens* (Paris 1899), fig. 483, a copy of which was held in UAAD's collection of anatomical atlases and textbooks.

63 Testut, *Traité d'anatomie humaine*, p. 388.

64 Nora Macdonald, 'Manners and Customs of the Ancient Egyptians', *PAAS*, 1900–1902, pp. 18–34, Plate V, Fig. 2, with caption: 'Mummy of Young Man from Koos, near Thebes, Showing Incision on Left Side (Archaeological Museum, University of Aberdeen)'. On Nora Macdonald see Helen Southwood, 'A Cultural History of Marischal Anthropological Museum in the Twentieth Century', PhD thesis, University of Aberdeen (2003).

65 On the removal of backgrounds from images of material objects in late nineteenth-century photographic practices, see Elizabeth Edwards, *Raw Histories: Photographs, Anthropology and Museums* (Oxford, 2001); Elizabeth Edwards, *The Camera as Historian: Amateur Photographers and Historical Imagination, 1885–1918* (Durham, NC, 2012).

66 'Ordinary Meeting', 30 January 1904, *PAAS* (1902–4), p. 99; Reid, 'Sagittal and Coronal Sections'.

67 Huntington, 'Morphological Museum', p. 606.

68 On lantern slides and their display, see Edwards, *Raw Histories*; Jennifer Tucker, *Nature Exposed: Photography as Eyewitness in Victorian Science* (Baltimore, MD, 2005).

69 'Report by Museum Committee, University of Aberdeen', 1906–1908, archive of UAMM.

70 Low, 'University of Aberdeen'.

71 Ibid., p. 210. Low, 'In Memoriam: Robert William Reid'.

72 Richard J. A. Berry, *A Clinical Atlas of Sectional and Topographical Anatomy*, (Edinburgh, 1911) p. 2, p. 7. On Richard Berry, see Ross L. Jones, *Humanity's Mirror: 150 Years of Anatomy in Melbourne* (Melbourne, 2007).

73 On mechanical objectivity see, Daston and Galison, *Objectivity*.

74 Berry, *Clinical Atlas*, p. 5, p. 12. Low, 'University of Aberdeen'.

75 Berry, *Clinical Atlas*, p. 12.

76 David Waterston, ed., *The Edinburgh Stereoscopic Atlas of Anatomy* (Edinburgh, 1905–06). For analysis of stereoscopic images, see Jonathan Crary, *Techniques of the Observer: On Vision and Modernity in the Nineteenth Century* (Cambridge, MA, 1992); Roberta McGrath, *Seeing Her Sex: Medical Archives and the Female Body* (Manchester, 2002); John Plunkett, 'Feeling Seeing: Touch, Vision and the Stereoscope', *History of Photography*, XXXVII (2013), pp. 389–96.

77 Review of '*The Edinburgh Stereoscopic Atlas of Anatomy*. Edited by David Waterston, MD, Lecturer and Demonstrator in the Department of Anatomy, University of Edinburgh. T. C. & E. C. Jack, Edinburgh, 1905', *Journal of Anatomy and Physiology*, XXXIX (1905), pp. 368–9. On trained judgement in scientific practices, see Daston and Galison, *Objectivity*.

78 Arthur Thomson, *The Anatomy of the Human Eye as Illustrated by Enlarged Stereoscopic Photographs* (Oxford, 1912).

79 Bruno Latour refers to cascades of 'ever-simplified inscriptions' in the practice of science, from three-dimensional objects to two-dimensional images, which make phenomena

increasingly intelligible; see Bruno Latour, 'Drawing Things Together', in *Representations in Scientific Practice*, ed. Lynch and Woolgar, pp. 19–68. For historical studies of three-dimensional models, rather than the reduction of three dimensions to two dimensions in science, see Nick Hopwood and Soraya de Chadarevian, eds, *Models: The Third Dimension of Science* (Stanford, CA, 2004).

80 Reid, 'Sagittal and Coronal Sections', p. 99.

81 'Report by Museum Committee, University of Aberdeen' (1905–10), archive of UAMM.

82 Anatomy Act Committee Minutes, vol. I, pp. 133–299. Old Machar Poor House and St Nicholas Poor House (referred to as West Poor House and East Poor House respectively from 1896) became Oldmill Poor House in 1907. Aberdeen Royal Lunatic Asylum became Aberdeen Royal Mental Hospital in 1933.

83 On museum collecting in colonial contexts, see Nélia Dias, 'From French Indochina to Paris and Back Again: The Circulation of Objects, People and Information, 1900–1932', *Museum & Society*, XIII (2015), pp. 7–21; Gosden and Knowles, *Collecting Colonialism: Material Culture and Colonial Change* (Oxford, 2001); Michael O'Hanlon and Robert Louis Welsch, *Hunting the Gatherers: Ethnographic Collectors, Agents and Agency in Melanesia, 1870s–1930s* (Oxford, 2000); Ricardo Roque, *Headhunting and Colonialism: Anthropology and the Circulation of Human Skulls in the Portuguese Empire, 1870–1930* (Basingstoke, 2010); Southwood, 'Cultural History of Marischal'; Wintle, *Colonial Collecting and Display*; see also Chapter Three (this volume) note 5.

84 Alexander J. F. Reid to R. W. Reid, 6 July 1895, MS letter, archive of UAAD; human skull, museum label dated 1895, collection of University of Aberdeen, Anatomy Museum (UAAM). The skull was obtained during the 1895 Chitral Relief Expedition in northwest British India (northern Pakistan).

85 Alexander Ogston to R. W. Reid, 8 December 1893, MS letter, archive of UAAD.

86 'Aberdeen University Museums', *Aberdeen Journal*, p. 4.

87 Reid, 'Presidential Address'.

88 Ibid.; R. W. Reid, 'The Development of Anthropology in the University of Aberdeen' (Aberdeen, 1934). Edward Burnett Tylor visited Aberdeen as Gifford Lecturer, 1889–91. On Tylor and developments in anthropology during the late nineteenth and early twentieth centuries, see Chris Gosden and Frances Larson with Alison Petch, *Knowing Things: Exploring the Collections at the Pitt Rivers Museum, 1884–1945* (Oxford, 2007); Henrika Kuklick, ed., *A New History of Anthropology* (Oxford, 2008); George W. Stocking, *After Tylor: British Social Anthropology, 1888–1951* (Madison, WI, 1995).

89 Edward B. Tylor, *Anthropology: An Introduction to the Study of Man and Civilization* (London, 1881), p. 60, p. 56.

90 Ibid.

91 W. H. Flower ,'Presidential Address to the Department of Anthropology, at the British Association for the Advancement of Science (York meeting), 1 September 1881', in *Essays in Museums*, ed. Flower, pp. 235–48, p. 246. On the collecting of human skulls during the second half of the nineteenth century and early twentieth century, see Nélia Dias, 'Nineteenth-century French Collections of Skulls and the Cult of Bones', *Nuncius*, XXVII (2012), pp. 330–47; Simon Harrison, 'Skulls and Scientific Collecting in the Victorian Military: Keeping the Enemy Dead in British Frontier Warfare', *Comparative Studies in Society and History*, L (2008), pp. 285–303; Elise Juzda, 'Skulls, Science and the Spoils of War: Craniological Studies at the United States Army Medical Museum, 1868–1900', *Studies in the History and Philosophy of Biological and Biomedical Sciences*, XL (2009), pp. 156–67; Roque, *Headhunting and Colonialism*; Fenneke Sysling, '"Not Everything That Says Java is from Java": Provenance and the Fate of Physical Anthropology Collections', in *The Fate of Anatomical Collections*, ed. Rina Knoeff and Robert Zwijnenberg (Farnham, 2015), pp. 195–210.

92 For analysis of the geographically widespread social relations of museums, see Gosden and Larson, with Petch, *Knowing Things*.

93 John D. Hargreaves, *Academe and Empire: Some Overseas Connections of Aberdeen*

University (Aberdeen, 1994); 'Report by Museum Committee, University of Aberdeen' (1909–11, 1912–13), archive of UAMM.

94 Human skulls, collection of UAAM.

95 R. W. Reid, 'Exhibition and Description of the Skull of a Microcephalic Hindu', *Journal of the Anthropological Institute*, XXIV (1895), pp. 105–8 (with plates XII, XIII), p. 105. R. W. Reid, *Illustrated Catalogue of the Anthropological Museum, University of Aberdeen* (Aberdeen, 1912).

96 W. H. Flower, *Catalogue of the Specimens Illustrating the Osteology and Dentition of Vertebrated Animals, Recent and Extinct, Contained in the Museum of the Royal College of Surgeons of England, Part I*, 2nd edn (London, 1907), p. xii. See Alberti, *Morbid Curiosities*; Roque, *Headhunting and Colonialism*.

97 'Report by Museum Committee, University of Aberdeen' (1904–5), archive of UAMM.

98 Allen J. Craigen to R. W. Reid, 14 April 1902, MS letter, archive of UAAD.

99 R. H. Spittal, 'Observations on Fourteen New Guinea Skulls', PAAS (1904–6), pp. 88–95 (with plates IV–VII), p. 89. On cultural representations of cannibalism in colonial discourse, see Annie E. Coombes, *Reinventing Africa. Museums, Material Culture and Popular Imagination in Late Victorian and Edwardian England* (New Haven, CT, 1994); Patrick Brantlinger, *Taming Cannibals: Race and the Victorians* (Ithaca, NY, 2011); Shirley Lindenbaum, 'Thinking About Cannibalism', *Annual Review of Anthropology*, XXXIII (2004), pp. 475–98.

100 Spittal, 'Observations', p. 89;

101 For discussion of how skull collectors represented indigenous displays of human heads and skulls, see Thomas, *Entangled Objects*.

102 Spittal, 'Observations', p. 93, p. 89, p. 91, p. 94.

103 W.R.C. Middleton to R. W. Reid, 11 October 1904, MS letter, archive of UAAD.

104 W.R.C. Middleton to R. W. Reid, 27 August 1902, MS letter, archive of UAAD.

105 W.R.C. Middleton to R. W. Reid, 11 October 1904, MS letter, archive of UAAD. James Clark, 'Description of the Distorted Feet of a Chinese Female', PAAS (1904–6), pp. 40–45 (with Plate I).

106 Clark, 'Description', p. 43.

107 Ibid., p. 43.

108 Hallam, 'Laboratoire anthropométrique'.

109 Paul Topinard, 'Observations upon the Methods and Process of Anthropometry', *Journal of the Anthropological Institute*, X (1881), pp. 212–24, p. 212.

110 Reid, 'Presidential Address', pp. 12–13.

111 For example, see R. W. Reid and J. H. Mulligan, 'Relation of Cranial Capacity to Intelligence', *Journal of the Royal Anthropological Institute*, LIII (1923), pp. 322–31.

112 J. Gray and J. F. Tocher, 'The Physical Characteristics of the Population of West Aberdeenshire', *Journal of the Anthropological Institute*, XXX (1900), pp. 86–8, p. 86. See Elizabeth Edwards, ed., *Anthropology and Photography, 1860–1920* (New Haven, CT, 1992); Christopher Morton and Elizabeth Edwards, eds, *Photography, Anthropology and History: Expanding the Frame* (Farnham, 2009); James Urry, *Before Social Anthropology: Essays on the History of British Anthropology* (Chur, Reading, 1993).

113 John George Garson and Charles Hercules Read, eds, *Notes and Queries on Anthropology* (for the Council of the Anthropological Institute), 2nd edn (London, 1892).

114 Francis Galton, 'On the Anthropometric Laboratory at the Late International Health Exhibition', *Journal of the Anthropological Institute*, XIV (1885), pp. 205–18 (with plates XII, XIII).

115 D. J. Cunningham and A. C. Haddon, 'The Anthropometric Laboratory of Ireland', *Journal of the Anthropological Institute*, XXI (1892), pp. 35–9, p. 36. See Elizabeth Edwards, 'Photographic "Types": The Pursuit of Method', *Visual Anthropology*, III (1990), pp. 235–58.

116 Reid, 'Presidential Address'.

117 A. Low, 'Aberdeen University Anatomical and Anthropological Society', p. 334.

118 Walker and Munro, *University of Aberdeen*; Visit to the Anatomical and Anthropometrical Museums, 1902, clippings of reports from local newspapers, UASC (MS 3753/2/6).

119 Aberdeen University Museums, *Aberdeen Journal*, p. 4.

120 Low, 'Aberdeen University Anatomical and Anthropological Society', p. 334. On William MacGregor and the wider context in which he collected, see Susan Cochrane and Max Quanchi, eds, *Pacific Collections in Australian Museums, Galleries and Archives* (Newcastle-upon-Tyne, 2007); Hargreaves, *Academe and Empire*; R. B. Joyce, *Sir William MacGregor* (Oxford, 1971); O'Hanlon and Welsch, *Hunting the Gatherers*; Southwood, 'Cultural History of Marischal'.

121 Walker and Munro, *University of Aberdeen*, p. 101.

122 'Reid, 'Presidential Address', p. 10; Topinard, 'Observations upon the Methods', p. 217, p. 216.

123 Topinard, 'Observations upon the Methods', p. 213, p. 213.

124 Reid, 'Development of Anthropology', p. 9.

125 James Adams, 'The Characteristics of Five Wa Kamba Skulls', *PAAS*, 1902–4, pp. 56–8; A. Elmslie Campbell, 'A Description of Six East African Skulls, With Measurements, Indices, and Tracings of the Same', *PAAS* (1908–14), pp. 24–9 (with plates I–III); Spittal, 'Observations'.

126 C. T. Andrew, 'Description of Four Decorated Skulls from New Guinea', *PAAS* (1899–1900), pp. 29–34 (with plates III, IV).

127 Reid, 'Presidential Address', p. 11, p. 12; Andrew, 'Description of Four Decorated Skulls', p. 29, p. 30. On anatomical methods, including dissection, used to study material objects, see Frances Larson, 'Anthropology as Comparative Anatomy? Reflecting on the Study of Material Culture during the Late 1800s and the Late 1900s', *Journal of Material Culture*, XII (2007), pp. 89–112.

128 Andrew, 'Description of Four Decorated Skulls', p. 33, p. 34.

129 R. W. Reid and C. T. Andrew, 'Comparison between a Skeleton of a Chinese Coolie from Singapore, a Skull of a Boxer from North China, and a Skeleton of a European', *PAAS* (1902–4), pp. 2–7, p. 2.

130 Ibid. p. 4.

131 'Ordinary Meeting', 30 June 1900, *PAAS* (1899–1900), pp. 39–43 (with plates V, VI), p. 39.

132 Ibid., p. 42, p. 41.

133 Ibid., plate V. For analysis of the display of indigenous people, see Roslyn Poignant, *Professional Savage: Captive Lives and Western Spectacle* (New Haven, CT, 2004); Sadiah Qureshi, *Peoples on Parade: Exhibitions, Empire, and Anthropology in Nineteenth-century Britain* (Chicago, IL, 2011).

134 C. G. Seligman, 'Anthropological Notes from British New Guinea', *PAAS* (1906–8), pp. 22–31 (with plates III, IV), p. 29. On Charles Seligman see Gosden and Larson, with Petch, *Knowing Things*.

135 Seligman, 'Anthropological Notes'.

136 Edwards, *Raw Histories*, p. 69. See also Elizabeth Edwards, 'Evolving Images: Photography, Race and Popular Darwinism', in *Endless Forms: Charles Darwin, Natural Science and the Visual Arts*, ed. Diana Donald and Jane Munro, exh. cat., Fitzwilliam Museum, Cambridge (New Haven, CT, 2009), pp. 167–92; Martin Kemp and Marina Wallace, *Spectacular Bodies: The Art and Science of the Human Body from Leonardo to Now*, exh. cat., Hayward Gallery, London (2000), p. 165.

137 'Aberdeen University Museums', *Aberdeen Journal*, p. 4.

138 Reid, 'Presidential Address', p. 14.

139 Reid, *Illustrated Catalogue*, p. v.

140 Ibid., p. iii, p. 301; A. Low, 'Aberdeen University Anatomical and Anthropological Society', p. 334.

141 Reid, *Illustrated Catalogue*, p. iii. Charles Michie, *Catalogue of Antiquities in the Archaeological Museum of King's College, University of Aberdeen* (Aberdeen, 1887);

'Report by Museum Committee, University of Aberdeen', 1906–7, archive of UAMM. Reid was curator of the Anthropological Museum until autumn 1938, when Low took the position until 1 January 1939; see Low, 'In Memoriam: Robert William Reid'.

142 Reid, 'Presidential Address', p. 11; Reid, 'Development of Anthropology', p. 8. In adopting this 'classification', Reid stated that he followed William Flower, see Reid, 'Presidential Address', p. 14.

143 The Anatomy Museum's collection of human skulls was referred to as one part of the 'Anthropological Collection' in Reid, *Illustrated Catalogue*, p. iii.

144 Anthropometrical Laboratory Register of Observations, 6 vols, 1896–1938, UASC (MSU 1332/5/1); Anthropometrical Registers of Fingerprints, 7 vols, 1896–1938, UASC (MSU 1332/5/2).

145 See R. W. Reid and John H. Mulligan, 'Communications from the Anthropometric Laboratory of the University of Aberdeen', *Journal of the Royal Anthropological Institute*, LIV (1924), pp. 287–315.

146 See Nélia Dias, 'The Visibility of Difference: Nineteenth-century French Anthropological Collections', in *The Politics of Display: Museums, Science, Culture*, ed. Sharon Macdonald (London, 1998), pp. 36–52, p. 42.

147 See Edwards, *Raw Histories*.

148 Anthropometrical Laboratory Register of Observations, vol. 1, 1896–1905, UASC (MSU 1332/5/1/1).

149 Ibid.; 'In Memoriam: The Staff, Students, and Alumni of the University who Laid Down Their Lives during the Wars 1914–18 and 1939–45', University of Aberdeen, www.abdn.ac.uk, accessed 10 November 2014.

150 'Lectures on Anatomy', *Aberdeen Journal*, 2 February 1891, p. 4. R. W. Reid, Popular Lectures on Anatomy, MS lecture notes, 1891–1902, UASC (MS 3753/2/1).

151 'Aberdeen University Museums', *Aberdeen Journal*, p. 4.

152 Ibid., p. 4.

153 See; Alberti, *Morbid Curiosities*; Billings, 'Medical Museum'; Maritha Rene Burmeister, 'Popular Anatomical Museums in Nineteenth-century England', PhD thesis, Rutgers University (2000).

154 'Aberdeen: An Exhibition Prohibited', *Aberdeen Journal*, 3 March 1883, p. 4; 'Contravention of Indecent Advertisements Act', *Aberdeen Journal*, 23 May 1895, p. 4; 'Museum of Science', *Aberdeen Weekly Journal*, 18 October 1895, p. 2.

155 Reid, 'Presidential Address', p. 15; Reid, *Illustrated Catalogue*. See Southwood, 'Cultural History of Marischal'.

156 For analysis of how museums and their collections of objects have shaped university disciplines, see Alberti, *Morbid Curiosities*; Samuel J.M.M. Alberti, *Nature and Culture: Objects, Disciplines and the Manchester Museum* (Manchester, 2009); Gosden and Larson, with Petch, *Knowing Things*; Frances Larson, 'Anthropological Landscaping'.

Six Living Anatomy

1 By 1923 the 1858 *Anatomy, Descriptive and Surgical* by Henry Gray with illustrations by Henry Vandyke Carter was in its 22nd edition, entitled *Anatomy Descriptive and Applied*, with Robert Howden as editor; see Ruth Richardson, *The Making of Mr Gray's Anatomy: Bodies, Books, Fortune, Fame* (Oxford, 2008).

2 R. D. Lockhart, 'The Anatomist's Dream', typescript poem, University of Aberdeen, Special Collections (UASC) (MS 3270/1/7/1/10). The poem was sung at a student dinner, University of Aberdeen, 1923. With reference to a psychoanalyst, Lockhart was probably alluding, humorously, to Sigmund Freud's *The Interpretation of Dreams* (English translation published 1913). On the reception of Freud's work in early twentieth-century Britain, see Natalya Lusty and Helen Groth, *Dreams and Modernity: A Cultural History* (London, 2013).

3 Lockhart, 'The Anatomist's Dream'.

4 F. W. Fyfe, 'In Memoriam, R. D. Lockhart', *Journal of Anatomy*, CLV (1987), pp. 203–8; R. D. Lockhart, 'The Regius Chair of Anatomy in the University of Aberdeen: Application, References and Testimonials of Robert D. Lockhart', 14 April 1938, printed/typescript document, UASC (MS 3270/1/4/5/1). Lockhart was curator of the Anthropological Museum from 1 January 1939 to 1979, see Helen Southwood, 'A Cultural History of Marischal Anthropological Museum in the Twentieth Century', PhD thesis, University of Aberdeen (2003).

5 'Additions to Anatomy Museum and Laboratories', 1908–38, MS notebook, archive of UAAD; 'Report by Museum Committee, University of Aberdeen', 1904–46, archive of University of Aberdeen, Marischal Museum (UAMM).

6 On poetics in museum display, and in science, see Ivan Karp and Steven D. Lavine, eds, *Exhibiting Cultures: The Poetics and Politics of Museum Display* (Washington, DC, 1991); Henrietta Lidchi, 'The Poetics and Politics of Exhibiting Other Cultures', in *Representation: Cultural Representations and Signifying Practices*, ed. Stuart Hall (Milton Keynes, 1997); James J. Bono, 'Making Knowledge: History, Literature, and the Poetics of Science', *Isis*, CI (2010), pp. 555–9.

7 R. D. Lockhart, 'The Art of Leaning Anatomy', *The Lancet*, 27 August 1927, pp. 460–61, p. 460.

8 Lorriane Daston and Peter Galison, *Objectivity* (New York, 2007). On the necessity of 'imaginative reflection' in science, see C. R. Bardeen, 'The Value of the Roentgen-ray and the Living Model in Teaching and Research in Human Anatomy', *Anatomical Record*, XIV (1918), pp. 337–40, p. 338. A negative evaluation of the 'unimaginative study of the human body' is made in, for example, 'Reviews: The New Anatomy', *British Medical Journal*, 26 June 1915, p. 1085.

9 Samuel J.M.M. Alberti, *Morbid Curiosities: Medical Museums in Nineteenth-century Britain* (Oxford, 2011); Jonathan Reinarz, 'The Age of Museum Medicine: The Rise and Fall of the Medical Museum at Birmingham's School of Medicine', *Social History of Medicine*, XVIII (2005), pp. 419–37. By 1950, in addition to the anatomical collections at the royal colleges in Edinburgh and London, and at several London teaching hospitals, anatomy museums were kept at the universities of Aberdeen, Birmingham, Cambridge, Cardiff (University College), Dundee (University College), Edinburgh, Glasgow, Leeds, Manchester, Sheffield, St Andrews (Bute Medical School), as well as at Queen's University Belfast, and Trinity College Dublin, see C. J. Hackett, 'A List of Medical Museums of Great Britain (1949–50)', *British Medical Journal*, 16 June 1951, pp. 1380–83.

10 A. E. Barclay, 'Models of the Human Stomach Showing Its Form Under Various Conditions', *Journal of Anatomy and Physiology*, LIV (1920), pp. 258–69, p. 258. Dr Rainy, 'Discussion', in *An Inquiry into the Medical Curriculum by the Edinburgh Pathological Club*, ed. Edinburgh Pathological Club (Edinburgh, 1919), pp. 67–8, p. 68. On trust invested in X-rays, see Bernike Pasveer, 'Representing or Mediating: A History and Philosophy of X-ray Images in Medicine', in *Visual Cultures of Science: Rethinking Representational Practices in Knowledge Building and Science Communication*, ed. Luc Pauwels (Hanover, NH, 2006).

11 On the practice of science as performance, see Iwan Rhys Morus, 'Placing Performance', *Isis*, CI (2010), pp. 775–8.

12 See, for example, 'Modern Anatomical Teaching', *The Lancet*, 9 December 1922, p. 1232; 'Teaching of Anatomy', *The Lancet*, 18 February 1928, pp. 348–9, p. 348; John C. McLachlan and Debra Patten, 'Anatomy Teaching: Ghosts of the Past, Present and Future', *Medical Education*, XL (2006), pp. 243–53.

13 G. Elliot Smith, 'The Teaching of Anatomy', in *Inquiry into the Medical Curriculum*, ed. Edinburgh Pathological Club, pp. 49–56, p. 53.

14 Ibid., p. 50.

15 Ibid., p. 54.

16 David Waterston, 'The Teaching of Anatomy', in *Inquiry into the Medical Curriculum*, ed. Edinburgh Pathological Club, pp. 57–62, p. 59; Alexis Thomson, 'Systematic Surgery',

in *Inquiry into the Medical Curriculum*, ed. Edinburgh Pathological Club, pp. 223–6, p. 226; G. Grey Turner, 'The Essentials of Surgical Teaching', in *Inquiry into the Medical Curriculum*, ed. Edinburgh Pathological Club, pp. 209–18; p. 215.

17 Elliot Smith, 'Teaching of Anatomy', p. 56.

18 'Teaching of Anatomy', *The Lancet*, 18 February 1928, pp. 348–9, p. 348.

19 T. Wingate Todd (1912), quoted in Wilton Marion Krogman, 'Fifty Years of Physical Anthropology: The Men, The Material, The Concepts', *Annual Review of Anthropology*, v (1976), pp. 1–14, p. 2.

20 R. D. Lockhart, G. F. Hamilton and F. W. Fyfe, *Anatomy of the Human Body* (London, 1959), p. 11.

21 The Chapel was destroyed in 1942, during the Second World War.

22 Annotated postcard, 20 February 1919, collection/papers of R. D. Lockhart, UASC (MS 3270).

23 Forty-six ex-servicemen returned to medical studies at Marischal College in 1918; see J. F. Fraser, *Doctor Jimmy: Some Reminiscences by Dr James Fowler Fraser, 1893–1979* (Aberdeen, 1980), p. 66.

24 Interview, with R. D. Lockhart, by Elizabeth Olson, 11 March 1985, UASC (MS 3620/1/18). See also Interview, with R. D. Lockhart, by Elizabeth Olson, 18 March 1985, UASC (MS 3620/1/19). On the treatment of soldiers' bodies, Joanna Bourke, *Dismembering the Male: Men's Bodies, Britain and the Great War* (London, 1996); Melissa Larner et al., eds, *War and Medicine* (London, 2008).

25 F. W. Fyfe, 'In Memoriam, R. D. Lockhart'; Lockhart, 'Art of Learning Anatomy'.

26 'Future of the Medical Museum', *The Lancet*, 24 March 1945, pp. 376–7, p. 377, p. 376. 'The Museum of the Royal College of Surgeons, London. Dispersal of Collections After Air-Raid Damage', *Museums Journal*, XLI (1942), pp. 287–8. This article reported on approximately 27,000 surviving specimens out of a pre air raid total of nearly 66,000.

27 'Air-raid Damage to Museums: London, Museum of Royal College of Surgeons', *The Museums Journal*, XLI (1941), p. 78; Cecil Wakely, 'The Hunterian Museum To-day', *Annals of the Royal College of Surgeons of England*, XXXVII (1965), pp. 329–45.

28 Arthur Keith, *An Autobiography* (London, 1950), p. 673.

29 'The Museum of the Royal College of Surgeons, London. Dispersal of Collections After Air-raid Damage', p. 288.

30 'Future of the Medical Museum', p. 376.

31 Ibid., p. 376.

32 Ibid., p. 376.

33 Ibid., p. 377. G. Grey Turner 'The Hunterian Museum Yesterday and Tomorrow', *The Lancet*, The Lancet, 24 March 1945, pp. 359–63; Wakeley, 'The Hunterian Museum Today'.

34 Hackett, 'List of Medical Museums'. Although possibly incomplete, this article recorded numbers of medical museums (pathological, anatomical and surgical museums) in 1949–50 as follows: London: 41, the provinces: 23, Scotland: 20, Wales: 2, Northern Ireland: 2, Eire: 2; these museums included 71 with founding dates as follows: before 1800: 4, 1800–1900: 29, 1900–1925: 19, 1925–1950: 19.

35 Lockhart, Hamilton and Fyfe, *Anatomy*, p. 1.

36 Elliot Smith, 'Teaching of Anatomy', p. 50.

37 'Review. *Cunningham's Manual of Practical Anatomy*. 9th edn. Revised and edited by J. C. Brash and E. B. Jamieson. In three volumes', *Journal of Anatomy*, LXX (1935), p. 185.

38 Lockhart, 'Art of Learning Anatomy', p. 460; Lockhart, Hamilton and Fyfe, *Anatomy*, p. 1.

39 Duncan Forbes, *An Exile's Eye: The Photography of Wolfgang Suschitzky*, exh. cat., Scottish National Portrait Gallery, Edinburgh (2002).

40 Ian A. Olson, 'Robert Douglas Lockhart (1894–1987), Regius Professor of Anatomy (1938–1965)', *Aberdeen University Review*, CLXXX (1988), pp. 330–34, p. 333. Fyfe, 'In Memoriam, R. D. Lockhart'; 'Anatomy Department, Inventory', 1969, typescript/MS list, archive of UAAD.

41 Anatomy Act Committee Minutes, Aberdeen, vol. I, 1856–1959, pp. 286–362, UASC
    (MSU 1332/4/1/1); Anatomy Act Committee Minutes, Aberdeen, vol. II, 1960–73,
    pp. 1–18, UASC (MSU 1332/4/1/2).

42 Lockhart, 'Art of Learning Anatomy', p. 460. James Howie, 'Professor Robert Douglas
    Lockhart, MD, FRSE (1894–1987)', *British Medical Journal*, 9 May 1987, pp. 1213.

43 Lockhart, 'Art of Learning Anatomy', p. 460; Lockhart, Hamilton and Fyfe, *Anatomy*,
    p. 1.

44 James Couper Brash, ed., *Cunningham's Manual of Practical Anatomy*, vol. III: *Head and
    Neck: Brain*, 11th edn (London, 1948), p. vi.

45 At Marischal College the number of female medical students rose rapidly during the
    1914–18 war, and just after the 1939 outbreak of war students at the London (Royal Free
    Hospital) School of Medicine for Women were taught in the Anatomy Department for
    about a year, see Fyfe, 'In Memoriam, R. D. Lockhart'; Lindy Moore, *Bajanellas and
    Semilinas: Aberdeen University and the Education of Women, 1860–1920* (Aberdeen, 1991).
    On gender in medical education, see Carol Dyhouse, *Students: A Gendered History*
    (London, 2006); Ruth Watts, *Women in Science: A Social and Cultural History* (London,
    2007).

46 See Jonathan Sawday, *The Body Emblazoned: Dissection and the Human Body in
    Renaissance Culture* (London, 1995); Martin Kemp and Marina Wallace, *Spectacular
    Bodies: The Art and Science of the Human Body from Leonardo to Now*, exh. cat., Hayward
    Gallery, London (2000).

47 Thomas Cooke and F. G. Hamilton Cooke, *Tablets of Anatomy, Dissectional and Scientific*,
    Part II: *Limbs, Abdomen, Pelvis*, 11th edn (London, 1898), p. 132dd.

48 Ibid., p. xxii.

49 Ibid., p. 132ee.

50 Elliot Smith, 'Teaching of Anatomy', pp. 50–51. On the unconscious in early twentieth-
    century science, see Daston and Galison, *Objectivity*.

51 G. Gordon-Taylor, 'In Defence of Eponyms', *Journal of the Royal College of Surgeons of
    Edinburgh*, IV (1959), pp. 105–20. See David Kachlik et al., 'Anatomical Terminology
    and Nomenclature: Past, Present and Highlights', *Surgical and Radiologic Anatomy*, XXX
    (2008), pp. 459–66.

52 Minutes of the Aberdeen University Anatomical and Anthropological Society (AUAAS),
    vol. II, 1947/48–1952/53, p. 34, UASC (MS U1332).

53 Minutes of the AUAAS, vol. III, n. pag. (October 1961).

54 Lockhart, Hamilton and Fyfe, *Anatomy*, p. 456, p. 458.

55 Ibid., p. 1; See Lockhart, 'Art of Learning Anatomy'.

56 Lockhart, Hamilton and Fyfe, *Anatomy*, p. 456, fig. 693.

57 Interview, with Dr Dorothy Younie (nee Mitchell), (1890–1999) (MB ChB 1921, MD
    1929), by Elizabeth Olson, 18 August 1986, UASC (MS 3620/1/51).

58 Interview, with retired member of teaching/research staff (A) from UAAD, by Elizabeth
    Hallam, 11 May 2007.

59 Elliot Smith, 'Teaching of Anatomy', p. 51.

60 Ibid., p. 56, p. 50.

61 Elliot Smith, 'Teaching of Anatomy', p. 50. Ivy Mackenzie, 'On the Teaching of
    Pathological Anatomy', in *Inquiry into the Medical Curriculum*, ed. Edinburgh
    Pathological Club, pp. 112–23, p. 118.

62 Waterston, 'Teaching of Anatomy', p. 58; 'Teaching of Anatomy', *The Lancet*,
    18 February 1928, pp. 348–9, p. 348.

63 The emphasis on 'coordination' is especially apparent in anatomical discourse during the
    first half of the twentieth century, see for example Lockhart, 'Art of Learning Anatomy';
    Elliott Smith, 'Teaching of Anatomy'; Royal College of Physicians of London, Planning
    Committee, *Report on Medical Education* (London, 1944).

64 Elliot Smith, 'Teaching of Anatomy', p. 52, p. 63.

65 Ibid., p. 53; Dr Sillar, 'Discussion', pp. 69–70, p. 69.

66 College of Physicians of London, Planning Committee, *Report on Medical Education*,
    p. 15.
67 R. D. Lockhart to H. J. Butchart, University Secretary, 25 July 1939, MS letter, UASC
    (MS 3270/2/1/2/1).
68 'The New Medical School at Aberdeen', *The Lancet*, 1 October 1938, p. 803; Fyfe, '
    In Memoriam, R. D. Lockhart', p. 204. See W. Hamish Fraser and Clive H. Lee,
    eds, *Aberdeen, 1800–2000: A New History* (East Linton, 2000); Elizabeth Hallam,
    'Disappearing Museums? Medical Collections at the University of Aberdeen', in *Medical
    Museums: Past, Present, Future*, eds Samuel J.M.M. Alberti and Elizabeth Hallam
    (London, 2013), pp. 44–59.
69 Hackett, 'List of Medical Museums'.
70 'Economy in the Museum', *The Lancet*, 28 February 1942, p. 267.
71 Fyfe, 'In Memoriam, R. D. Lockhart', p. 204. R. D. Lockhart to H. J. Butchart,
    University Secretary, 29 April 1939, MS letter, UASC (MS 3270/2/1/2/1).
72 R. D. Lockhart, 'Complete Double Aortic Arch', *Journal of Anatomy*, LXIV (1930), pp.
    189–93; 'Museum Material', 1959–69, MS/typescript list of *c.* 17 pages, archive of UAAD;
    Preserved, dissected specimen (hand), dated 1964, collection of University of Aberdeen,
    Anatomy Museum (UAAM). Adam,Rouilly purchased human skeletons from Reknas Ltd,
    in Calcutta, for supply to medical schools from the 1930s to 1985, see Adam,Rouilly,
    'The 90th Anniversary of Adam,Rouilly, 1918–2008' (company booklet, 2008).
73 John D. Hargreaves, *Academe and Empire: Some Overseas Connections of Aberdeen
    University, 1860–1970* (Aberdeen, 1994); Southwood, 'Cultural History of Marischal'.
    On museums and decolonization, see Claire Wintle, 'Decolonising the Museum: The
    Case of the Imperial and Commonwealth Institutes', *Museum and Society*, XI (2013),
    pp. 185–201.
74 'Report by Museum Committee, University of Aberdeen', 1939–40, archive of UAMM.
    On anatomical practices and the acquisition of deceased bodies in Australia, see Helen
    Macdonald, *Possessing the Dead: The Artful Science of Anatomy* (Melbourne, 2010)
75 Viscountess Stonehaven to R. D. Lockhart, 21 November 1941, MS letter, archive of UAMM.
76 See Charles Hunt, 'African Art at the University of Aberdeen', *African Arts*, XIX (1986),
    pp. 48–85.
77 R. D. Lockhart to Viscountess Stonehaven, 22 December 1941, MS letter, archive of
    UAMM, n. pag. 'Report by Museum Committee, University of Aberdeen', 1941–2, archive
    of UAMM.
78 R. D. Lockhart, 'The Medical School', in *The Fusion of 1860: A Record of the Centenary
    Celebrations and a History of the United University of Aberdeen, 1860–1960*, ed. W. Douglas
    Simpson (Edinburgh, 1963), pp. 242–8.
79 Fyfe, 'In Memoriam, R. D. Lockhart'.
80 Ibid., p. 204. The acquisition of the horse from George V is noted in: 'Medical School
    Tour, 1938' newspaper clipping, papers of R. D. Lockhart, University of Birmingham,
    Special Collections (GB 150, US 46).
81 'Museum Material', 1959–69, archive of UAAD.
82 Samuel J.M.M. Alberti, 'The Museum Affect: Visiting Collections of Anatomy and
    Natural History', in *Science in the Marketplace: Nineteenth-century Sites and Experiences*,
    eds Aileen Fyfe and Bernard Lightman (Chicago, IL, 2007), pp. 371–403, Alberti, *Morbid
    Curiosities*; Tony Bennett, *Pasts Beyond Memory: Evolution, Museums, Colonialism*
    (London, 2004).
83 R. D. Lockhart, 'The Circus of Life', 1931–4, p. 1, typescript lecture, UASC (MS
    3270/3/22); Lockhart, 'Regius Chair of Anatomy'.
84 Lockhart, 'Circus of Life', p. 1. On Virchow's work with performers in travelling shows,
    see Roslyn Poignant, *Professional Savage: Captive Lives and Western Spectacle* (New Haven,
    CT, 2004).
85 Interview, with R. D. Lockhart, by Elizabeth Olson, n. pag. Hengler's Circus ran from
    the 1860s to the 1920s in Glasgow.

86 On the circus, see Marius Kwint, 'The Legitimization of the Circus in Late Georgian England', *Past and Present*, CLXXIV (2002), pp. 72–115; Gillian Arrighi, 'The Circus and Modernity: A Commitment to "the Newer" and "the Newest"', *Early Popular Visual Culture*, X (2012), pp. 169–85; Paul Bouissac, *Circus As Multimodal Discourse: Performance, Meaning, and Ritual* (London, 2012).

87 For example, R. D. Lockhart, set of slides on anatomical, anthropological and horticultural themes, *c.* 1940–70, UASC (MS 3270/8/7/10).

88 'Pantomime Acrobats. Assistance in Scientific Investigation. X-ray and Cinema Records', *Birmingham Mail*, 20 January 1933, n. pag., newspaper clipping, collection/papers of R. D. Lockhart, UASC (MS 3270/3/22).

89 Lockhart, 'Circus of Life', p. 1.

90 'Pantomime Acrobats', *Birmingham Mail*, n. pag.

91 David Rutherford Dow (1889–1979), Biographical Information, GASHE: Gateway to Archives of Scottish Higher Education, online resource, www.gashe.ac.uk, accessed 10 November 2014. 'Anatomy Model: Boxer Pummelled But Does Not Hit Back', *Aberdeen Journal*, 11 April 1925, p. 8. 'In Memoriam, Thomas Yeates', *Journal of Anatomy*, XCVII (1963), pp. 289–90. 'Muscles of a Dancer; Leeds Theatre Royal Girl to be X-rayed', *Yorkshire Evening Post*, 6 February 1932, p. 8.

92 R. D. Lockhart, *Living Anatomy: A Photographic Atlas of Muscles in Action and Surface Contours* (London, 1960 [1948]), p. 60. 'In Memoriam, R. D. Lockhart'.

93 Lockhart, 'Regius Chair of Anatomy', p. ii.

94 Lockhart, 'Art of Learning Anatomy', p. 460.

95 Lockhart, *Living Anatomy*, p. 61.

96 '"The Circus of Life". Acrobat in Cinema and Radiogram. Prof. Lockhart's Lecture', *Evening Sentinel*, 18 May 1934, n. pag., newspaper clipping, collection/papers of R. D. Lockhart, UASC (MS 3270/3/22).

97 Lockhart, Hamilton and Fyfe, *Anatomy*, p. 54.

98 R. D. Lockhart, 'Show Business', set of slides for lecture, *c.* 1950s, UASC (MS 3270/3/17).

99 R. D. Lockhart, 'Movements of the Normal Shoulder Joint and of a Case with Trapezius Paralysis Studied by Radiogram and Experiment in the Living', *Journal of Anatomy*, LXIV (1930), pp. 288–302, p. 288. L. H. Hamlyn and Patricia Thilesen, 'Models in Medical Teaching with a Note on the Use of a New Plastic', *The Lancet*, 5 September 1953, pp. 472–75, p. 472.

100 Lockhart, Hamilton and Fyfe, *Anatomy*, p. 293, p. 305.

101 Ibid., epigraph, n. pag. Lewis Caroll, *Alice's Adventures in Wonderland* (London, 2003 [1865]). This section of this chapter develops an initial discussion in Elizabeth Hallam, 'Anatomists' Ways of Seeing and Knowing', in *Fieldnotes and Sketchbooks: Challenging the Boundaries between Descriptions and Processes of Describing*, ed. Wendy Gunn (Frankfurt, 2009), pp. 69–99.

102 Lockhart, Hamilton and Fyfe, *Anatomy*, p. vii.

103 On Alberto Morrocco, see Victoria Keller and Clara Young, *Alberto Morrocco* (Edinburgh, 1993).

104 Fyfe, 'In Memoriam, R. D. Lockhart'.

105 Ibid.; Lockhart, Hamilton and Fyfe, *Anatomy*, p. 307, fig. 487.

106 J. N. Aston, 'Book Reviews. *Anatomy of the Human Body*. By R. D. Lockhart, G. F. Hamilton and F. W. Fyfe. 1959. London: Faber and Faber', *Journal of Bone and Joint Surgery*, XLI (1959), pp. 893–4, p. 894. Fyfe, 'In Memoriam, R. D. Lockhart', p. 206. On colour in mid-twentieth-century three-dimensional sculptural forms, see Roberta Panzanelli, Eike D. Schmidt and Kenneth D. S. Lapatin, eds, *The Colour of Life: Polychromy in Sculpture from Antiquity to the Present*, exh. cat., J. Paul Getty Museum at the Getty Villa, Malibu (Los Angeles, 2008).

107 Howard Dickson, 'Obituary: Forest William Fyfe', *British Medical Journal*, 2 February 2002, p. 302

108 Lockhart, Hamilton and Fyfe, *Anatomy*, p. 1; Lockhart, 'Art of Learning Anatomy',

p. 460. Lockhart, 'Regius Chair of Anatomy'.

109 See S. H. Daukes, *The Medical Museum: Modern Developments, Organisation and Technical Methods Based on a New System of Visual Teaching*, London, 1929, p. 155, p. 16. This display technique was also used more recently for *The Visible Human Plexi-book: Male,* and *Female*, 2000, National Library of Medicine, see Michael Sappol, *Dream Anatomy*, exh. cat., National Library of Medicine (U.S.), Bethesda (Washington, DC, 2002).

110 Lockhart, *Living Anatomy*, Preface, n. pag.

111 Ibid., p. 8.

112 Ibid., p. 6, p. 9, p. 72.

113 Ibid., p. 10. For example, Lockhart appears in photographs on p. 11, pp. 18–21, p. 25, p. 28, p. 32.

114 Lockhart, *Living Anatomy*, p. 8. See E. M. Tansey, 'Keeping the Culture Alive: The Laboratory Technician in Mid-twentieth-century British Medical Research', *Notes and Records of the Royal Society*, LXII (2008), pp. 77–95.

115 Fyfe, 'In Memoriam, R. D. Lockhart', p. 205

116 Lockhart, *Living Anatomy*, dust jacket, n. pag.

117 Ibid., p. 61.

118 Lockhart, *Living Anatomy*, Preface, n. pag.

119 A. Low, 'University of Aberdeen, Department of Anatomy', *Methods and Problems of Medical Education*, 17th series (1930), pp. 207–12; p. 210.

120 Lockhart, 'Art of Learning Anatomy', p. 460. Lockhart, *Living Anatomy*, p. 14, p. 15.

121 J. Whillis, 'Review. *Living Anatomy. A Photographic Atlas of Muscles in Action and Surface Contours*. By R. D. Lockhart, London Faber and Faber', *Journal of Anatomy*, LXXXIII (1949), pp. 176–7, p. 176. On the early use of film in medical education, see for example 'Anatomical Films', *The Lancet*, 28 June 1919, p. 1125; 'The Cinematograph in Medicine', *The Lancet*, 16 April 1932, pp. 845–6. On film in medicine see Kirsten Ostherr, *Medical Visions: Producing the Patient Through Film, Television, and Imaging Technologies* (Oxford 2013); Leslie J. Reagan, Nancy Tomes and Paula A. Treichler, eds, *Medicine's Moving Pictures: Medicine, Health, and Bodies in American Film and Television* (Rochester, NY, and Suffolk, 2007.)

122 Lockhart, 'Regius Chair of Anatomy'. R. D. Lockhart, *The Action of Muscles, Vertebral Column, Hip and Shoulder Joints, in Living Subjects,* Part I: *The Living Anatomical Model*; Part II: *Five Male Acrobats*; Part III: *Four Female Acrobats*', films, 1933. Copies of the films are held at the Wellcome Library.

123 Lockhart, *Action of Muscles, Vertebral Column*.

124 On intermedial relations between cinematography and X-ray imaging *c.* 1900, see Solveig Jülich, 'Media as Modern Magic: Early X-ray Imaging and Cinematography in Sweden', *Early Popular Visual Culture*, VI (2008), pp. 19–34.

125 On the erosion of distinctions between the bodily interior and exterior in twentieth-century medicine, see Lisa Cartwright, *Screening the Body: Tracing Medicine's Visual Culture* (London, 1995).

126 E. Barclay-Smith, ed., 'Anatomical Society of Great Britain and Ireland, Proceedings, November 1933–Jun 1934', *Journal of Anatomy*, LXIX (1934), pp. 129–52, p. 151. R. D. Lockhart, 'Reviews. *The Human Figure in Motion*. By Eadweard Muybridge. Dover Publications Inc.' *Journal of Anatomy*, XCI (1957), p. 144. On Eadweard Muybridge, see Marta Braun, *Eadweard Muybridge* (London, 2010); Stephen P. Rice, 'Picturing Bodies in the Nineteenth Century', in *A Cultural History of the Human Body*, ed. Michael Sappol and Stephen P. Rice (London, 2014), pp. 213–35; Rebecca Solnit, *Motion Studies: Time, Space and Eadweard Muybridge* (London, 2004).

127 Minutes of the AUAAS, vol. I, p. 63, p. 155, p. 23, p. 26, p. 42. On cine-radiography, see James F. Brailsford, 'The Radiology of Living Anatomy', *British Medical Journal*, 2 June 1934, p. 984–6.

128 David MacDougall, *The Corporeal Image: Film, Ethnography, and the Senses* (Princeton,

NJ, and Oxford, 2006), p. 25. On perceivers' bodily involvement in visual images, see Michael Taussig, *Mimesis and Alterity: A Particular History of the Senses* (London, 1993).

129 Scottish Education Department, *Visual and Aural Aids: A Report of the Advisory Council on Education in Scotland* (Edinburgh, 1950), p. 16, p. 15. On entertainment and education via medical films see K. Ostherr, 'Medical Education Through Film: Animating Anatomy at the American College of Surgeons and Eastman Kodak', in *Learning with the Lights off: Educational Film in the United States*, ed. Devin Orgeron, Marsha Orgeron and Dan Streible (Oxford, 2012), pp. 168–92.

130 For example, on guidance for audiences of educational films, see Hannah Landecker, 'Microcinematography and the History of Science and Film', *Isis*, XCVII (2006), pp. 121–32, p. 129.

131 'The Cinematograph in Medicine', *The Lancet*, 16 April 1932, pp. 845–6, p. 845.

132 Lockhart, 'In Memoriam, Gilbert Frewin Hamilton', *Journal of Anatomy*, CXVIII (1974), pp. 611–12, p. 611.

133 'Filmstrip in Medical Teaching, *The Lancet*, 22 March 1947, p. 377.

134 Interview, with retired member of teaching/research staff (A) from UAAD, by Elizabeth Hallam, 11 May 2007.

135 F. W. Fyfe, 'The Teaching of Anatomy in Health Education', *Health Education Journal*, VII (1949), pp. 155–9, p. 155.

136 David L. Bassett, *A Stereoscopic Atlas of Anatomy*, Section II: *Head and Neck*, Reels 35–84 (Portland, OR, 1954). Photography for the atlas was by William Gruber, inventor of the View-Master stereoscope and reels.

137 W. Montague Cobb, 'Book Reviews, Bassett, David L. *A Stereoscopic Atlas of Human Anatomy*, Section II: *Head and Neck*, 5 v., Reels 35–84. Portland, Oregon, Sawyer's, 1954', *Bulletin of the Medical Library Association*, XLIII (1955), pp. 582–3, p. 582, p. 583

138 Lockhart, 'Art of Learning Anatomy'.

139 Cooke and Cooke, *Tablets of Anatomy*, p. xvii, p. xv.

140 For overviews of anatomical terminology, see Kachlik et al., 'Anatomical Terminology'; Ian Whitemore, 'Terminologia Anatomica: New Terminology for the New Anatomist', *Anatomical Record*, CCLVII (1999), pp. 50–53.

141 Lockhart, Hamilton and Fyfe, *Anatomy*, p. 2. The names for anatomical parts used in their book were those recommended by the International Congress of Anatomists in Paris, 1955. On metaphors in anatomy, see Elizabeth Hallam, 'Articulating Bones: An Epilogue', *Journal of Material Culture,* XV (2010), pp. 465–92.

142 Lockhart, Hamilton and Fyfe, *Anatomy*, p. 3, p. 42, p. 51, p. 77, p. 105, p. 95, p. 96, p. 264, p. 270, p. 325, p. 24, pp. 456–8, p. 494.

143 On metaphors in science, see S. Maasen and Peter Weingart, *Metaphors and the Dynamics of Knowledge,* (London, 2000); Laura Otis, 'Science Surveys and Histories of Literature: Reflections on an Uneasy Kinship', *Isis*, CI (2010), pp. 570–77.

144 For instance, André Breton referred to the phrase repeatedly, for example in a 1922 lecture, 'Caractères de l'évolution moderne et ce qui en participe', see André Breton, *The Lost Steps*, trans. Mark Polizzotti (Lincoln, NE, 1996 [1924]). The image is taken from Lautréamont's *Chants de Maldoror* (1868), see Lautréamont, *Maldoror and Poems*, trans. Paul Knight (London, 1978 [1868]), p. 217.

145 Lockhart, 'Art of Learning Anatomy', p. 460.

146 Christopher Tilley, *Metaphor and Material Culture* (Oxford, 1999), p. 261.

147 Lockhart was, for example, President of the Anatomical Society of Great Britain and Ireland 1955–7, and Dean of Medicine at the University of Aberdeen 1959–62; see Fyfe, 'In Memoriam, R. D. Lockhart'. *Living Anatomy*, and *Anatomy of the Human Body* received positive reviews in leading medical journals, including the *British Journal of Surgery* in 1948 (XXXVI, p. 223) and 1959 (XLVII, p. 208). On Surrealism, see Michael Sheringham, *Everyday Life: Theories and Practices from Surrealism to the Present* (Oxford, 2006); Julia Kelly, *Art, Ethnography and the Life of Objects: Paris, c. 1925–35* (Manchester, 2007).

148 Minutes of the AUAAS, vol. II, p. 192.

149 Ibid., p. 192, p. 193.
150 Ibid. Photograph of R. D. Lockhart, presenting his 'Lecture on the Ear', 1964, UASC (MS 3270/8/1/12).
151 R. D. Lockhart, 'Stepping in Society', 1926–7, p. 1, typescript lecture, UASC (MS 3270/3/22).
152 R. D. Lockhart, 'Other Tales of Mystery and Imagination', 1930s–1960s, typescript lecture, UASC (MS 3270/3/19); Interview, with R. D. Lockhart, by Elizabeth Olson, 11 March 1985, UASC (MS 3620/1/18).
153 On colour in anatomical display, see Elizabeth Hallam, 'Anatomopoeia', in *Making and Growing: Anthropological Studies of Organisms and Artefacts*, eds Elizabeth Hallam and Tim Ingold (Farnham, 2014), pp. 65–88.
154 Nan Shepherd, 'Professors and Students', in *The Fusion of 1860: A Record of the Centenary Celebrations and a History of the United University of Aberdeen, 1860–1960*, ed. W. Douglas Simpson (Edinburgh, 1963), pp. 140–45, p. 144–5.
155 Olson, 'Robert Douglas Lockhart', p. 334.
156 Fyfe, 'In Memoriam, R. D. Lockhart', p. 208.
157 Lockhart, Hamilton and Fyfe, *Anatomy*, p. 495, p. 40.
158 Anke te Heesen, 'News, Paper, Scissors: Clippings in the Sciences and Arts around 1920', in *Things that Talk: Object Lessons from Art and Science*, ed. Lorraine Daston (New York, 2004), pp. 297–327.
159 Lockhart, Hamilton and Fyfe, *Anatomy*, p. 248, fig. 372. R. D. Lockhart, 'Apes and Ivory, Skulls and Roses', 1950s–1960s, set of slides for lecture, UASC (MS 3270/3/22).
160 R. D. Lockhart, set of slides on anatomical, anthropological and horticultural themes, *c.* 1940–70, UASC (MS 3270/8/7/10). On '"cubist" visual culture' as manifested in medical images during the first half of the twentieth century, see Cartwright, *Screening the Body*, p. 91.
161 R. W. Reid, *Illustrated Catalogue of the Anthropological Museum, Marischal College, University of Aberdeen* (Aberdeen, 1912), p. 235, p. 240. Reid presented the 'distorted' feet of a 'Chinese female, along with plaster of Paris casts of the same to the Anthropological Museum in 1907; he also listed a 'Maori, head of, tattooed and mummified', see *Illustrated Catalogue*, p. 235, p. 240.

Seven Paper, Wax and Plastic

1 Throughout, I refer to 'plastic' (the everyday term that refers to a group of materials) and also to 'plastics', following the terms as used by the people in this study.
2 Thomas Cooke and F. G. Hamilton Cooke, *Tablets of Anatomy, Dissectional and Scientific*, Part II: *Limbs, Abdomen, Pelvis*, 11th edn (London, 1898), p. 132ee. Historical studies of anatomical models have tended to focus mainly on those made in wax, yet a wide range of further materials have also been used in three-dimensional modelling of the body. See S.J.M.M. Alberti, 'Wax Bodies: Art and Anatomy in Victorian Medical Museums', *Museum History Journal*, II (2009), pp. 7–35; Soraya de Chadarevian and Nick Hopwood, eds, *Models: The Third Dimension of Science* (Stanford, CA, 2004); Thomas N. Haviland and Lawrence Charles Paris, 'A Brief Account of the Use of Wax Models in the Study of Medicine', *Journal of the History of Medicine and Allied Sciences*, XXV (1970), pp. 52–75; Nick Hopwood, *Embryos in Wax: Models from the Ziegler Studio* (Cambridge and Bern, 2002); Pam Lieske, '"Made in Imitation of Real Women and Children": Obstetrical Machines in Eighteenth-century Britain', in *The Female Body in Medicine and Literature*, ed. Andrew Mangham and Greta Depledge (Liverpool, 2011), pp. 69–88; Anna Maerker, *Model Experts: Wax Anatomies and Enlightenment in Florence and Vienna, 1775–1815* (Manchester, 2011); Roberta Panzanelli, ed., *Ephemeral Bodies: Wax Sculpture and the Human Figure* (Los Angeles, CA, 2008); Jessica Riskin, 'Eighteenth-century Wetware', *Representations*, LXXXIII (2003), pp. 97–125; K. F. Russell, 'Ivory Anatomical Manikins', *Medical History*, XVI (1972), pp. 131–42.

3 George Blaine, 'Biological Teaching Models and Specimens', *The Lancet*, 25 August 1951, pp. 337–40, p. 337, p. 339.

4 'The Great Exhibition. Objects Connected with the Theory and Practice of Medicine and Surgery', Thirteenth Notice, *The Medical Times: A Journal of Medical Science, Literature, Criticism, and News*, III (New Series) (5 July–27 December 1851), pp. 210–11, p. 210.

5 Thomas Henry Huxley, 'Universities: Actual and Ideal', address delivered 27 February 1874, in *Rectorial Addresses delivered at the University of Aberdeen, 1835–1900*, ed. Peter John Anderson (Aberdeen, 1902), pp. 170–98, p.187, p. 188.

6 'The New Anatomical Buildings at Oxford', *The Lancet*, 21 October 1893, pp. 1025–9, p. 1027.

7 Ibid., p. 1027, p. 1028.

8 Ibid., p. 1027.

9 On passive observation in nineteenth-century science, see Lorriane Daston and Peter Galison, *Objectivity* (New York, 2007).

10 Ibid.

11 R. W. Reid, 'Presidential Address to the Aberdeen Anatomical and Anthropological Society', *University of Aberdeen Proceedings of the Anatomical and Anthropological Society* (*PAAS*), (1899–1900), pp. 6–15, p. 11; 'Teaching of Anatomy', *The Lancet*, 18 February 1928, pp. 348–9, p. 348.

12 'Teaching of Anatomy', *The Lancet*, p. 348.

13 Cooke and Cooke, *Tablets of Anatomy*, p. 132cc.

14 Ibid., p. 132cc, p. 132oo.

15 Ibid., p. 132hh, 108n.

16 Ibid., p. 108o, 132bb.

17 Ibid., p. 152s, p. 152u, p. 152w.

18 Ibid., p. xv.

19 George S. Huntington, 'The Morphological Museum as an Educational Factor in the University System', *Science*, New Series, XIII (1901), pp. 601–11, p. 604.

20 Cooke and Cooke, *Tablets of Anatomy*, p. 132bb.

21 Haviland and Parish, 'Brief Account of the Use of Wax Models'; Nick Hopwood, 'Artist Versus Anatomist, Models Against Dissection: Paul Zeiller of Munich and the Revolution of 1848', *Medical History*, LI (2007), pp. 279–308.

22 Elizabeth T. Hurren, *Dying for Victorian Medicine: English Anatomy and its Trade in the Dead Poor, c. 1834–1929* (Basingstoke, 2012); Fiona Hutton, *The Study of Anatomy in Britain, 1700–1900* (London, 2013); Ruth Richardson, *Death, Dissection and the Destitute*, 2nd edn (London, 2001).

23 Cooke and Cooke, *Tablets of Anatomy*, p. vii, p. 132ff.

24 Ibid., p. 132dd; Thomas Cooke, 'The Teaching of Anatomy: Its Aims and Methods', *The Lancet*, 4 November 1893, pp. 1153–5, p. 1153.

25 On the concept of transparency in early nineteenth-century anatomy see Michel Foucault, *The Birth of the Clinic: An Archaeology of Medical Perception*, trans. A. M. Sheridan (London, 2003 [1963]). The ideal of transparency, as a cultural construct, is analysed in José van Dijck, *The Transparent Body: A Cultural Analysis of Medical Imaging* (Seattle, 2005).

26 J. Arthur Thomson, *Introduction to Science*, (London, 1911), pp. 27–8.

27 Ibid., p. 20, p. 27, p. 34.

28 For discussion of a recent annotated English translation of Vesalius' *Fabrica*, see www.vesaliusfabrica.com, accessed 9 March 2015.

29 Helkiah Crooke, *Mikrokosmographia: A Description of the Body of Man* (London, 1615), pp. 26–7. Andreas Vesalius, *De humani corporis fabrica* (Basel, 1543). On dissecting instruments in the *Fabrica*, see Elizabeth Hallam, 'Articulating Bones: An Epilogue', *Journal of Material Culture*, XV (2010), pp. 465–92

30 Crooke, *Mikrokosmographia*, p. 649, p. 729. See Katharine Rowe, '"God's Handy Worke":

Divine Complicity and the Anatomist's Touch', in *The Body in Parts: Fantasies of Corporeality in Early Modern Europe*, ed. David Hillman and Carla Mazzio (London, 1997), pp. 285–309.

31 Jonathan Goldberg, *Writing Matter: From the Hands of the English Renaissance* (Stanford, CA, 1990).

32 James Scratchley, *The London Dissector; Or System of Dissection Practised in the Hospitals and Lecture Rooms of the Metropolis*, 7th edn (London, 1826), p.1.

33 Richard Quain, *The Anatomy of the Arteries of the Human Body with its Applications to Pathology and Operative Surgery in Lithographic Drawings with Practical Commentaries* (London, 1844).

34 Quain, *Anatomy of the Arteries*, title page.

35 Henry Lonsdale, *A Sketch of the Life and Writings of Robert Knox, the Anatomist* (London, 1870), p. 153, p. 154. On Knox's work, see Isobel Rae, *Knox, the Anatomist* (Edinburgh, 1964); A. W. Bates, *The Anatomy of Robert Knox: Murder, Mad Science and Medical Regulation in Nineteenth-century Edinburgh* (Eastbourne, 2010).

36 For analysis of atlases in the practice of science, see Daston and Galison, *Objectivity*.

37 Martin Kemp and Marina Wallace, *Spectacular Bodies: The Art and Science of the Human Body from Leonardo to Now*, exh. cat., Hayward Gallery, London (2000); Ruth Richardson, *The Making of Mr Gray's Anatomy: Bodies, Books, Fortune, Fame* (Oxford, 2008).

38 F. G. Parsons and William Wright, *Practical Anatomy: The Student's Dissecting Manual*, (London, 1912), p. xv; James Couper Brash, ed., *Cunningham's Manual of Practical Anatomy*, vol. III. *Head and Neck: Brain*, 11th edn (London, 1948). On the adaptation of anatomy tools from other domains of work, see Hallam, 'Articulating Bones'.

39 Parsons and Wright, *Practical Anatomy*, p. xv.

40 Brash, *Cunningham's Manual*.

41 Cooke and Cooke, *Tablets of Anatomy*, p. xiv. See E. B. Jamieson, *Illustrations of Regional Anatomy, Complete Volume, Seven Sections*, 5th edn (Edinburgh, 1944 [1934–6]). This textbook comprising mainly illustrations was originally published as a series of seven separate sections with removable plates. For discussion of textbooks in the practices of science, see Marga Vicedo, 'Introduction: The Secret Lives of Textbooks', *Isis*, CIII (2012), pp. 83–7, and articles in this themed issue.

42 E. B. Jamieson, *Illustrations of Regional Anatomy. Section II, Head and Neck (Containing 61 Plates)* (Edinburgh, 1934), Preface, n. pag.

43 'Artificial Anatomy', *Caledonian Mercury*, 26 June 1826, p. 4.

44 'Westminster Medical Society, Saturday, February 4, 1832 . . . Extraordinary Anatomical Machine', *The London Medical and Surgical Journal*, 11 February 1832, in Michael Ryan, ed., *The London Medical and Surgical Journal*, vol. I (London, 1832), pp. 56–60; Anna Maerker, 'Anatomizing the Trade: Designing and Marketing Anatomical Models as Medical Technologies, ca. 1700–1900', *Technology and Culture*, LIV (2013), pp. 531–62; Anna Maerker, 'User-developers, Model Students and Ambassador Users: The Role of the Public in the Global Distribution of Nineteenth-century Anatomical Models', in *The Fate of Anatomical Collections*, eds, Rina Knoeff and Robert Zwijnenberg (Farnham, 2015), pp. 129–42.

45 *Catalogue of the Clastic Anatomical Models of Dr Auzoux* (London, 1851). Audrey B. Davis, 'Louis Thomas Jerôme Auzous and the Papier Maché Anatomical Model', in *La ceroplastica nella scienza e nell'ate: atti del i congresso internationale Firenze, 3–7 giugno 1975* (Florence, 1977); Michel Lemire, *Artistes et mortels* (Paris, 1990).

46 'Académie Royale de Médicine, Rapport sur une pièce d'anatomie clastique du Docteur Auzoux' (1835), quoted in Christopher Hoolihan, *An Annotated Catalogue of the Edward C. Atwater Collection of American Popular Medicine and Health Reform*, vol. I: *A–L*, (Rochester, NY, 2001), p. 5.

47 Louis Auzoux, *Catalogue des préparations d'anatomie clastique du Dr Auzoux, 1858* (Paris, 1858); 'Foreign Intelligence. France', *Aberdeen Journal*, 25 July 1855, p. 6; Gustave

Flaubert, *Bouvard and Pécuchet*, trans. A. J. Krailsheimer (Harmondsworth, 1976 [1881]), pp. 71–3. See Julie K. Brown, *Health and Medicine on Display: International Expositions in the United States, 1876–1904* (Cambridge, MA, 2009); Maerker, 'Anatomizing the Trade'; Michael Sappol, *A Traffic of Dead Bodies: Anatomy and Embodied Social Identity in Nineteenth-Century America* (Princeton, NJ, 2002).

48 Louis Auzoux, *Anatomie clastique du Docteur Auzoux, Catalogue de 1869* (Paris, 1869). On Auzoux's botanical models, see Margaret Maria Cocks, 'Dr Louis Auzoux and His Collection of Papier-mâché Fowers, Fruits and Seeds', *Journal of the History of Collections*, XXVI (2014), pp. 229–48; Margaret M. Olszewski, 'Designer Nature: The Papier-mâché Botanical Teaching Models of Dr Auzoux in 19th-century France, Great Britain and America', PhD thesis, University of Cambridge (2010).

49 'Westminster Medical Society', *London Medical and Surgical Journal*, ed. Ryan, p. 56; 'Anatomy, *Artificial*', *Museum of Foreign Literature and Science*, XXV (1834), p. 381–2, p. 382; 'Westminster Medical Society', *The Times*, 6 February 1832, p. 6.

50 'Westminster Medical Society', *London Medical and Surgical Journal*, ed. Ryan, p. 56.

51 'A Bill for Regulating Schools of Anatomy', *Westminster Review*, XVI (1832), pp. 482–96, p. 489.

52 Ibid., pp. 488–9.

53 'London, February 13', *Newcastle Courant*, 18 February 1832, p. 2.

54 'Artificial Anatomy', *Literary Gazette and Journal of Belles Lettres, Arts, Sciences, &c.* (London 1826), p. 202. On the term 'artificial anatomy', see Renato G. Mazzolini, 'Plastic Anatomies and Artificial Dissections', in *Models: The Third Dimension of Science*, ed. de Chadarevian and Hopwood, pp. 43–70.

55 'Artificial Anatomy', *Caledonian Mercury*, p. 4; Samuel D. Gross, *A System of Surgery; Pathological, Diagnostic, Therapeutic, and Operative*, vol. 1 (Philadelphia, PA, 1859), p. 422.

56 R. Temple Wright, *Medical Students of the Period* (Edinburgh, 1867), p. 21.

57 Wright, *Medical Students*, p. 25. On the association of anatomy and cannibalism see Bates, *Anatomy of Robert Knox*.

58 Richardson, *Death, Dissection*; Wright, *Medical Students*.

59 'Saturday, November 8th, 1845', *Medical Times: A Journal of English and Foreign Medicine*, XIII (27 September 1845– 28 March 1846), pp. 138–9, p. 138. Wright, *Medical Students*.

60 'Saturday, November 8th, 1845', p. 138.

61 Ibid., p. 138, p. 139. On dissection and the formation of professional medical identity, see Sappol, *Traffic of Dead Bodies*.

62 For a history of the manicule, see William H. Sherman, *Used Books: Marking Readers in Renaissance England* (Philadelphia, PA, 2008).

63 A 'complete model of a woman', with a set of fourteen uteri at various stages of gestation which could be removed and changed was available, see *Catalogue of Anatomical Models, Made by Dr Auzoux* (Albany, 1844), p. 4. See Tatjana Buklijas and Nick Hopwood, 'Making Visible Embryos' website, www.hps.cam.ac.uk/visibleembryos, accessed 19 October 2015.

64 Maerker, *Model Experts*; Mazzolini, 'Plastic Anatomies and Artificial Dissections'.

65 Cocks, 'Dr Louis Auzoux and His Collection'; Maerker, 'Anatomizing the Trade'; Jean-Jacques Motel, *L'anatomie clastique et le musée de l'écorché d'anatomie du Neubourg* (Brac, 2004).

66 Bart Grob, *The World of Auzoux: Models of Man and Beast in Papier-mâché* (Leiden, 2000); Motel, *L'anatomie clastique*; permanent exhibition of Auzou'x models at Musée de l'Écorché d'Anatomie, Le Neubourg, France; Smithsonian National Museum of American History, 'Artificial Anatomy: Papier-Mâché Anatomical Models', www.americanhistory.si.edu, accessed 10 November 2014.

67 'Anatomical Model', *The Hull Packet and Humber Mercury*, 14 February 1832, p. 4. See Maerker, *Model Experts*.

68 'Anatomy, *Artificial*', p. 382.

69 On Towne's models, see Samuel J.M.M. Alberti, 'Wax Bodies: Art and Anatomy in Victorian Medical Museums', *Museum History Journal*, II (2009), pp. 7–36; R. Ballestriero, 'Anatomical Models and Wax Venuses: Art Masterpieces or Scientific Craft Works?', *Journal of Anatomy*, CCXVI (2010), pp. 223–34.

70 'The Great Exhibition', *Medical Times*, p. 210.

71 de Chadarevian and Hopwood, *Models*; Hopwood, *Embryos in Wax*.

72 'Report by Museum Committee, University of Aberdeen', 1920–21, archive of University of Aberdeen, Marischal Museum.

73 'Westminster Medical Society', *London Medical and Surgical Journal*, Ryan, p. 56

74 On flap anatomy, see Andrea Carlino, *Paper Bodies: A Catalogue of Anatomical Fugitive Sheets, 1538–1687*, trans. Noga Arikha (London, 1999)

75 U.S. National Library of Medicine, 'The Visible Human Project', www.nlm.nih.gov, accessed 10 November 2014. For analysis of the Visible Human Project, see Thomas J. Csordas, *Body/Meaning/Healing* (Basingstoke, 2002); Catherine Waldby, *The Visible Human Project: Informatic Bodies and Posthuman Medicine* (London, 2000).

76 See Carlino, *Paper Bodies*; Eric Faden, 'Movables, Movies, Mobility: Nineteenth Century Looking and Reading', *Early Popular Visual Culture*, V (2007), pp. 71–89; Michael Sappol, *Dream Anatomy*, exh. cat., National Library of Medicine (U.S.), Bethesda (Washington, DC, 2002); Jonathan Sawday, *The Body Emblazoned: Dissection and the Human Body in Renaissance Culture* (London, 1995).

77 Cooke and Cooke, *Tablets of Anatomy*, p. 1080.

78 G.-J. Witkowski, *Human Anatomy and Physiology. Part IV. A Movable Atlas Showing the Mechanism of Vision. (The Eye)* (London, 1880?–1889).

79 G.-J. Witkowski, *Human Anatomy and Physiology. Part V. A Movable Atlas Showing the Mechanism of Hearing and Mastication by Means of Superimposed Coloured Plates. (The Ear and Teeth)* (London, 1880?–1889).

80 William S. Furneaux, ed., *Philips' Popular Mannikin or Model of the Human Body. An Illustrated Representation with Full and Descriptive Letterpress* (London, 1900?).

81 J. E. Cheesman, *Baillière's Synthetic Anatomy. A Series of Drawings on Transparent Sheets for Facilitating the Reconstruction of Mental Pictures of the Human Body* (London, 1926–36), Part I, 'Author's Introduction to the Series', n. pag.; J. Ernest Frazer, 'Forward', n. pag.; 'Instructions for Use', Part XIII, n. pag. 'Reviews and Notices of Books', *British Journal of Surgery*, XXIV (1937), p. 633.

82 Cheesman, *Baillière's Synthetic Anatomy*, 'Author's Introduction to the Series', Part I, n. pag.; 'Instructions for Use', Part I, n. pag.

83 Ibid., 'Instructions for use', Part VII, n. pag; 'Instructions for Use', Part IV, n. pag.

84 'Reviews. *Baillière's Synthetic Anatomy*. By J. E. Cheesman. Part XIII. The Eye and Orbit. 1936. London: Baillière, Tindall & Cox', *British Journal of Surgery*, XXIV (1937), p. 633. 'Review. *Baillière's Synthetic Anatomy*. By J. E. Cheesman. Part I, The Shoulder and Arm. Part II, The Forearm. Part III, The Hand. London: Baillière, Tindall & Cox, 1926', *Journal of Anatomy*, LXI (1927), p. 386; 'Anatomical Illustration', *The Lancet*, 4 December 1936, p. 1324.

85 Cooke and Cooke, *Tablets of Anatomy*, p. xx.

86 Jamieson, *Illustrations of Regional Anatomy, Section II, Head and Neck*, Preface, n. pag.

87 E. B. Jamieson, *Illustrations of Regional Anatomy, Section VII, Lower Limb, (Containing 52 Plates.)* (Edinburgh, 1936), Preface, n. pag.

88 Ibid., n. pag.

89 Jamieson, *Illustrations of Regional Anatomy, Complete Volume, Seven Sections*.

90 The blackboard version of the head in illus. 151 relates to the 'Sagital Section of Head' illustration on paper, see Jamieson, *Illustrations of Regional Anatomy. Complete Volume, Seven Sections*, Section II.– Head and Neck, 53. For an anthropological analysis of colour, see Diana Young, 'The Colours of Things', in *Handbook of Material Culture*, ed. Chris Tilley et al. (London, 2006), pp. 173–85.

91 Jamieson, *Illustrations of Regional Anatomy, Section II, Head and Neck*, Preface, n. pag.

92   Ibid., n. pag.

93   Jamieson, *Illustrations of Regional Anatomy, Section VII, Lower Limb*, Preface, n. pag.

94   Goyder's Clinical Stencil Plates, Instruction card, n. pag. The stencils were reviewed in 'New Inventions. Goyder's Clinical Stencil Plates, (Registered)', *The Lancet*, 4 June 1881, p. 918.

95   Wright, *Medical Students*, p. 23.

96   See Tobias Cheung, 'Omnis Fibra Ex Fibra: Fibre Oeconomies in Bonnet's and Diderot's Models of Organic Order', in *Transitions and Borders Between Animals, Humans and Machines, 1600–1800*, ed. Tobias Cheung (Leiden, 2010); Hisao Ishizuka, '"Fibre Body": The Concept of Fibre in Eighteenth-century Medicine, *c.* 1700–40', *Medical History*, LVI (2012), pp. 562–84; Matthew Landers and Brian Muñoz, eds, *Anatomy and the Organization of Knowledge, 1500–1850* (London, 2012).

97   Cooke and Cooke, *Tablets of Anatomy*, p. xxvii, p. xxi

98   Ibid., p. xxvii, p. xxi.

99   Wendell J. S. Krieg, *A Polychrome Atlas of the Brain Stem* (Evanston, IL, 1960), p. 1.

100 David G. Whitlock, 'The Cajal Club: Its Origin, Originator and Benefactor, Wendell J. S. Krieg', *Brain Research Reviews*, LV (2007), pp. 450–62.

101 F. N. Low, 'Review, *Brain Mechanisms in Diachrome*, by Wendell J. S. Krieg. Brain Books, Evanston, 1955', *Quarterly Review of Biology*, XXXII (1957), pp. 73–4, p. 74.

102 Elizabeth Hallam, 'Anatomopoeia', in *Making and Growing: Anthropological Studies of Organisms and Artefacts*, ed. Elizabeth Hallam and Tim Ingold (Farnham, 2014), pp. 65–88.

103 The making of dermatome models in medical schools is discussed in Simon Knepper, Johan Kortenray and Antoon Moorman, eds, *Forces of Form: The Vrolik Museum* (Amsterdam, 2009).

104 'Knitted Anatomy', Museum label, n.d., University of Edinburgh, Anatomical Museum.

105 Wright, *Medical Students*, p. 40.

106 J. Bell Pettigrew, 'Anatomical Preparation-making as Devised and Practiced at the University of Edinburgh and at the Hunterian Museum of the Royal College of Surgeons of England', *The Lancet*, 23 November 1901, pp. 1399–1403, p. 1401.

107 See Elizabeth Hallam and Tim Ingold, eds, *Creativity and Cultural Improvisation* (Oxford, 2007)

108 F. J. Shepherd, 'Notes of a Visit to some of the Anatomical Schools and Surgical Clinics of Europe in 1887', *Canadian Medical Association Journal*, XIV (1924), pp. 59–65, p. 62.

109 Henry H. Donaldson, 'Notes on Models of the Brain', *American Journal of Psychology*, IV (1891), pp. 130–31; Susanna Phelps Gage, 'The Method of Making Models from Sheets of Blotting Paper', *The Anatomical Record*, I (1907), pp. 166–9; R. M. Strong, 'An Inexpensive Model of the Principal Spinal Cord and Brain Stem', *Anatomical Record*, XIX (1920), pp. 35–8.

110 For example, models made at Marischal College by John Davidson, museum attendant in botany, *c.* 1893–1911, see James Trail, Testimonial for John Davidson, 17 March 1911, in John Davidson manuscripts, University of British Columbia Archives.

111 R. D. Lockhart, 'The Art of Learning Anatomy', *The Lancet*, 27 August 1927, pp. 460–61.

112 Blaine, 'Biological Teaching Models', p. 338. On plastics see Susan Mossman, *Fantastic Plastic: Product Design and Consumer Culture* (London, 2008); Jennifer Gabrys, Gay Hawkins and Mike Michael, eds, *Accumulation: The Material Politics of Plastic* (London, 2013).

113 Elena Canadelli, '"Scientific Peep Show": The Human Body in Contemporary Science Museums', *Nuncius*, XXVI (2011), pp. 159–84; Karen A. Rader and Victoria E. M. Cain, *Life on Display: Revolutionizing U.S. Museums of Science and Natural History in the Twentieth Century* (Chicago, 2014); Klaus Vogel, 'The Transparent Man: Some Comments on the History of a Symbol', in *Manifesting Medicine: Bodies and Machines*, ed. Robert Bud et al. (Amsterdam, 1999), pp. 31–61.

114 Vogel, 'Transparent Man', p. 43.

115 Rader and Cain, *Life on Display*.

116 See Michelle Henning, 'Legibility and Affect: Museums as New Media', in *Exhibition Experiments*, eds Sharon Macdonald and Paul Basu (Oxford, 2007), pp. 25–46; Mary Anne Staniszewski, *The Power of Display: A History of Exhibition Installations at the Museum of Modern Art* (Cambridge, MA, 1998). On interactivity in current museums see Christian Heath and Dirk vom Lehn, 'Configuring 'Interactivity': Enhancing Engagement in Science Centres and Museums', *Social Studies of Science*, XXXVIII (2008), pp. 63–91.

117 L. H. Hamlyn and Patricia Thilesen, 'Models in Medical Teaching with a Note on the Use of a New Plastic', *The Lancet*, 5 September 1953, pp. 472–5, p. 472, p. 473.

118 Somso, *Catalogue of Anatomical Models* (company catalogue, 1928); Somso, *Catalogue of Anatomy, Zoology, Botany, Skeletons, Skulls* (company catalogue, 1954).

119 Paul J. Cannon, J. T. Fitzgerald and J. Sheehan, 'A Schematic Model of the Spinal Cord and Brain Stem', *The Lancet*, 31 August 1957, p. 409.

120 Adam,Rouilly, 'Adam,Rouilly, The 90th Anniversary, 1918–2008' (company booklet, 2008).

121 Tom Fisher, 'A World of Colour and Bright Shining Surfaces: Experiences of Plastics after the Second World War', *Journal of Design History*, XXVI (2013), pp. 285–303.

122 Roland Barthes, 'Plastic', *Perspecta*, XXIV (1988), pp. 92–3, p. 92. Originally published in Roland Barthes, *Mythologies* (Paris, 1957).

123 Ibid., p. 93.

124 Umberto Eco, *The Open Work*, trans. Anna Cancogni (London, 1989 [1962]).

125 Anna Dezeuze, ed., *The 'Do-It-Yourself' Artwork: Participation from Fluxus to New Media* (Manchester, 2010).

126 'The Teaching of Anatomy', *The Lancet*, 31 August 1946, pp. 308–09, p. 308, p. 309.

127 Ibid., p. 308.

128 Cannon, Fitzgerald and Sheehan, 'A Schematic Model'.

Eight Relocations and Memorials

1 Interview, with R. D. Lockhart, by Elizabeth Olson, 11 March 1985, UASC (MS 3620/1/18).

2 R. D. Lockhart, G. F. Hamilton and F. W. Fyfe, *Anatomy of the Human Body* (London, 1959), p. 1.

3 On material and spatially located memory practices, see for example Susan A. Crane, ed. *Museums and Memory* (Stanford, CA, 2000); Susan A. Crane, 'The Conundrum of Ephemerality: Time, Memory, and Museums', in *A Companion to Museum Studies*, ed. Sharon Macdonald (Oxford, 2011); pp. 98–109; Greg Dickinson, Carole Blair and Brian L. Ott, eds, *Places of Public Memory: The Rhetoric of Museums and Memorials* (Tuscaloosa, AL, 2010); Elizabeth Hallam and Jenny Hockey, *Death, Memory and Material Culture* (Oxford, 2001); Francis A. Yates, *The Art of Memory* (London, 1966).

4 In an earlier publication I suggested that this transformation of the Anatomy Museum at Marischal College took place during the 1950s, see Elizabeth Hallam, 'Anatomy Display: Contemporary Debates and Collections in Scotland', in *Anatomy Acts: How We Come to Know Ourselves*, eds Andrew Patrizio and Dawn Kemp (Edinburgh, 2006), pp. 119–35. With subsequent archival research and interviews I have revised this to the late 1960s. Interview, with retired member of teaching/research staff (C) from University of Aberdeen, Anatomy Department (UAAD), by Elizabeth Hallam, 11 May 2007; 'Anatomy Department, Inventory', 1969, typescript/MS list, archive of UAAD.

5 I derive the term 'necro-topography' from the term 'necrogeography' which was used in 1960s and 1970s to refer to geographical studies concerned with the dead, see Richard V. Francaviglia, 'The Cemetery as an Evolving Cultural Landscape', *Annals of the Association of American Geographers*, LXI (1971), pp. 501–9. For analysis of death and memorialization

in spatial contexts, see Jenny Hockey, Kate Woodthorpe and Carol Komaromy, eds, *The Matter of Death: Space, Place and Materiality* (Basingstoke, 2010); Avril Maddrell and James D. Sidaway, eds, *Deathscapes: Spaces for Death, Dying, Mourning and Remembrance* (Farnham, 2010).

6   Adrian Forty, 'Introduction', in Adrian Forty and Susanne Küchler, eds, *The Art of Forgetting* (Oxford, 1999), p. 13.

7   Catalogue, University of Aberdeen, Anatomy Museum (UAAM), *c.* 1969, typescript, archive of UAAD.

8   Robert Reid, for instance, catalogued the Anthropological Museum at Marischal College, see R. W. Reid, *Illustrated Catalogue of the Anthropological Museum, University of Aberdeen* (Aberdeen, 1912).

9   David Jenkins, 'Object Lessons and Ethnographic Displays: Museum Exhibitions and the Making of American Anthropology', *Comparative Studies in Society and History*, XXXVI (1994), pp. 242–70, p. 253. See Samuel J.M.M. Alberti, *Morbid Curiosities: Medical Museums in Nineteenth-century Britain* (Oxford, 2011), Tricia Close-Koenig, 'Cataloguing Collections: The Importance of Paper Records of Strasbourg's Medical School Pathological Anatomy Collection', in *The Fate of Anatomical Collections*, ed. Rina Knoeff and Robert Zwijnenberg (Farnham, 2015), pp. 211–27. For a survey of textual practices in medicine, see Volker Hess and J. Andrew Mendelsohn, 'Case and Series: Medical Knowledge and Paper Technology, 1600–1900', *History of Science*, XLVIII (2010), pp. 287–314.

10   Bruno Latour, 'Drawing Things Together', in *Representations in Scientific Practice*, ed. Lynch and Woolgar, pp. 19–68.

11   For analysis of lists from perspectives in the history of science, see the articles in the themed issue, 'Focus: Listmania', *Isis*, CIII (2012), pp. 710–52.

12   J. Struthers, 'The Progress of the Medical School', in *Aurora Borealis Academica: Aberdeen University Appreciations, 1860–1889*, ed. P. J. Anderson (Aberdeen, 1899), pp. 212–36, p. 227.

13   Ibid., p. 229.

14   'Additions to Anatomy Museum and Laboratories', MS notebook, archive of UAAD.

15   Ibid., n. pag.

16   'Museum Material', 1959–69, MS/typescript list *c.* 17 pages, archive of UAAD.

17   'An Unrelated Cranium', noted ibid.

18   Alison Shaw, 'Obituary: Professor David Sinclair, Educator and Anatomist', *The Scotsman*, www.scotsman.com, 8 May 2013.

19   J. J. Edwards and M. J. Edwards, *Medical Museum Technology* (London, 1959), p. 3.

20   D. C. Sinclair, 'The Place of Anatomy in the Medical Curriculum', *Postgraduate Medical Journal*, XXXIII (1957), pp. 160–64, p. 161.

21   Denis Dooley, 'A Dissection of Anatomy', *Annals of the Royal College of Surgeons of England*, LIII, 1973, pp. 13–26.

22   D. C. Sinclair, 'The Two Anatomies', *The Lancet*, 19 April 1975, pp. 875–8.

23   Alberti, *Morbid Curiosities*; Samuel J.M.M. Alebrti and Elizabeth Hallam, eds, *Medical Museums: Past, Present, Future* (London, 2013). For discussion of anatomical collections in Europe, see Rina Knoeff and Robert Zwijnenberg, eds, *The Fate of Anatomical Collections* (Farnham, 2015).

24   'Anatomy Department, Inventory', 1969, archive of UAAD; Interview, with retired member of teaching/research staff (B) from UAAD, by Elizabeth Hallam, 17 July 2003; Interview, with retired member of teaching/research staff (C) from UAAD, by Elizabeth Hallam, 11 May 2007.

25   Interview, with retired member of teaching/research staff (C) from UAAD, by Elizabeth Hallam, 11 May 2007.

26   Ibid.

27   Edwards and Edwards, *Medical Museum Technology*, p. 148.

28   W. H. Flower, 'Modern Museums', in W. H. Flower, *Essays on Museums and Other*

Subjects Connected with Natural History (London, 1898 [1893]), pp. 30–53, p. 41.

29 'Future of the Medical Museum', *The Lancet*, 24 March 1945, pp. 376–7, p. 376.

30 D. C. Sinclair, *A Student's Guide to Anatomy* (Oxford, 1961), p. 21.

31 'Anatomy Department, University of Aberdeen, Bequest to Zoology Department, February 1966, Preliminary Catalogue Nos'. MS notebook, archive of University of Aberdeen, Zoology Museum (UAZM).

32 Viscountess Stonehaven to Robert D. Lockhart, 21 November 1941, MS letter, archive of University of Aberdeen, Marischal Museum.

33 'Anatomy Department, University of Aberdeen, Bequest to Zoology Department', archive of UAZM.

34 For analysis of changing practices and perceptions relating to preserved animals, see Samuel J.M.M. Alberti, *The Afterlives of Animals: A Museum Menagerie* (Charlottesville, VA, 2011); Joan B. Landes, Paula Young Lee and Paul Youngquist, eds, *Gorgeous Beasts: Animal Bodies in Historical Perspective* (University Park, PA, 2012); Rachel Poliquin, *The Breathless Zoo: Taxidermy and the Cultures of Longing* (University Park, PA, 2012).

35 See E. M. Tansey, 'Keeping the Culture Alive: The Laboratory Technician in Mid-twentieth-century British Medical Research', *Notes and Records of the Royal Society*, LXII (2008), pp. 77–95.

36 J Struthers, 'On the Rudimentary Hind-limb of a Great Fin-whale (*Balænoptera musculus*) in Comparison with those of the Humpback Whale and Greenland Right-whale', *Journal of Anatomy and Physiology*, XXVII (1893), pp. 291–335 (With Plates XVII–XX).

37 Interview, with retired member of staff (technician) from UAAD, by Elizabeth Hallam, 19 August 2003; Interview, with retired member of teaching/research staff (C) from UAAD, by Elizabeth Hallam, 11 May 2007.

38 In 1979 professional anthropologist Charles Hunt was appointed as museum curator, see Helen Southwood, 'A Cultural History of Marischal Anthropological Museum in the Twentieth Century', PhD thesis, University of Aberdeen (2003). On the divergence of anatomy and anthropology at the University of Oxford in the 1930s, see Chris Gosden and Frances Larson with Alison Petch, *Knowing Things: Exploring the Collections at the Pitt Rivers Museum, 1884–1945* (Oxford, 2007).

39 The plaster casts had been transferred to the Anthropological Museum by 1971, see annotated photograph of the casts, archive of University of Aberdeen, Marischal Museum (UAMM).

40 Plaster casts of blocks of Parthenon frieze, dated *c.* 1881, slip catalogue, 3 and 10 July 1975, archive of UAMM.

41 R. D. Lockhart (1960), quoted in Southwood, '*Cultural History of Marischal*', p. 263.

42 Human skulls from Anatomy Museum, slip catalogue, dated July 1967–18 January 1972, archive of UAMM. Some skulls were temporarily returned to the Anatomy Department for a display, 12 March 1971.

43 Charles Hunt to E. J. Clegg, 6 September 1979, 20 September 1979, MS letters, Museums and Galleries Committee papers, 1978–87, n. pag., UASC (MSU 1332/6).

44 On museum collections and the definition of university disciplines, see Samuel J.M.M. Alberti, *Nature and Culture: Objects, Disciplines and the Manchester Museum* (Manchester, 2009); Gosden and Larson, with Petch, *Knowing Things*; Lawrence Keppie, *William Hunter and the Hunterian Museum in Glasgow, 1807–2007* (Edinburgh, 2007).

45 'Anatomy Department, Inventory', 1969, archive of UAAD.

46 R. N. Mackie to Anatomy Department, 16 May 1972, MS letter; photographs and correspondence relating to the retirement of William Anderson in June 1972, UASC (MS 3750/4).

47 Medical museums organised by anatomical subdivisions were noted in C. J. Hackett, 'A List of Medical Museums of Great Britain (1949–50)', *British Medical Journal*, 16 June 1951, pp. 1380–83; Derek Martin, 'Medical Museums', *Medical and Biological Illustration*, I (1951), pp. 144–51.

48 For example, E. B. Jamieson, *Illustrations of Regional Anatomy, Complete Volume, Seven*

Sections, 5th edn (Edinburgh, 1944 [1934–36]). See also Sinclair, *Student's Guide to Anatomy*.

49 See Keppie, *William Hunter*.

50 See 'Edinburgh University, Anatomy Museum', Museums Galleries Scotland website, www.museumsgalleriesscotland.org.uk, accessed 11 November 2014.

51 Edwards and Edwards, *Medical Museum Technology*, p. 143, p. 144.

52 Sophie Forgan, 'The Architecture of Display: Museums, Universities, and Objects in Nineteenth-century Britain', *History of Science*, XXXII (1994), pp. 139–62; Thorsten Opper, 'Ancient Glory and Modern Learning: the Sculpture-decorated Library', in *Enlightenment: Discovering the World in the Eighteenth Century*, ed. Kim Sloan with Andrew Burnett (London, 2003), pp. 58–67.

53 'Anatomy Department, Inventory', 1969, archive of UAAD.

54 Ibid.

55 Interview, with retired member of staff (technician) from UAAD, by Elizabeth Hallam, 19 August 2003.

56 Edwards and Edwards, *Medical Museum Technology*; L. W. Proger, 'The Preparation of Museum Specimens', *Annals of the Royal College of Surgeons of England*, VIII (1951), pp. 388–91; D. H. Tompsett, *Anatomical Techniques*, 2nd edn (Edinburgh, 1970).

57 Edwards and Edwards, *Medical Museum Technology*, p. 144.

58 Andreas Vesalius, *De humani corporis fabrica* (Basel, 1534); Lockhart, Hamilton and Fyfe, *Anatomy*. See Michael Sappol, *Dream Anatomy*, exh. cat., National Library of Medicine (U.S.), Bethesda (Washington, DC, 2002).

59 Jessie Dobson, 'Conservators of the Hunterian Museum: IV. William Henry Flower', *Annals of the Royal College of Surgeons of England*, XXX (1962), pp. 383–91; Keppie, *William Hunter*.

60 W. H. Flower, 'Museum Organisation', in Flower, *Essays on Museums* (London, 1898 [1889]), pp. 1–29, p. 13.

61 S. H. Daukes, *The Medical Museum: Modern Developments, Organisation and Technical Methods Based on a New System of Visual Teaching* (London, 1929), p. 20.

62 Interview, with retired member of staff (technician) from UAAD, by Elizabeth Hallam, 19 August 2003

63 Catalogue, UAAM, *c.* 1969, archive of UAAD.

64 Ibid., n. pag.

65 D. C. Sinclair, 'An Experiment in the Teaching of Anatomy', *The Journal of Medical Education*, XL (1965), pp. 401–13; Dooley, 'A Dissection of Anatomy'.

66 Sinclair, *Student's Guide to Anatomy*, p. 17. Requirements regarding students' dissection in medical schools were reduced in 1958 by the General Medical Council, which was formed in 1858 to oversee medical education.

67 Sinclair, *Student's Guide to Anatomy*, p. 20, p. 21.

68 Ibid., p. 20.

69 Ibid., p. 20.

70 Sinclair, 'Place of Anatomy', p. 162.

71 Sinclair, *Student's Guide to Anatomy*, p. 18.

72 Catalogue, UAAM, *c.* 1969, archive of UAAD.

73 Ibid., catalogue entries for TM 1. Model of the larynx, and TM 2. Model of the pulmonary lobule, n. pag.

74 Martin, 'Medical Museums', p. 144.

75 This display was probably partly based on former medical student and anatomist in Manchester, G.A.G. Mitchell's articles that discussed the history of anatomy in Scotland, especially G.A.G. Mitchell, 'Anatomical and Resurrectionist Activities in Northern Scotland', *Journal of the History of Medicine and Allied Sciences*, IV (1949), pp. 417–30. The mortsafe was from the Quaker Burial Ground, Kinmuck, *c.* 1800–1830; it was given on permanent loan by the Society of Friends in Aberdeen in December 1939, and formerly housed in the Old Meeting House, Kinmuck. See Martyn L. Gorman, 'Scottish

Echoes of the Resurrection Men', M.Litt. thesis, University of Aberdeen (2010).

76 Dissections (for example of the hand and foot) preserved in 1964 appear to have been the last dated and currently extant specimens to have been obtained for the Anatomy Museum.

77 Elizabeth Hurren, *Dying for Victorian Medicine: English Anatomy and Its Trade in the Dead Poor, c. 1834–1929* (London, 2012); Fiona Hutton, *The Study of Anatomy in Britain, 1700–1900* (London, 2013); Ruth Richardson, *Death, Dissection and the Destitute*, 2nd edn (London, 2001).

78 Anatomy Act Committee Minutes, Aberdeen, vol. I, 1856–1959, p. 56, University of Aberdeen, Special Collections (UASC), (MSU 1332/4/1/1).

79 Anatomy Act Committee Minutes, vol. I, p. 2. See Pennington, *The Modernisation of Medical Teaching at Aberdeen in the Nineteenth Century* (Aberdeen, 1994); Richardson, *Death, Dissection*.

80 Ibid., pp. 1–2.

81 Pat Jalland, *Death in the Victorian Family* (Oxford, 1996); Richardson, *Death, Dissection*; Julie-Marie Strange, *Death, Grief and Poverty in Britain, 1870–1914* (Cambridge, 2005).

82 Anatomy Act Committee Minutes, vol. I, p. 1.

83 Register of Bodies Brought to the Parochial Burying House, Aberdeen, 1843–1944, 2 vols, UASC (MSU 1332/4/3).

84 Anatomy Act Committee Minutes, vol. I, p. 5–6.

85 Ibid., p. 8. William Turner, Evidence, 3 July 1876, in *Report of the Royal Commissioners Appointed to Inquire into the Universities of Scotland, with Evidence and Appendix*, vol. III: *Evidence – Part II* (Edinburgh 1878), pp. 303–11, p. 304.

86 'An Act for Regulating Schools of Anatomy', 1 August 1832, (2&3 Gul. IV c.75).

87 Anatomy Act Committee Minutes, vol. I, p. 80.

88 Ibid., p. 80; p. 158. On the Nellfield Cemetery superintendent's malpractices regarding graves, see 'Nellfield Cemetery Dispute: Alleged Tampering with Graves', *Aberdeen Journal*, 23 May 1899, p. 7. Among newspaper reports of problems in burial practices at the cemetery were suggestions that dissected human remains had been inappropriately buried in walk-ways (rather than in a plot), and in a private grave that contained a number of coffins, see 'Nellfield Cemetery Scandal: The Trial of Coutts', *Aberdeen Journal*, 9 September 1899, pp. 6–7.

89 Anatomy Act Committee Minutes, vol. I, p. 197.

90 Ibid., p. 252, p. 258.

91 Anatomy Act Committee Minutes, Aberdeen, vol. II, 1960–73, p. 36, UASC (MSU 1332/4/1/2); D. C. Sinclair to J. Gray Kilgour, typescript letter, 10 November 1969, archive of UAAD.

92 Anatomy Act Committee Minutes, vol. I, p. 196, p. 206.

93 Ibid., p. 208.

94 Ibid., p. 220. In 1915–19 the Oldmill Poorhouse (built in 1904–7 to replace St Nicholas and Old Machar poorhouses) was evacuated for use as a military hospital, the inmates transferred to other poorhouses in the area.

95 Anatomy Act Committee Minutes, vol. I, pp. 286–362; Anatomy Act Committee Minutes, vol. II, pp. 1–20.

96 Anatomy Act Committee Minutes, vol. II, p. 39.

97 Richardson, *Death, Dissection*, p. 419.

98 Ibid., p. 260. See Douglas J. Davies, 'The Sacred Crematorium', *Mortality*, I (1996), pp. 83–94; Pat Jalland, *Death in War and Peace: A History of Loss and Grief in England, 1914–1970* (Oxford, 2010); Peter Jupp, *From Dust to Ashes: The Development of Cremation in England, 1820–1997* (New York, 2006); David Prendergast, Jenny Hockey, Leonie Kellaher, 'Blowing in the Wind? Identity, Materiality, and the Destinations of Human Ashes', *Journal of the Royal Anthropological Institute*, XII (2006), pp. 881–98.

99 Richardson, *Death, Dissection*, p. 260; Ruth Richardson, 'Human Dissection and Organ Donation: A Historical and Social Background', *Mortality*, XI (2006), pp. 151–65.

100 Laurence Dopson, 'Bequeathing Bodies For Dissection', *Scots Law Times*, 11 October 1958, pp. 189–92. For example, only one of the 610 bodies received by the University College, Dundee from 1888 to 1954 was bequeathed. It was not until the 1970s that the increase in body donations was marked enough for the anatomy department at Dundee to become 'self-sufficient', see R. R. Sturrock, 'The Anatomy Department At University College, Dundee, 1888–1954', *Medical History*, XXI (1977), pp. 310–15, p. 310.

101 Anatomy Act Committee Minutes, vol. I, p. 315.

102 Ibid., p. 347.

103 'Widow's Body for Research: A Fine Cause', *The Press and Journal*, 6 December 1960, n. pag., newspaper clipping, archive of UAAD. Further press articles were published in 1965 and television coverage was also considered, see Anatomy Act Committee Minutes, vol. II, p. 22.

104 Correspondence regarding requests to bequeath bodies to the University of Aberdeen, 1965–72, UASC (MSU 1332/4/4/17).

105 Anatomy Act Committee Minutes, vol. II, p. 3, p. 7.

106 Correspondence regarding requests to bequeath bodies, 1965–72, UASC.

107 Intending donor letters to D. C. Sinclair, 12 June 1971, 31 January 1967, Correspondence regarding requests to bequeath bodies, 1965–72, UASC. See Sturrock, 'Anatomy Department'.

108 Anatomy Act Committee Minutes, vol. II, p. 39.

109 Ibid., typescript insert p. 3.

110 F. W. Fyfe, 'In Memoriam, R. D. Lockhart', *Journal of Anatomy*, CLV (1987), pp. 203–8; Records relating to the receipt of bodies at UAAD, 1953 (counterfoils with notes); 'Bequests Which Aid Medical Science', *Press and Journal*, 6 December 1958, n. pag., newspaper clipping, archive of UAAD. To date I have found no reference to an anatomy memorial service prior to this in Britain. The memorial service in Aberdeen inspired a similar service of thanksgiving first held in May 1982 for donors to medical schools at the University of London, see Eric Tinker, 'An Unusual Christian Service: For Those Who Have Donated Their Bodies for Medical Education and Research', *Mortality*, III (1998), pp. 79–82. On services in further medical schools in Britain and the USA by the 1990s, see Maralyn Druce and Martin H. Johnson, 'Human Dissection and Attitudes of Preclinical Students to Death and Bereavement', *Clinical Anatomy*, VII (1994), pp. 42–49; Susan E. Weeks, Eugene E. Harris, and Warren G. Kinzey, 'Human Gross Anatomy: A Crucial Time to Encourage Respect and Compassion in Students', *Clinical Anatomy*, VIII (1995), pp. 69–79.

111 Fyfe, 'In Memoriam, R. D. Lockhart', p. 205. 'Bequests Which Aid Medical Science', UAAD.

112 Records relating to the receipt of bodies at UAAD, 1953, 1955, 1960, 1965 (counterfoils with notes), archive of UAAD.

113 Ibid., 1958; Correspondent to R. D. Lockhart, 1957, n. pag., MS letter, archive of UAAD.

114 Interview, with Chaplain at the University of Aberdeen, by Elizabeth Hallam, 28 August 2006.

115 Ibid.

116 Anatomy Act Committee Minutes, Aberdeen, vol. II, p. 21.

117 Fieldnotes, UAAD, 23 May 2008.

118 For analysis of the social and cultural significance of names, see Gabriele vom Bruck and Barbara Bodenhorn, eds, *An Anthropology of Names and Naming* (Cambridge, 2009).

119 See Alan Thomson, 'Conferred in the Spirit of Good Relations', www.timeshighereducation.co.uk, 17 June 2005.

120 For analysis of war memorials, see for example Jalland, *Death in War and Peace*; Nicholas J. Saunders, ed., *Matters of Conflict: Material Culture, Memory and the First World War* (London, 2004); Michael Rowlands, 'Remembering to Forget: Sublimation as Sacrifice in War Memorials', in *The Art of Forgetting*, ed. Forty and Küchler, pp. 129–46.

121 Since 2009 the memorial book has been in a display case at the Anatomy Department at the Suttie Centre for Teaching and Learning Healthcare, Foresterhill, Aberdeen.

122 Anatomy Act Committee Minutes, vol. II, p. 26.

123 Ibid., p. 29.

124 The memorial is composed of a stone facing, synthetic granite and a concrete 'feature beam' with white marble chips for the inscription, as noted in: Doric Construction Company to W. Coutts Youngson, typescript letter, 26 February 1974, archive of UAAD. On the significance of materials in generating affective responses to memorials, see Zachary Beckstead et al., 'Collective Remembering Through the Materiality and Organization of War Memorials', *Journal of Material Culture*, XVI (2011), pp. 193–213.

125 D. C. Sinclair to the Town Clerk – Aberdeen, 19 March 1974, typescript letter; 'Memorial Area', *The Press and Journal*, 17 May 1974, newspaper clipping; 'Memorial', Aberdeen newspaper clipping 1974; all archive of UAAD. Tinker, 'Unusual Christian Service'.

126 For example, 286 completed bequest forms were received by the Anatomy Department in 1967: Anatomy Act Committee Minutes, vol. II, p. 28; on the cremation and burial of donors, and Sinclair's proposal for a memorial: Anatomy Act Committee Minutes, vol. II, p. 33.

127 Ibid., p. 33.

128 D. C. Sinclair to E. M. Wright, Principal and Vice-Chancellor of the University of Aberdeen, typescript letter, 19 June 1972, archive of UAAD.

129 D. C. Sinclair to the Town Clerk – Aberdeen, 19 March 1974, typescript letter, archive of UAAD.

130 Anatomy Act Committee Minutes, vol. II, p. 36; D. C Sinclair to J. Gray Kilgour, typescript letter, 10 November 1969, archive of UAAD.

131 Anatomy Act Committee Minutes, vol. II, p. 36–7, p. 40; File of letters regarding the memorial at Trinity Cemetery, 1969–8, archive of UAAD.

132 Anatomy Act Committee Minutes, vol. II, p. 36.

133 Ibid., p. 37.

134 Ibid., p. 41.

135 Ibid. p. 41, D. C. Sinclair to J. Gray Kilgour, typescript letter, 10 November 1969, archive of UAAD.

136 File of sketches and notes relating to the memorial at Trinity Cemetery, 1969–8, archive of UAAD.

137 Ibid.

138 See Paul Connerton, *How Modernity Forgets* (Cambridge, 2009); Forty, 'Introduction', *The Art of Forgetting*, ed. Forty and Küchler.

139 See Thomas W. Laqueur, 'Memory and Naming in the Great War', in *Commemorations: The Politics of National Identity*, ed. John R. Gillis (Princeton, NJ, 1994), pp. 150–67. For discussion of similarities in treatment of bodies of men who died in war and bodies of the poor dying in workhouses, both having been buried in communal graves, see Bourke, *Dismembering the Male: Men's Bodies, Britain and the Great War* (London, 1996); Strange, *Death, Grief*.

140 On the history of crematoria design, see Hilary J. Grainger, 'Ambiguity, Evasion and Remembrance in British Crematoria', in *Lest We Forget: Remembrance and Commemoration*, eds, Maggie Andrews, with Charles Bagot Jewitt and Nigel Hunt (Stroud, Gloucestershire, 2011), pp. 124–27; Hilary J. Grainger, *Death Redesigned: British Crematoria, History, Architecture and Landscape* (Reading, 2006).

141 Letter, James Kelman, 24 June, 1974; Letter, W. Coutts Youngson, 7 July 1974. Anatomy Department Archive.

142 W. Coutts Youngson to D. C. Sinclair, 8 June 1972, typescript letter; D. C. Sinclair to E. M. Wright, Principal and Vice-Chancellor of the University of Aberdeen, typescript letter, 19 June 1972, archive of UAAD.

143 Anatomy Act Committee Minutes, vol. II, insert of minutes 11 June 1973.

144 W. Coutts Youngson to James (Kelman?), 7 July 1974, typescript letter, archive of UAAD.

145 Keith Ross to Alan Main, 9 December 1976, typescript letter, archive of UAAD.

146 Ibid.; E. J. Clegg to Ross Naylor, 20 February 1978, typescript letter, archive of UAAD.

147 See Maurice Bloch and Jonathan Parry, eds, *Death and the Regeneration of Life* (Cambridge, 1982); Doris Francis, Leonie A. Kellaher and Georgina Neophytou, *The Secret Cemetery* (Oxford, 2005); Hallam and Hockey, *Death, Memory*.

148 Letter, David Sinclair, 19 March 1974.

149 Daukes, *Medical Museum*, p. 26, p. 58.

150 Report on Anatomy Department Museum, October 1986, Museums and Galleries Committee papers, 1978–87, n. pag., UASC (MSU 1332/6).

151 Elizabeth Hallam, 'Disappearing Museums? Medical Collections at the University of Aberdeen', in *Medical Museums: Past, Present, Future*, ed. Samuel J.M.M. Alberti and Elizabeth Hallam (London, 2013), pp. 44–59.

SELECT BIBLIOGRAPHY

Alberti, Samuel J.M.M., *Morbid Curiosities: Medical Museums in Nineteenth-century Britain* (Oxford, 2011)
—, and Elizabeth Hallam, eds, *Medical Museums: Past, Present, Future* (London, 2013)
Åhrén, Eva, *Death, Modernity, and the Body: Sweden, 1870–1940*, trans. D. W. Olson (Rochester, NY, 2009)
Candlin, Fiona, *Art, Museums and Touch* (Manchester, 2010)
Chaplin, Simon, 'John Hunter and the "Museum Oeconomy", 1750–1800', PhD thesis, King's College, London (2009)
Coopmans, Catelijne, et al., eds, *Representation in Scientific Practice Revisited* (Cambridge, MA, 2014)
Cunningham, Andrew, *The Anatomist Anatomis'd: An Experimental Discipline in Enlightenment Europe* (Farnham, 2010)
Daston, Lorraine, and Peter Galison, *Objectivity* (New York, 2007)
de Chadarevian, Soraya, and Nick Hopwood, eds, *Models: The Third Dimension of Science* (Stanford, CA, 2004)
Dudley, Sandra, ed., *Museum Materialities: Objects, Engagements, Interpretations* (London, 2010)
Eco, Umberto, *The Open Work*, trans. Anna Cancogni [1962] (London, 1989)
Edwards, Elizabeth, Chris Gosden and Ruth B. Phillips, eds, *Sensible Objects: Colonialism. Museums and Material Culture* (Oxford, 2006)
Farnell, Brenda, *Dynamic Embodiment for Social Theory: 'I Move Therefore I Am'* (London, 2012)
Good, Byron, *Medicine, Rationality and Experience* (Cambridge, 1994)
Gosden, Chris, and Frances Larson with Alison Petch *Knowing Things: Exploring the Collections at the Pitt Rivers Museum, 1884–1945* (Oxford, 2007)
Hahn, Cynthia, *Strange Beauty: Issues in the Making and Meaning of Reliquaries, 400–circa 1204* (University Park, PA, 2012)
Hallam, Elizabeth, 'Anatomopocia', in *Making and Growing: Anthropological Studies of Organisms and Artefacts*, ed. Elizabeth Hallam and Tim Ingold (Farnham, 2014), pp. 65–88
—, and Jenny Hockey, *Death, Memory and Material Culture* (Oxford, 2001)
—, Jenny Hockey and Glennys Howarth, *Beyond the Body: Death and Social Identity* (London, 1999)
Harvey, Penny, et al., eds, *Objects and Materials: A Routledge Companion* (London, 2014)
Hockey, Jenny, Kate Woodthorpe and Carol Komaromy, eds, *The Matter of Death: Space, Place and Materiality* (Basingstoke, 2010)
Hopwood, Nick, *Embryos in Wax: Models from the Ziegler Studio* (Cambridge and Bern, 2002)
Hurren, Elizabeth H., *Dying for Victorian Medicine: English Anatomy and its Trade in the Dead Poor, c. 1834–1929* (Basingstoke, 2012)
Hutton, Fiona, *The Study of Anatomy in Britain, 1700–1900* (London, 2013)
Ingold, Tim, *Making: Anthropology, Archaeology, Art and Architecture* (London, 2013)
Kemp, Dawn, with Sara Barnes, *Surgeons' Hall: A Museum Anthology* (Edinburgh, 2009)
Kemp, Martin, and Marina Wallace, *Spectacular Bodies: The Art and Science of the Human Body from Leonardo to Now*, exh. cat., Hayward Gallery (London, 2000).
Keppie, Lawrence, *William Hunter and the Hunterian Museum in Glasgow, 1807–2007* (Edinburgh, 2007)
Klestinec, Cynthia, *Theatres of Anatomy: Students, Teachers, and Traditions of Dissection in Renaissance Venice* (Baltimore, MD, 2011)

Lambert, Helen, and Maryon McDonald, eds, *Social Bodies* (Oxford, 2009)

Lock, Margaret, *Twice Dead: Organ Transplants and the Reinvention of Death* (Berkeley, CA, 2002)

—, and Judith Farquhar, eds, *Beyond the Body Proper: Reading the Anthropology of Material Life* (Durham, NC, 2007)

—, and Vinh-Kim Nguyen, *An Anthropology of Biomedicine* (Chichester, 2010)

MacDonald, Helen, *Possessing the Dead: The Artful Science of Anatomy* (Melbourne, 2010)

Macdonald, Sharon, *Behind the Scenes at the Science Museum* (Oxford, 2002)

Maerker, Anna, *Model Experts: Wax Anatomies and Enlightenment in Florence and Vienna, 1775–1815* (Manchester, 2011)

Messbarger, Rebecca, *The Lady Anatomist: The Life and Work of Anna Morandi Manzolini* (Chicago, IL, 2010)

Park, Katharine, *Secrets of Women: Gender, Generation, and the Origins of Human Dissection* (New York, 2006)

Patrizio, Andrew, and Dawn Kemp, eds, *Anatomy Acts: How We Come to Know Ourselves* (Edinburgh, 2006)

Pauwels, Luc, ed., *Visual Cultures of Science: Rethinking Representational Practices in Knowledge Building and Science Communication* (Hanover, NH, 2006)

Prentice, Rachel, *Bodies in Formation: An Ethnography of Anatomy and Surgery Education* (Durham, NC, 2013)

Richardson, Ruth, *Death, Dissection and the Destitute*, 2nd edn (London, 2001)

Sappol, Michael, *A Traffic of Dead Bodies: Anatomy and Embodied Social Identity in Nineteenth-century America* (Princeton, NJ, 2002)

—, *Dream Anatomy*, exh. cat., National Library of Medicine, Bethesda, MD (Washington, DC, 2002)

Seremetakis, C. Nadia, *The Last Word: Women, Death and Divination in Inner Mani* (Chicago, IL, 1991)

Shapin, Steven, *Never Pure: Historical Studies of Science as if It Was Produced by People with Bodies, Situated in Time, Space, Culture, and Society, and Struggling for Credibility and Authority* (Baltimore, MD, 2010)

Smith, Pamela H., Amy R. W. Meyers and Harold J. Cook, eds, *Ways of Making and Knowing: The Material Culture of Empirical Knowledge* (Ann Arbor, MI, 2014)

Stephens, Elizabeth, *Anatomy as Spectacle: Public Exhibitions of the Body from 1700 to the Present* (Liverpool, 2011)

Thomas, Nicholas, *Entangled Objects: Exchange, Material Culture, and Colonialism in the Pacific* (Cambridge, MA, 1991)

Tilley, Christopher, *Metaphor and Material Culture* (Oxford, 1999)

ACKNOWLEDGEMENTS

Research for this book began in 1999 when I was teaching anthropology at the University of Aberdeen, in northeast Scotland. I had the privilege of holding classes on material culture, working with the inspiring collection artefacts and display spaces in Marischal Museum (formerly the Anthropological Museum) at Marischal College. It was there that I first heard of the Anatomy Museum, which was part of the Anatomy Department in the back quadrangle of the same college where medical students were taught human anatomy. These two museums, of anthropology and of anatomy, were the last of nine that had flourished at this site during the nineteenth and early twentieth century; the other seven had long been evacuated along with their departments, some to premises elsewhere in the university's buildings, leaving a cavernous empty complex of college rooms. I arranged to visit the unusually resilient Anatomy Museum and so I initiated what was to become an intensive and at times very challenging project. This museum seemed at the time to offer me fascinating ways to develop my previous research on the anthropology of death and the body, yet it was to take me in many unanticipated directions and to present me with many questions and issues that I am still working through.

To investigate the contemporary uses of the Anatomy Museum, as an anthropologist, and to trace aspects of its history I frequently visited the Anatomy Department to conduct fieldwork, observing the work of staff and medical students in the Museum and its surrounding rooms, talking with people about their learning and their teaching, interviewing retired staff, devising two questionnaires, studying objects on display and in storage, photographing anatomical atlases and three dimensional models of the human body. This research, at Marischal College until 2009 (and subsequently at the new teaching facility), was made possible by the permission granted by the then Licensed Teacher of Anatomy at the University of Aberdeen in consultation with the then Her Majesty's Inspector of Anatomy, the government-appointed person who at the time oversaw the teaching of anatomy in England, Scotland and Wales. Much of what I have been able to explore and write about has depended on the access I was given to the spaces where medical teaching was taking place.

Staff and students in the Anatomy Department among whom I conducted my fieldwork have preferred to remain anonymous in my account and to be referred to instead by the titles of their professional posts/ positions in the university. For this reason their names do not appear in this book, but I thank them all sincerely for their incredible generosity; they have taken time to explain and to show me their work and studies relating to anatomy. They have helped me to learn how they themselves learn, and in doing so they have contributed enormously to my understanding of this book's subject-matter.

Alongside – indeed, central to – the fieldwork for this project, was museum-based study of material objects and associated archival research. Closely studying, and sometimes handling, museum objects has been integral to my approach and has greatly enriched my interpretations. To further analyse the Anatomy Museum's holdings, I traced their links with textual records and visual images in Aberdeen, and in museums and archives in Scotland and England. Through these methods, I came to understand material objects, and bodies, in the early twenty-first-century Anatomy Museum as part of social and cultural processes that extend across a much wider geographical space and longer period of time; this book charts some of my journey in moving toward this understanding. My research with the museum and archive collections listed in the acknowledgements to follow was especially fruitful and rewarding.

This project received funding from the British Academy (grant no. SG-39337), the University of Aberdeen's College of Arts and Social Sciences, and the Principal's Fund, as well as the University of Oxford; these resources have been essential in producing this book. I have benefitted hugely from the help and support of many at the University of Aberdeen: in particular I thank Arnar Arnason, Alison Brown, Caroline Craig, Mike Craig, Neil Curtis, Martyn Gorman, Tim Ingold, Alan Knox, Ben Marsden, Easter Smart, Claire Smith, Nancy Wachowich, and Margo Wright. At the University of Oxford, the School of Anthropology and Museum Ethnography has provided a very stimulating and supportive environment for my research; I thank, especially, Marcus Banks, Inge Daniels, Clare Harris, Elisabeth Hsu, Chris Morton and Laura Peers.

For their assistance with my research and their valuable insights, I am very grateful to Caroline Morris and Anthony Payne at the University of Glasgow's Museum of Anatomy; Gordon Findlater at the University of Edinburgh's Anatomy Department; Simon Chaplin, when at the Royal College of Surgeons of England; Dawn Kemp, when at the Royal College of Surgeons of Edinburgh; staff at the University of Birmingham Special Collections, and at the Science Museum's store, Blythe House in London.

Photographers Norman Little and Wolfgang Suschitzky have very kindly provided me with images, and John McIntosh has spent many hours producing expert photographs for my research. Working with John in photographic sessions helped me to interpret many of the material objects in this study. Ray Lucas at the Manchester School of Architecture generously produced a meticulous floor plan (in Chapter One, illus. 21).

Artists Christine Borland and Jodie Carey have provided photographs of their work, which I very much appreciate. Jenny Whitebread and Michael Whitebread at Adam,Rouilly have been very generous in granting access to their company's archive and in supplying permission to use images of anatomical models in my research. Ann Philip has generously shared with me many memories of anatomist Robert Lockhart's work, which have helped my interpretations of his anatomical practice.

Colleagues and friends who read earlier drafts of chapters have given me invaluable comments and advice, so many thanks – as ever – go to Sam Alberti, Elizabeth Edwards, Jenny Hockey and Anna Maerker. At Reaktion I thank Marquard Smith who advised me in the very early stages of this book, and especially Michael Leaman who gave me such wise and incisive feedback on the entire first draft (when it was double the length of its published version) and who has been wonderfully patient during this book's revision.

Through all of my research and writing, my family – especially Ian – has sustained me with much love, food, laughter and encouragement, for which I give them all deeply heartfelt thanks.

PHOTO ACKNOWLEDGEMENTS

The author and publishers wish to express their thanks to the below sources of illustrative material and/or permission to reproduce it.

Aberdeen Art Gallery & Museums (photo Aberdeen Art Gallery & Museums Collections): 79; Aberdeen Medico-Chirurgical Society: 70; photo Harry Bedford Lemere: 74; from Richard J. A. Berry, *A Clinical Atlas of Sectional and Topographical Anatomy* (Edinburgh, 1911): 105; Bibliothèque du Saulchoir, Paris, France/Archives Charmet: 47; from *Bon-Accord*, 13 November 1886: 77; photos The Bridgeman Art Library: 45, 46, 47, 55; photo © Stanley B. Burns, MD and the Burns Archive: 15; photo Jodie Carey: 9; Church of St Foy, Conques, France: 46; photo Alan Dimmick, reproduced courtesy Christine Borland and Fabric Workshop & Museum, Philadelphia: 8; Gemäldegalerie Alte Meister, Kassel/© Museumslandschaft Hessen Kassel/Arno Hensmanns: 55; photo Getty Images: 5; photos Elizabeth Hallam: 3, 4, 11, 12, 13, 20, 23, 26, 27, 28, 29, 36, 37, 41, 43, 44, 59, 62, 67, 68, 69, 72, 73, 78, 82, 99, 101, 105, 106, 107, 108, 110, 111, 113a–d, 121, 139, 145, 147, 148, 149, 150, 151, 153, 155, 161, 162, 164, 166, 170; photos © The Hunterian Museum and Art Gallery, University of Glasgow: 7, 60; photos The Hunterian Museum at the Royal College of Surgeons of England, London: 1, 6, 18, 19, 75, 117, 118, 163; from Edward B. Jamieson, *Illustrations of Regional Anatomy*, 5th edn (Edinburgh, 1944): 150; from Wendell J. S. Krieg, *A Polychrome Atlas of the Brain Stem* (Evanston, IL, 1960): 153; photos Norman Little: 31, 35, 42, 100, 132; from Robert D. Lockhart, *Living Anatomy: A Photographic Atlas of Muscles in Action and Surface Contours*, 5th edn (London, 1960): 128; from Robert D. Lockhart, Gilbert F. Hamilton and Forest W. Fyfe, *Anatomy of the Human Body* (London, 1959): 126; photo London Metropolitan Archives, reproduced by kind permission of Guy's and St Thomas' Charity: 95; from Alexander Low, 'University of Aberdeen Department of Anatomy', in *Methods and Problems of Medical Education* (New York, 1930): 93 (right); Ray Lucas: 21; photos John McIntosh: 2, 22, 32, 33, 34, 38, 39, 40, 63, 64, 65, 66, 80, 83, 84, 98, 141, 142, 143, 146, 165; Rijksmuseum, Amsterdam/Giraudon: 45; photo © Royal Commission on the Ancient and Historical Monuments of Scotland. Licensor www.scran.ac.uk: 74; Science Museum, London (photos Science and Society Picture Library): 58, 152; from *Somso Models: Anatomy*, commercial catalogue, 1970: 156; photo © Succession Picasso/DACS, London 2007: 135; photographed with permission of Surgeons' Hall Museums, Royal College of Surgeons of Edinburgh: 78, 82; photo Wolfgang Suschitzky: 119; photographed with permission of University of Aberdeen, Anatomy Department: 2, 4, 11, 12, 13, 20, 22, 23, 26, 27, 28, 29, 31, 32, 33, 34, 35, 38, 39, 40, 42, 62, 67, 68, 69, 72, 73, 83, 84, 98, 99, 100, 101, 105, 106, 107, 108, 110, 111, 113a–d, 121, 132, 139, 141, 142, 143, 146, 147, 149, 150, 153, 158, 159, 161, 162, 164, 165, 167; photographed with permission of University of Aberdeen, Anatomy Department, and reproduced courtesy Somso® models from Adam,Rouilly: 26, 28, 32; University of Aberdeen, Marischal Museum: 16, 65, 66, 76, 81, 85, 102, 103, 136, 137; University of Aberdeen, Natural Philosophy Collection: 63, 64; University of Aberdeen, Special Collections: 10, 17, 24, 25, 30, 51, 54, 87, 88, 89, 90, 91, 92, 94, 96, 97, 104, 109, 112, 114, 115, 116, 120, 122, 124, 125, 126, 127, 128, 130, 131, 133, 134, 140, 154, 160, 168, 169; from *University of Aberdeen Proceedings of the Anatomical and Anthropological Society, 1900* (Aberdeen, 1900): 113a–d (Pl. III); from *University of Aberdeen Proceedings of the Anatomical and Anthropological Society, 1904–06* (Aberdeen, 1906): 99 (Pl. VIII), 110 (Pl. VI), 111 (Pl. I); University of Birmingham, Special Collections: 123; photographed with permission of University of Edinburgh, Anatomical Museum: 37, 43, 44, 145, 151, 155;

photographed with permission of University of Glasgow, Museum of Anatomy: 3, 36, 59; from Robert Walker (and A. M. Munro), *University of Aberdeen, Quatercentenary Celebrations, September 1906: Handbook to City and University* (Aberdeen, 1906): 93 (left); from David Waterston, *The Edinburgh Stereoscopic Atlas of Anatomy* (Edinburgh, 1905–6): 106, 107, 108; photo Wellcome Library, London: 14, 48, 49, 50, 53, 56, 57, 61, 86, 129, 138, 144; University of Aberdeen, Zoology Museum: 71, 80, 157.

INDEX

Illustration numbers are in *italics*

Aberdeen, Anatomical Museum formation
(*c.* 18th to mid-19th century) 133–56
 anatomy, study 143–52
 antiquities and curiosities 137–43
 bodies of executed criminals and 'bodies
 of the poorer sort', legal acquisition of
 145, 146
 dissecting room, and hygiene concerns
 143
 funeratory 146
 illustrated lectures *67*, 147, 148–9
 natural philosophy apparatus collection
 63–4, 139–41
 preparations, anatomical 147
 preservation of human skeletons and
 tissue 146
 public opposition to practice of anatomy
 145–6
 rebuilding, Marischal College 141, 146,
 147–8
 skulls, donation 137
 skulls, importance of study of 146–7
 student note-taking 149–52
 topographic anatomy 147
Aberdeen, Anatomical Museum growth
(1860s–90s) Struthers's professorship
157–98
 anatomical actualities, observation
 of 162–7
 Anatomical Department, creation
 of 160–61
 architectural structure 159–62, 169–70
 articulated skeletons *76*, 170, 182
 authority structure and division
 of labour 185–91
 'Bush-woman' and 'Bushman' plaster
 casts 20–21, *85*, *112*, 193–4, 203,
 232, 325
 classical sculpture, plaster casts 161–2
 codes of conduct 189
 collection gathering 158, 171–7, 183
 comparative anatomy 173–4
 display, importance of 188–90

dissections and body supply 163–4,
171–2
foetal displays *78*, 173
former students' gifts to 158, 183
funeratory, bodies obtained from 164,
172–3
international museum expansion,
effects of 159
labelling, importance of *82*, 163, 188–90
live shows 192–8
museum 'models', or prototypes 167–70
naturalists and taxidermists, collaboration
with 177–82
practical learning, encouragement
of 162–7
preparations, anatomical *82*, 158, 188–9
racial differences, study of 183–4
Struthers's anatomical list 318–19
Struthers's international connections
and reciprocity 182–4
Struthers's private collection *78*, 172,
173–4, 188, 203, 255
Struthers's public lectures 196–7
Struthers's social relationships, and
museum collecting 177–84
vertebrate animals for comparative
anatomy *89–90*, 174–5, 182–4, 186–7,
189, 190, 192–3, 201–2, 321
visual instruction and anatomical
wallcharts 164–7
whale study and dissection *87–9*, *159*,
175–8, 182, 201, 202, 255, 270,
323, 324
see also Struthers, John
Aberdeen, Anatomy Museum development
(1890s–1930s), Reid's professorship
199–237
anthropometric laboratory *see*
anthropometric
laboratory/Anthropological Museum,
Aberdeen
apes in tree exhibit *123*, *158*, 252,
322–3, 324

colonial power relations and body
acquisitions 20–21, 37–8, 222–6, 232,
234–5, 254
'digital eye' 207, 221
dissecting room 94, 205–6, 207–14
education, continuity and staff 204–5
electric lighting 205–6
expert drawings of sectioned specimens,
display of 211–14
floor plans 93, 205–7
funerary and poor house, bodies
acquired 222
ground floor and gallery exhibits 87–90,
200–203
imaging techniques and framing 224–5,
226
labelling techniques 210, 211–12, 224
lantern slides 102–4, 215, 216, 217–18,
232
lecture theatre 205–6
Marischal College extension (1895) 92,
205–6
microscopes and magnification 100,
214–15
obscene advertisements charge 236
photography 102–3, 215, 216–17,
218–19, 225, 232
racial differences, study of 109, 223–5,
227–37
Reid's museum acquisitions book 319
Reid's professional relationships and
human and animal body acquisitions
222–4
Reid's public lectures 235–6
skeletal specimens 200–204
skulls 110, 113a–d, 223, 224–5, 229–31,
232, 326
stereoscopic photographs 106–8, 219–21,
298
X-ray images 111, 218, 226
see also Reid, Robert William
Aberdeen, Anatomy Museum and living
anatomy (1920s–60s), Lockhart's
professorship 238–77
anatomical collections, display of 253–9
anatomical eponyms, use of 120, 249–50
anatomical poetics see anatomical poetics
anatomical wayfinding 248–52
annual inventories 319
bodies, acquisition of 247, 254, 338
dissecting room 119, 140, 246–50, 287
First World War effects on students 243
'giant' and 'dwarf' skeleton contrasts 123,
252, 259
illustrated textbooks, importance of
images 260–65
Lockhart's lectures 131, 250, 256, 257,
270, 272, 274
magazine and newspaper clippings, use
of 133, 272–4

narratives as mnemonic devices 250–51
non-human remains, acquisition of
123–4, 252–3, 254–5, 322
popular performance and entertainment
links 255–9, 265
student drawings, encouragement of 251
students as 'living models' in anatomy
classes 265, 266
study of dead and living bodies together
240, 241–6
visual aids see visual aids
wall 'book' 127, 261, 263, 264
X-ray images 240, 242, 257–8, 265–6
see also Lockhart, Robert Douglas
Aberdeen, Anatomy Museum,
reconfiguration (1960s–70s), Sinclair's
professorship
anatomical illustrations, wall-mounted
161, 328–9
Anatomy in Aberdeen historical narrative
34, 80, 81, 334
animal skeletons, removal to Zoology
Museum 157, 321, 322–3
annual inventories 319–20
'bay system', museum layout 85–6,
327–9, 331–2
cataloguing and anatomical lists 318–20,
332, 333–4
curricular change effects 320
ethnographic artefacts to Anthropological
Museum 160, 323–7
ground-floor exhibits as anatomical
regions 321, 327–9
material inscriptions (labels and signs),
use of (1965) 319–20, 330–32, 333–4
memorial book, creation 165, 342–3
Perspex cases replacing glass 163, 329,
330
reframing and rewording 327–34
specimens, reframing 162, 164, 329–30,
332
Trinity Cemetery memorial 166–70,
343–8, 349, 350–52
see also Sinclair, David C.
Aberdeen Mechanics' Institution exhibition
137–8
Aberdeen Medico-Chirurgical Society (AMCS)
137, 139, 145
anatomical preparations 152–3, 154–5,
160
contact-building and collection expansion
153
crocodile skeleton 71, 153–4, 158, 174,
255, 322–3, 324
medical 'case' discussions 152–3, 154
resurrectionists, graves 145
Aberdeen, Natural History Museum 143,
147, 155, 170, 255
Aberdeen Natural History Society 180
Aberdeen, Pathological Museum 169

Aberdeen Recreation Grounds, whale exhibits
175, 176
Aberdeen Royal Infirmary 155, 160
Aberdeen Trinity Cemetery memorial *166–70*,
343–8, 349, 350–52
Aberdeen University Anatomical and
Anthropological Society (AUAAS) 212–13,
231–2, 250–51, 270
Aberdeen University, Archaeological Museum
102, 214, 215, 233
Aberdeen University King's College Chapel
340
Adair, Dr Frederick, Anatomical Museum
195, 196
'Adam and Eve at the Tree of Knowledge'
(Amman) *52*, 114, 115
Adam, Rouilly 254
Somso models *26, 28, 32*, 61, 62, 63, 73,
86, *156*, 312–13
advertisements, obscene advertisements
charge 236
Alcock, Alfred William 222
Alice's Adventures in Wonderland (Carroll) 260
AMCS *see* Aberdeen Medico-Chirurgical
Society (AMCS)
Amsterdam surgeons' guild 97–8
Anatomia humani corporis (Bidloo) *56*,
120–21
anatomical actualities, observation of 162–7
anatomical display *see* display methods
anatomical division, Anatomy Museum's
ground floor and gallery *35*, 82–3,
84–6, 321
anatomical eponyms, use of *120*, 249–50
anatomical illustrations *see* illustrations
anatomical intermediality *see* intermediality
anatomical knowledge 13, 45, 47, 48–9, 90,
104–6, 160
see also anatomical models; dissecting
rooms; individual anatomy museums;
labelling; lectures; living bodies;
preparations; textbooks; visual aids
anatomical lists 318–20, 332, 333–4
anatomical models
and classical sculpture 123–4
dermatomes, models showing *3*, 14,
15–16, *29*, 67, 68, *154*, 161, 203,
308, 309
disassembling and assembling 42, 92–5,
141–4, 289–98
papier mâché *see* Auzoux, Dr Louis
three-dimensional 91–6, 250, 261, 282–3
wooden 60, 178, 295
see also demonstrations
anatomical models, plastic 280, 283–4, 312–14
anatomical visualization, models as
'stepping stones' 91–2
Cellon 312
Deutsches Hygiene Museum, Dresden *28*,
63, 312

as intermediaries 74–5, 82, 89, 91–5
labelling 89, 90
Plasticine 261, 311
replacing specimens 86
robustness of 91–5
Somso *26, 28, 32*, 61, 62, 63, 73, 86, *156*,
312–13
anatomical models, wax 261, 295–8
Calenzuoli, Francesco 27, *58*, 124–5
depths of 'living' bodily interior, portrayal
of 121–6
heart 27, 62, 63
Maison Tramond *see* Maison Tramond
Morandi Manzolini, Anna 122–3
Rouppert, N. *see* Rouppert, N.
Susini, Clemente *57*, 123–4, 125
Weisker, Dr Rudolf *84*, 191
anatomical plates, *A System of Anatomical
Plates of the Human Body* (Lizars) *69*,
149, 150, 287
anatomical poetics (means of making
anatomical meaning) 239, 241, 268–72
and juxtaposition 272–7
references to popular and literary
culture 270
rhododendron flowers and Lockhart's
professorship *130–31*, 271–2
terminology and metaphors 268–71, 283
anatomical practices 12–13, 15, 17, 37, 49
memorials and public visibility *see*
memorials
see also articulation; anatomical models;
demonstrations; display; dissections;
drawings; intermediaries; living anatomy;
preparations; specimens; photography
anatomical preparations *see* preparations
anatomical regions, Anatomy Museum
ground-floor exhibits as 321, 327–9
anatomical terms 51–2, 88–9, 211, 249, 259
see also labelling
anatomical visualization, embodied 48–53,
77, 84–5
involving mental work 49, 52, 71, 91, 163,
251–2, 278–9, 296, 301, 310, 315, 332
plastic models as 'stepping stones' 91–2
relating three-dimensional bodies to
two-dimensional illustrations 91–6
see also intermediality
visual memory 332–3
anatomical wayfinding 248–52
'The Anatomist's Dream' (poem) (Lockhart)
238, 240
Anatomy in Aberdeen historical narrative
34, 80, 81, 334
Anatomy Act (1832) 81, 133, 146, 283,
335, 336
Anatomy Act (1871) amendment 164
Anatomy Act (1984) 66
Anatomy of the Arteries of the Human Body
(Quain) *68, 139*, 147–8, 149, 285–7, 296

anatomy atlases
  *Clinical Atlas of Sectional and
    Topographical Anatomy* (Berry) *105*, 218,
    219, 302
  *The Edinburgh Stereoscopic Atlas of
    Anatomy* (Waterston) *106–7*, 221
  A Polychrome Atlas of the Brain Stem
    (Krieg) *153*, 307–8
  The Descriptive Atlas of Anatomy
    (Osborne-Walker) J. *73*, 165–6
  see also maps; visual aids
The Anatomy of the Bones of the Human Body
    (Barclay) *67*, 147, 148
Anatomy Class (Suschitzky) *119*, 247
anatomy colouring books 90
Anatomy of the Human Body (Lockhart) 68,
    126–7, *132*, 240, 251, 259, 260–63,
    268–9, 270, 273, 274, 305, 329
Anatomy of the Human Eye (Thompson) 221
The Anatomy Lesson of Dr Nicolaes Tulp
    (Rembrandt) *23*, 54–5
*The Anatomy Lesson of Professor Frederik
    Ruysch* (Van Neck) *45*, 98–9
anatomy theatres *48*, 103–8
  authoritative books, use of 106
  Bologna University 122
  carnival celebrations 104
  collections of preserved human and
    animal remains (17th century) 108–13
  criminals' bodies, use of 104, 110,
    130–31, 142
  dead as memento mori 109–10
  Hunterian Museum of the Royal College
    of Surgeons, London 130
  Leiden University *50*, 109–10, 112,
    114–15
  male body as 'generic human body' 106
  mirrors and acquisition of self-knowledge
    112
  Padua University 104
  religious relevance 104
  self-dissection images 104, 108
  gender of dissected bodies 106–7
  Theatre of Anatomy (Pugin) *61*, 131, 132
  uterus dissection, significance of *48*,
    105, 106–7
  see also dissecting room and dissections
Anderson, William 254, 327
Andrew, Charles T. 229–31
animals
  apes *see* apes
  crocodile skeleton *71*, 153–4, *158*, 174,
    255, 322–3, 324
  elephants *75*, *90*, 153, 167, 169, 183,
    189, 191, 192, 202, 255, 323
  flamingo *79–80*, 179, 180
  Galen and animal dissection 106
  non-human remains, acquisition of
    62, 65, 85, *123–4*, 222, 252–3, 254–5,
    322

The Rearing Horse with Rider (Von
    Hagens) *5*, 23
  skeletons, removal of to Zoology Museum
    157, 321, 322–3
  vertebrate animals for comparison
    purposes *89–90*, 174–5, 182, 183, 184,
    186–7, 189, 190, 192–3, 201–2, 321
  whale study and dissection *87–9*, *159*,
    175–8, 182, 201, 202, 255, 270, 323,
    324
  see also comparative anatomy; insect
    collection (Sim); Natural History
    Museum, Aberdeen; Zoology Museum,
    Aberdeen
animated corpse illustration (Vesalius) *49*,
    107, 108
animated nervous system in 'The Anatomist's
    Dream' 238, 240
Anthropological Institute of Great Britain and
    Ireland 182, 227, 228
Anthropological Map (Tylor) *109*, 223
Anthropological Museum (later Marischal
    Museum), Aberdeen 21, 43, 45, 206,
    228, 236, 255
  Lockhart as curator 239, 323–5
  relocation (1907) 207, 233, 235–6
  photographic collection of curiosities
    (Ogston) *16*, 38, 40–41
  temporary displays *137*, 274–5, 277
anthropometric laboratory, Aberdeen *112*,
    114, 206, 207, 227–37
  living bodies, study of 229, 231–2, 233–4
antiquities 111, 133, 137–8, 142, 155–6, 233
apes
  skeletons *76*, 170, 182, 200
  in tree exhibit *123*, *158*, 252, 322–3, 324
  see also animals
archaeological excavations, Anatomy
    Museum, Aberdeen 45
architectural structure, Anatomical Museum,
    Aberdeen 159–62, 169–70
archives *20*, 44, 319, 338, 340, 341
arms *see under* limbs
arteries *see under* blood vessels
articulation
  apes *see* apes
  exploded skull *2*, 9, 10, 11, 12
  hand models 75
  human skeleton *31*, 72, 73, 95
  instructions (Auzoux) *144*, 293–4
  museum articulator, Royal College of
    Surgeons *19*, 42, 43
  Vesalius' articulated skeletons 108
  see also display methods
artists and artworks 21–3, 26–8, 261, 305,
    312, 342
  see also individual artists
Asclepius, Greek god of medicine 107, 347
assembling
  anatomical models, disassembling and

assembling *42*, 92–5, *141–4*, 289–98
as collecting *see* collecting
atlases *see* anatomy atlases
AUAAS (Aberdeen University Anatomical and
    Anthropological Society) 212–13, 231–2,
    250–51, 270
Audubon, John James 147
authority structure and division of labour
    185–91
Auzoux, Dr Louis 62, 289–96, 313
    anatomical model with detachable parts
        91–2, *141–4*, 191, 290–92, *293–4*
    eardrum model *83*, 190, 191, 215
    kidney, enlarged model *40*, 87, 88, 203,
        215
    'Ovologie' model *145*, 294, 295

Baillière's Synthetic Anatomy 149, 299–302
Barclay, John 68, 144, 161, 167
    *The Anatomy of the Bones of the Human
        Body* 67, 147, 148
Bartlett, Sydney *163*, 330
'bay system', museum layout 85–6, 327–9,
    331–2
Bell, Charles 144, 285
    A System of Dissections 13, 32, 33
Bell, John and Charles 126
Berlin Adorante dermatome figure (Brucciani)
    29, 67, 68, *154*, 161, 203, 308, 309
Berlin Aquarium 192
Berry, Richard, *Clinical Atlas of Sectional and
    Topographical Anatomy* 105, 218, 219, 302
Bidloo, Govard, *Anatomia humani corporis 56*,
    120–21
blackboard diagram (Jamieson) *151*, 303–5
blood vessels
    arm (Maclise) *68*, 148, 149
    arteries, *Anatomy of the Arteries of the
        Human Body* (Quain) *68*, *139*, 147–8,
        149, 285–7, 296
    leg (Maclise) *139*, 285, 286
    neck (Cameron) *126*, 261, 330
    veins *60*, 65, 77, 129, *146*, 203, 295, 297,
        298, 301
body acquisition 47, 51, 57–9, 247, 254, 338
    Anatomy Act Committee 338, 342, 344,
        345, 347
    anonymity, preservation of 69–70
    body availability 163–4, 171–2, 208–9
    burial practices 336, 343–50
    and colonial power relations 222, 223–6,
        232, 234–5, 254
    executed criminals and 'bodies of the
        poorer sort' 145, 146
    funerary and Funeratory Committee
        335–8, 345
    payments for unclaimed bodies 336
    resurrectionists, graves *34*, 81, 145
    scarcities 208–9, 336–7
    unclaimed bodies 335–7, 346

body donation 337–9
    and cremation 36, 47, 57, 58, 61, 66,
        317, 337, 348–9, 350
    donors' instructions for burial 339–40
    memorial book *165*, 341, 342–3
    memorial service 339–41
    memorials *see* memorials
    publicity 338
Body Worlds exhibitions (Von Hagens) 22,
    23–4
    The Rearing Horse with Rider 5, 23
Bologna University
    Archiginnasio Anatomy Theatre, wooden
        anatomical sculptures (Lelli) 122
    dissection coinciding with carnival
        celebrations 104
    wax models (Morandi) 122
Bon-Accord, caricature of John Struthers *77*,
    171–2, 197
bones
    in artwork *9–10*, 29–30
    Czech Republic, Sedlec Ossuary *10*, 29,
        30
    Malta, Chapel of Bones, Valletta *116*,
        242–3
    ossuaries *10–11*, 30, 31–2, 33, *116*, 242–3
    sculptures *see* Carey, Jodie
    see also skeleton
books *see* textbooks
Borges, Jorge Luis, 'The Circular Ruins' 7
Borland, Christine, *Bullet Proof Breath 8*, 27,
    28
botany 33, *116*, 152, 155, 156, 180, 289
Brady and Martin, clinical stencil plates 306
brain
    models (Hamilton) 311
    stem fibre drawings *153*, 307–8, 330
    see also head
Brain Books, publications 308
Braune, Wilhelm 212
British Association for the Advancement
    of Science 176, 178, 197, 227
Brookes, Joshua, museum 144, 152
Brucciani, Domenico 161, 162
    Berlin Adorante, dermatome figure *29*,
        67, 68, *154*, 161, 203, 308, 309
    'Bush-woman' and 'Bushman' plaster
        casts *20–21*, *85*, *112*, 193, 194, 203, 232,
        325
burial practices 47, 57, 58, 61, 66, 317, 336,
    343–50
    bodies, donors' instructions 339–40
    see also cremation; embalming; memorials
Burke, William 145
Bush, Charles *19*, 42, 43
'Bush-woman' and 'Bushman' plaster casts
    20–21, *85*, *112*, 193–4, 203, 232, 325
Byron, Lord 270

cabinets of curiosities
    anatomical collections 116–18
    mirrors and acquisition of self-knowledge
    112–13
    prestige and value 111–12
    see also curiosities
Cain, Alexander 264
Calenzuoli, Francesco, wax anatomical model
    27, *58*, 124–5
Cambridge University, *Theatre of Anatomy*
    (Pugin) *61*, 131, 132
Cameron, Gordon S., neck nerves and blood
    vessels illustration *126*, 261, 330
cannibalism 224, 292
Carey, Jodie, *Untitled 9*, 29
Carlini, Agostino, *Smugglerius* 161
Casino Royale (film) 22
cataloguing and anatomical lists 318–20, 332
Cathcart, Charles Walker 212
Cave, Dr A.J.E. 258
Cellon (plastic) 312
cemetery
    Trinity Cemetery memorial *166–70*,
    343–8, 349, 350–52
    see also burial practices; memorials
ceroplasty *see* anatomical models, wax
Cheesman, Dr John Eric, forearm layering
    sheets *149*, 301–2
Chiara of Montefalco, healing miracles 99
Chinese female foot *65*, *111*, 141, 226, 275
circus performance, slide *125*, 256, 257
classical sculpture, and models' postures
    123–4
cleaner, Hunterian Museum of the Royal
    College of Surgeons, London *18*, 41, 43
Clegg, Edward J. 55, 326, 348
Clinical Atlas of Sectional and Topographical
    Anatomy (Berry) *105*, 218, 219, 302
clinical stencil plates *152*, 305–6
clippings, magazine and newspaper, use of
    133, 272–4
clothing *17*, 39, 40, 66, 247
codes of conduct 47, 66, 189
Coleridge, Samuel Taylor 270
collecting
    colonial power and travel 20–21, 37–8,
    222, 223–6, 232, 234–5, 254
    as museum-making 8–9, 10–11, 15–16,
    19
    preserved human and animal remains
    (17th century) 108–13
    Struthers's private collection *78*, 172,
    173–4, 188, 203, 255
    Struthers's professorship 171–7
    see also detail, and museum creation
colonialism 20–21, 37–8, 222, 223–6, 232,
    234–5, 254
colour use 90, 121, 261, 308–10
commercial exhibitions for public viewing
    195–6

comparative anatomy 62, 63–4, 144, 147,
    152, 162, 167–70, 173–4, 222, 236
    Aberdeen Zoology Museum *157*, 321,
    322–3
    Dublin, Trinity College Museum of
    Comparative Anatomy 228
    see also animals
conceptual work 15, 212, 233, 280, 284, 298,
    302, 314
Cooke, Thomas 207–8, 214, 248, 268,
    281–2, 283, 288, 302, 307
Copland, Patrick 139–40
    'Head of Despair' *63*, 140
correlation techniques 52, 75, 76, 79, 86, 91
    see also anatomical models; dissections;
    living bodies; visual aids
corridor (entrance), Anatomy Museum,
    Aberdeen 22, 54–5, *89*, *159*, *165*, 175,
    201, 202, 255, 270, 323, 324, 342
Craigen, Allan James 224
cremation 36, 47, 57, 58, 61, 66, 317, 337,
    348–9, 350
    see also burial practices; memorials
criminals' bodies, use of 104, 110, 130–31, 142
crocodile skeleton *71*, 153–4, *158*, 174, 255,
    322–3, 324
    see also animals
Crooke, Helkiah, *Mikrokosmographia 138*,
    284–5
Cruickshank, William 261
Cunningham, Daniel 228
Cunningham's Manual of Practical Anatomy
    287–8
curator responsibilities 184–5
    Lockhart as curator of Anthropological
    Museum 323–5
curiosities 110, 111, 121, 129, 133, 137–43,
    155–6, 192
    'artificial curiosities' 141–2
    cabinets *see* cabinets of curiosities
    categorization 142
    collection (Rackstrow) 121–2, 130
    'natural curiosities' 142–3
    photographic collection (Ogston) *16*, 38,
    40–41
    preservation of (Hunter) 129
    theatres of anatomy, displays in 110–11
curricular change effects 320
cutting instruments 62–3, 64, *138*, 284–9
    see also dissecting room and dissections
Cuvier, Georges 68, 161, 173–4
Czech Republic, Sedlec Ossuary, Kutná Hora,
    human bones display *10*, 29, 30

Dance of Death imagery 114
dark room for photographic work 207
    see also photography
Darwin, Charles 181–2
    On the Origin of Species 157–8
Daukes, Sidney 330–31

De la Croix, François 121
Death: A Self-portrait exhibition, Wellcome
    Collection 26, 29
death, memento mori *see* memento mori
deathbed portraits 42
decay and decomposition 27, 31, 40, 57–8,
    60, 113–14, 145, 153, 155, 176, 336
    see also embalming; memento mori;
    preservation
demonstrations 19, 50, 54, 69, 75, 77, 98–9,
    106, 108, 130, 140, 152–3, 218
    room 206
    see also anatomical models; illustrations;
    living bodies
dermatomes 3, 14, 15–16, 29, 67, 68, *154*,
    161, 203, 308, 309
    see also nerves; skin
design
    anatomy museums 45, 146, 167, 253,
    255, 317, 320, 327
    memorial *166–70*, 343–8, 349, 350–52
Desnoues, Guillaume 121
detachable parts, anatomical model with
    (Auzoux) 91–2, *141–4*, 191, 290–92,
    293–4
detail, and museum creation 185–91
    see also collecting; labelling
diagrams *4*, 17, 18, 70–71, 79, 89, 90, 92–3
    blackboard diagram (Jamieson) *151*,
    303–5
    Diagrams of the Nerves of the Human Body
    (Flower) *62*, 135–6
    embryo 18
    masking of background *101–3*, 214,
    215–17
    see also illustrations; labelling
diamond engraving, Hunter, William 330
digital eye 207, 221
disassembling *see* assembling
display, methods 19, 20, 188–90, 253–9
    lighting 24–6, 65, 74, 205, 257, 264, 330
    Perspex cases replacing glass *163*, 329,
    330
    reciprocal shaping 46–7
    tactile display dynamics 46–8, 76–7
    see also anatomical practices
dissecting room and dissections *29–30*, 55,
    56, 57, 59, 65–80
    advantages to learning 281–2
    anatomical images and three-dimensional
    models, use of 282–3
    body acquisition *see* body acquisition
    cleanliness and tidiness 143, 247, 293
    clothing 66, 247
    codes of conduct 47, 66, 189, 292–3
    concealment of body areas 71
    cutting instruments 62–3, 64, *138*,
    284–9
    expert drawings of sectioned specimens,
    display of 211–14

first incision 70–71
injuries sustained 292
journey, dissecting as 246–53
learning process and skills 247–9
Lockhart's professorship *119, 140*,
    246–50, 287
manual training and mnemonics of the
    body 76–7
mistakes, learning from 74
multi-sensory learning 48–9
'normal variation' of anatomical structures
    71, 75
note-taking, shift towards 79
observation of students' own living bodies
    47, 75–6, *see also* living bodies
patterns of reference 73–5
plastic models, relating to 74–5, 82, 89
portrait busts and plaster casts *29*, 67,
    68–9, *89*, 161, 202
prosections as guides 74, 78–80
reduction in allocation of hours
    (1945–70) 320
Reid's professorship *94, 97, 99*, 205–6,
    207–14, 298
servant role 188
skin removal 71
surface anatomy study 75–6, 79
A System of Dissections (Bell) *13*, 32, 33
'variations' and 'abnormalities', drawings
    of *97*, 209–11
visual memory cultivation 332–3
wayfinding through the body *120*,
    248–50
    see also anatomy theatres
Doctor Death exhibition, Wellcome Collection
    26
Don, Alexander, head and neck watercolour
    98, 211, 212, 298
Dooley, Denis 342
Dow, David Rutherford 258
drawings
    expert drawings of sectioned specimens,
    display of 211–14
    photographs of drawings of anatomical
    sections *99*, 212–14, 298
    student drawings, encouragement of 251
    'variations' and 'abnormalities', drawings
    of *97*, 209–11
    see also illustrations; visual aids
Dresden, Deutsches Hygiene Museum 28, 63,
    312
dress code *17*, 39, 40, 66, 247
Dublin, Trinity College Museum of
    Comparative Anatomy 228
Dublin University, Rackstrow collection 122
Dundee Museum, Tay Whale 175–7, 178
Dyce, Robert, curiosities collection 138–9,
    154–5
Dyce, William 138–9, 152–3

ear
  eardrum model (Auzoux) *83*, 190, 191,
    215
  giant scale *121*, *131*, 250, 270, 271, 272
  preparations of the middle and inner
    39, 87
  'schematic representation inner ear'
    100, 214, 215
  student drawing *122*, 251
Edinburgh, City Art Centre, *Anatomy Acts*
  exhibition 27
Edinburgh, Royal Society of Surgeons of
  Edinburgh (RCSEd)
  'Bush-woman' and 'Bushman' plaster
    casts *85*, 193, 194
  expansion (early 19th century) 144
  intermedial displays 212
  as model for Aberdeen Anatomical
    Museum 167
  Struthers's private collection 172
  Surgeons' Hall 26, 138, 144
The Edinburgh Stereoscopic Atlas of Anatomy
  106–7, 221
Edinburgh University Anatomical Museum
  18, *37*, *74*, 84, 168, 305, 327
  authority structure and division of labour
    187
  expansion (1884) 168
  eye, wax model (Maison Tramond) *43*,
    94–5
  Fabrica (De humani corporis fabrica)
    (Vesalius) display *44*, 97, 98
  knitted anatomy *155*, 308–10
  as model for Aberdeen Anatomical
    Museum 167–8
Edinburgh University medical school, Burke,
  William, dissection 145
Edwards, John 320, 321, 327, 330
electric lighting 205–6
electrostatic demonstrations (Copland) *63*,
  140
elephants 75, *90*, 153, 167, 169, 183, 189,
  191, 192, 202, 255, 323
  see also animals
Elliot Smith, Grafton 241–2, 252
embalming 47, 57–8, 69–70, 99, 137
  see also burial practices
embodied practices 9, 11–12, 40, 51–2, 77,
  79–80, 159, 279–80, 310–11, 314–15,
  333
  see also living bodies
embroidery 308
embryology 18, 49, 83, 86, 204, 233, 267,
  327
  see also foetus
emotional responses 31, 33, 34, 36, 66, 100,
  340, 341
empire *see* colonialism
entry restrictions
  Anatomy Museum, Aberdeen 53–4, 66

Glasgow University, Hunterian Museum
  144
Essential Clinical Anatomy (Moore and Agur)
  41, 89
ethnographic artefacts to Anthropological
  Museum 160, 323–7
Ethnographic Survey of the British Isles 227
Ewing, Alexander 143–4, 152
Exquisite Bodies exhibition, Wellcome
  Collection 26
eye
  Anatomy of the Human Eye (Thompson)
    221
  paper layers (Witkowski) *147*, 299
  with spectacles model (Jones) *64*, 140,
    141
  wax model (Maison Tramond) *43*, 94–5
Fabrica (De humani corporis fabrica) (Vesalius)
  20, 44, *48–9*, 97, 104–8, 114
  animated corpse illustration *49*, 107, 108,
    330
  Edinburgh University Anatomical
    Museum display *44*, 97, 98
  title page *48*, 104–7
Fairland, William *Medical Anatomy* (Sibson)
  72, 164–5
feet, Chinese female foot *65*, *111*, 141, 226,
  275
female body
  anatomical section *99*, 212–13
  Chinese female foot *65*, *111*, 141, 226,
    275
  female dissection in *Fabrica* (Vesalius) *48*,
    104–6
  Italian wax tableau of female head *53*,
    115, 116
  photographed pencil drawing of woman's
    body *99*, 212–13
  plaster cast of woman's torso (Hunter) *59*,
    127–8
  wax anatomical model (Susini) *57*, 123–4,
    125
  see also foetus; male body; uterus
film
  Casino Royale 22
  as visual aid 265–7
flamingo *79–80*, 179, 180
  see also animals
Flaubert, Gustave 289
floor plans *21*, *49–50*, *93*, 205–7
Florence University, 'La Specola' museum 27,
  123
Flower, William Henry 169, 178, 182, *184–5*,
  188–9, 193, 203, 212, 223, 224, 321
  Diagrams of the Nerves of the Human Body
    62, 135–6
  inks and printing experiments 330
flowers
  in European reliquaries 32–3, *47*, 102

rhododendron flowers and Lockhart
130–31, 271–2
Still-life of Flowers on Woodland Ground
(Ruysch) *55*, 118, 119
foetus
for baptism (Italy) 99
embryology 18, 49, 83, 86, 204, 233,
267, 327
foetal displays *78*, 173
skeletons (Maison Tramond) *78*, 173
see also female body; uterus
Fontana, Felice 123, 294–5
formaldehyde 20, 58, 65–6, 204
see also preservation
framing, and imaging techniques 224–5, 226
France
display reliquaries, convents producing
102–3
Paris, Académie royale des sciences 121
St George Reliquary, Conques *46*, 101
Fraser, Angus, pancreas drawing *70*, 149, 151
funerals *see* burial practices; cemetery;
cremation; memorials
funerary 146, 164, 172–3
Fyfe, Forest William 260, 261, 264

Galen and animal dissection 106
Galton, Francis 227–8
gasserian ganglion model *62*, 84, 135–6
see also nerves
gender of dissected bodies, theatres of
anatomy 106–7
George Washington Wilson & Co. *17*, 39,
40, *92*, 175, 176, 206
Germanicus statue 161
gesture 77, 106, 108, 188
Gibb, Robert *91*, 175–6, 180, 188, 203, 206
Glasgow, Hunterian Museum *see* Hunterian
Museum, Glasgow University
Glasgow University, Museum of Anatomy
36, 83
Fabrica (De humani corporis fabrica)
(Vesalius) 97
memorial book 342–3
models showing dermatomes *3*, 14,
15–16
plaster cast of woman's torso (Hunter)
59, 127–8
preserved human foetus 129
glass, Perspex replacing glass cases *163*, 329,
330
Gordon-Taylor, Gordon 249–50
grave, resurrectionists *34*, 81, 145
Gravid Uterus (Hunter) 126, 128
Gray, David 177–8
Gray's Anatomy 165, 238
ground floor and gallery, Aberdeen Anatomy
Museum *34–5, 42*, 80–86, *87–90*, 93,
200–203, 321, 327–9, 334
Gunn, Dr John 189

Haddon, Alfred 228
hair
'Head of Despair' *63*, 140
models with *53, 57*, 115, 116, 122, 123,
124
in mourning jewellery *14*, 33–4
removal 58, 69
Hamilton, D. J., brain models 311
Hamilton, Gilbert Frewin 260, 261, 267
Hamlyn, L. H. 312
hands 32, 73, 74, 75
Handyside, Peter 173
Hare, William 145
Harvey, William *29*, 67, 68, 109, 161
head
'Decorated skulls from New Guinea' *110,
113a–d*, 225, 230, 275
dissection 17, *136*, 261, 274, 276
exploded skull (Rouppert) *2*, 9, 10, 11,
12, 191
For the Love of God (Hirst) 27–8
historical skulls 62, 63
Maori *toi moko* (preserved tattooed heads)
21, 275, 326
plaster model (Steger) *38, 85*
'Sagittal section of head' (Jamieson) *151*,
303–5
skull and spine preparation *82*, 188–9
skulls and Anatomy Museum interior
adaptation *110, 113a–d*, 223, 224–5,
229–31, 232, 326
skulls' donation (Thomson) 137
skulls, importance of study of 146–7
watercolour (Don) *98*, 211, 212, 298
see also brain
'Head of Despair' (Copland) *63*, 140
Head of a Woman (Picasso) *135*, 274, 276
heart *1*, 6, *69*, 77, 149, 150
A Necessary Change of Heart (Isaacs) 27
plastic models *28*, 63
respiration and circulation depiction *72*,
165
wax model *27*, 62, 63
Hirst, Damien 27–8
historical, anatomical material defined as
62–3, 80, 85–6, 90, 91–2, 94–5, 96
Houdon, Jean-Antoine, *L'Écorché* 161
Human Anatomy and Physiology (Witkowski)
147, 299
human body
dead *see* body acquisition; body donation
living *see* living bodies
Human Tissue Act (2004), Human Tissue
(Scotland) Act (2006) 35–6, 66
Hunt, Charles 326
Hunter, John *29*, 67, 68, *75*, 131, 135, 161,
169
Hunter, William
dead bodies as essential requirement
130–31

diamond, engraving with 330
dissection for Royal Academy of Arts, London 161
Glasgow University museum bequest 144
placenta preservation *60*, 129–30
plaster cast of woman's torso *59*, 127–8
preparations, preservation of *60*, 126, 128–30, 144
private anatomy school 126, 130
rarities, preservation of 129
uterus study *59–60*, 126–30
on wax figures 125–6
Hunterian Museum, Glasgow University
    A Healing Passion exhibition *7*, 25, 26
    entry restrictions 144
    Hall of Anatomy, opening of 144
Hunterian Museum of the Royal College of Surgeons, London *18–19*, 41, 42–3, *42*
    Bush, Charles, museum articulator *19*, 42, 43
    cleaner *18*, 41, 43
    Company of Surgeons anatomy theatre 130
    Crystal Gallery *6*, 24–6
    as 'great ship' (Keith) 135
    as model for Aberdeen Anatomical Museum 168–9
    museum employees resident in 41
    reciprocity with Aberdeen Anatomical Museum 182
    reconstruction 246
    Second World War bombing *117–18*, 243–5
    'Skeleton Jacket' and 'Organ Waistcoat' 16
    stereoscopic photographs *75*, 169, 192
Huntly, Marquis of 142
Huxley, Thomas Henry 279

illustrations
    arm blood vessels and muscles (Maclise) *68*, 148, 149
    faithful illustration of dissections, call for 126
    illustrated lectures *67*, 147, 148–9
    illustrated textbooks, importance of images 260–65
    leg blood vessels and tendons (Maclise) *139*, 285, 286
    lower leg muscles (Morrocco) *132*, 273, 274
    wall-mounted *161*, 328–9
    see also demonstrations; diagrams; drawings; textbooks; tracing
Illustrations of Regional Anatomy (Jamieson) *150*, 288, 302–3
imagination, use of 126, 240, 241, 250
imaging techniques and framing 224–5, 226
inscriptions 11, 78–80, 106, 117, 285
    cataloguing and anatomical lists 318–20, 332

material inscriptions (labels and signs), use of 319–20, 330–32, 333–4
    memorial book *165*, 342–3
    see also labelling
insect collection (Sim) *81*, 180, 181
    see also animals
intermediality 17–18, *42*, 53, 74, 85, 90, 91–5, 212, 239, 258–9, 264, 333
intermuseality 20, 159, 351
International Health Exhibition (1884) 227–8
intestine *1*, 6, 16, *69*, 77, 124–5, *146*, 149–50, *155*, 172, 203, 297–8, 308–10
inventories 319–20
Isaacs, John, *A Necessary Change of Heart* 27

Jamieson, Edward Bald
    blackboard diagram *151*, 303–5
    Illustrations of Regional Anatomy *150*, 288, 302–3
Jones, W. & S., eye with spectacles model *64*, 140, 141
journey, dissecting as 246–53

Kahn, Dr Joseph, Anatomical Museum 195
Keith, Arthur 42–3, *94*, 135, 208, 223, 244
Kellas, Arthur *115*, 234, 235
kidney
    cross-section (Jamieson) *150*, 303, 304
    enlarged model (Auzoux) *40*, 87, 88, 203, 215
kin 31, 35, 57, 58, 99, 134, 205, 340, 350
King, George 183
King, John 139
Knight, William, model of a Chinese lady's foot *65*, 141
knitted anatomy *155*, 308–10
Knox, Robert 145, 173–4, 287
Krieg, Wendell J. S., *A Polychrome Atlas of the Brain Stem 153*, 307–8

labelling
    importance of *82*, 163, 188–90
    need for clear 32, 73, 88–90, *98*, 211, 212
    plastic anatomical models 89, 90
    problems, and overseas transportation 153
    reframing and rewording 327–34
    techniques 210, 211–12, 224
    Wellcome Collection 330–31
    see also anatomical terms; detail, and museum creation; diagrams; inscriptions; signage
laboratory
    anthropometric *see* anthropometric laboratory, Aberdeen
    embryological 207
    science/general *21*, 49, 50, 78, *93*, *127*, 160, 205–7, 261, 262, 264
language *see* anatomical terms
lantern slides *see* slides

layering practices 298–302

learning
dissecting rooms, learning process and skills 247–9, 281–2
learning to 'think anatomically' about living body 252–3
multi-sensory learning 48–9
practical learning, encouragement of 162–7
shaping 310–15

lecture theatre 22, 54, *93*, *104*, 130, 137, 161, 205–6, 217, 218, 242, 267

lectures
'The Circus of Life' 256, 257
illustrated *67*, 147, 148–9
Lockhart's lectures *131*, 250, 256, 257, 270, 272, 274
Reid's public lectures 235–6
Struthers's public lectures 196–7

legs *see under* limbs

Leiden University, anatomy theatre *50*, 109–10, 112, 114–15

Lelli, Ercole 122

Leonardo da Vinci 298

library 140, 161, 327–9

lighting 205–6

limbs
arm blood vessels and muscles illustration (Maclise) *68*, 148, 149
arms, forearm layering sheets (Cheesman) *149*, 301–2
deletion, practice of 125, 128
leg blood vessels and tendons illustration (Maclise) *139*, 285, 286
legs in the act of walking (newspaper clipping) *133*, 274
legs, lower leg muscles illustration (Morrocco) *132*, 273, 274

Lister, Arthur Hugh 212

live shows 192–8

liver *1*, 6, *69*, *146*, 149, 150, *155*, 297, 298, 308–10

Liverpool Museum of Anatomy, plaster casts of human bodies *86*, 193–4

Living Anatomy (Lockhart) *128*, 258, 259, 263–5

living bodies 229, 231–2, 251, 258
observation of students' own 47, 75–6, 265, 266
observation of racial differences 193
study of dead and living bodies together 52–3, 240, 241–6
see also embodied practices

'living' bodily interior, portrayal of 119–32
coloured wax anatomical models 121
deletion of limbs, practice of 125, 128
dissection of bodies, comparison with 120–21
double view (inside and outside) 124–5
faithful illustration of dissections, call for 126

models' postures and classical sculpture 123–4
plaster casts 127–8
as teaching resource 120
wax modelling 121–5
wax modelling, criticism of 125–6

Lizars, Alexander Jardine 55, 147, 154, 160

Lizars, John 147
A System of Anatomical Plates of the Human Body *69*, 149, 150, 287

Lizars, William Home, lymphatic vessels and organs illustration *69*, 149, 150

Lockhart, Robert Douglas 11, 12, 30, 41–2, 55, *128*, 204, 238–9, 264, 311
'The Anatomist's Dream' 238, 240
Anatomy of the Human Body 68, *126–7*, *132*, 240, 251, 259, 260–63, 268–9, 270, 273, 274, 305, 329
Anatomy Museum *see* Anatomy Museum and living anatomy, Lockhart's professorship
circus performance slide *125*, 256, 257
as curator of the Anthropological Museum 323–5
ear, giant scale *121*, *131*, 250, 270, 271, 272
gasserian ganglion model *62*, 84, 135–6
head dissection showing cranial nerves *136*, 261, 274, 276
Living Anatomy *128*, 258, 259, 263–5
postcard from Chapel of Bones, Valletta, Malta *116*, 242–3
on shared memories 316

London, Guy's Hospital Anatomical Museum 144, 296

London, Hayward Gallery, *Spectacular Bodies* exhibition 26, 27

London, Hunterian Museum *see* Hunterian Museum of the Royal College of Surgeons, London

London, Royal Academy of Arts, Hunter, William dissection 161

London, St Thomas's Hospital *95*, 161, 204, 209

London, University College 163, 286–7, 312

Lonsdale, Henry 173

Low, Alexander 55, 136, 204

lungs *1*, 6, 27, *72*, 76, *163*, 165, 329, 330

lymphatic vessels and organs illustration (Lizars) *69*, 149, 150

Macdonald, Nora *102*, 215, 216–17

MacGillivray, William 147

MacGregor, William 228

Mackenzie, William 158

Maclise, Joseph
arm blood vessels and muscles illustration *68*, 148, 149
leg blood vessels and tendons illustration *139*, 285, 286

magazine and newspaper clippings, use of *133*, 272–4

magnification
  lantern slides *102–4*, 215, 216, 217–18, 232
  microscopes *100*, 214–15

Maison Tramond 180, 191, 296–8, 313
  eye, wax model *43*, 94–5
  foetal skeletons *78*, 173
  torso, wax model *33*, 77
  see also Rouppert, N.

male body
  anatomical model with detachable parts (Auzoux) 91–2, *141–4*, 191, 290–92, 293–4
  as 'generic human body' 106
  layers in *Philips' Popular Mannikin 148*, 299, 300
  see also female body

Malta, Chapel of Bones, Valletta *116*, 242–3

Manzolini, Giovanni 122

Maori *toi moko* (preserved tattooed heads) 21, 275, 326

maps
  anatomical 91, 248, 251, 281–2
  Anthropological Map (Tylor) *109*, 223
  see also anatomy atlases

masking of background *101–3*, 214, 215–17

material inscriptions *see* inscriptions; labelling

material relationships 52–3, 85, 91, 307

material and visual culture, of anatomy 36–43

materials, anatomical bodies *see* anatomical bodies

Matthews, R. W. 261, 305

maze, museum as synoptic 43–5

Medical Anatomy (Sibson) *72*, 164–5, 166–7, 287

memento mori 113–19
  in anatomical books 114–15
  bodily decay, depiction of 113–14
  Dance of Death imagery 114
  dead as, theatres of anatomy 109–10
  funerary sculpture 113–14
  Italian wax tableau of female head *53*, 115, 116
  Leiden University, anatomy theatre 114–15
  objects in the shape of skeletons and skulls 114
  printed images 114
  private anatomical collections 115–17
  Ruysch, Frederik collection *54*, 117–18
  transi tombs 113–14, *115*
  vanitas imagery 115–16
  see also decay

memorials
  books for body donors *11–12*, 31, 32–3, 54, *165*, 342–3
  ossuaries *10–11*, 30, 31–2, 33, *116*, 242–3
  and ritualized disposal 31–6, 99

Trinity Cemetery memorial *166–70*, 343–8, 349, 350–52
  see also burial practices

menageries 175, 192–3, 322
  see also animals

mental visualization 49, 52, 71, 91, 163, 251–2, 278–9, 296, 301, 310, 315, 332
  see also anatomical visualization

metaphors
  and anatomical poetics 268–71, 283
  museum as 'ganglion in education' 62, 135–6
  museum as 'great ship' 135
  tree *see* Aberdeen, Anatomical Museum growth, Struthers's professorship

Meursius, Johannes, Leiden anatomy theatre engraving *50*, 109

microscopes and magnification *100*, 214–15

Middleton, William 225–6, 231

mirrors and acquisition of self-knowledge 112

mistakes, learning from 74, 75

mnemonics 76–7, 250–51

models *see* anatomical models

Moir, Andrew 145

Moir, James *91*, 205

Monro, Alexander 120

Moore Brothers 174

Morandi Manzolini, Anna, anatomical waxes 122–3

Morris, Caroline, dermatomes, models showing *3*, 14, *15–16*

Morrocco, Alberto 42, 261, 329
  lower leg muscles illustration *132*, 273, 274

mortsafe with padlock and key 81

mortuary 23, 56, 57–9, 160, 206

mourning jewellery *14*, 33–4

MRI and CT scans 49

mummies
  embalming techniques 137
  in painted coffin *66*, 142, 143
  unwrapped *102*, 215, 216–17

muscle anatomy *128*, 263–4

museum attendant's role 187–8

museum dynamics 18–21

museum-making *see* Aberdeen, Anatomical Museum formation (*c.* 18th to mid-19th century); Aberdeen, Anatomical Museum growth, Struthers's professorship

Muybridge, Eadweard, man performing a forward flip *129*, 266

name, body donors to anatomy *see under* memorials

narratives as mnemonic devices 250–51

Natural History Museum, Aberdeen 143, 147, 155, 170
  see also animals

natural philosophy apparatus collection (18th century) *63–4*, 139–41

naturalists and taxidermists, collaboration with 177–82
neck
head and neck watercolour (Don) *98*, 211, 212, 298
nerves 17, *82*, 85, *126*, *136*, 188–9, 240–41, 261, 274, 276, 330
nerves
brain stem *153*, 307–8
chains of 269
gasserian ganglion model *62*, 84, 135–6
neck 17, *82*, 85, *126*, *136*, 188–9, 240–41, 261, 274, 276, 330
portrayal in *Baillière's Synthetic Anatomy* *149*, 301
see also dermatomes
newspaper clippings, use of *133*, 272–4
non-human specimens *see* animals

obscene advertisements charge 236
Obscene Publications Act 196
Ogston, Alexander 222
photographic collection of curiosities *16*, 38, 40–41
open objects 13–18, 280, 314
'Organ Waistcoat' (Sheffield) *1*, 6, 16
Osborne-Walker, J., *The Descriptive Atlas of Anatomy* 73, 165–6
ossuaries *10–11*, 30, 31–2, 33, *116*, 242–3
outlining techniques 302–6
'Ovologie' model (Auzoux) *145*, 294, 295
Owen, Richard *118*, 244, 245
Oxford anatomy school, collection of rarities (17th century) 110–11
Oxford University, Pitt Rivers Museum 19

PAAS (*University of Aberdeen Proceedings of the Anatomical and Anthropological Society*) *99*, *102*, 212–13, 215, 216, 231
Padua University, anatomy theatre 104
painting *see* artists and artwork; illustrations
pancreas *1*, 6, *70*, 149, 151
paper anatomy *see under* textbooks
paper and cardboard brain models 311
papier mâché models *see* Auzoux, Dr Louis
Paris, Académie royale des sciences 121
pathology 7, 25, 26, 144, 154, 167, 169–70, 209, 246, 311, 320
Pauw, Pieter 109
Payne, Anthony, dermatomes, models showing *3*, 14, *15–16*
performative work 18, 19, 40, 241, 246, 256
Perspex cases replacing glass *163*, 329, 330
see also transparent displays
Philip, J. M. 305
Philips' Popular Mannikin 148, 299, 300
photography
advantages 218–19, 225
background masking *102–3*, 215, 216–17
dark room 207

photographic collection of curiosities (Ogston) *16*, 38, 40–41
photographs of drawings of anatomical sections *99*, 212–14, 298
popular body displays 255–9
post-mortem *15*, 34–5
prohibition in dissecting rooms 66
stereoscopic *106–8*, 219–21, 267–8, 298
physiology 115, *147*, 158, 190, 299
Picasso, Pablo, *Head of a Woman 135*, 274, 276
Pierce, Charles E. 305
Pirrie, William 138
placenta preservation (Hunter) *60*, 129–30
see also foetus
plaster casts *29*, 67, 68–9, *89*, 161, 202
'Bush-woman' and 'Bushman' plaster casts 20–21, *85*, *112*, 193–4, 203, 232, 325
depths of 'living' bodily interior, portrayal of 127–8
Glasgow University, Museum of Anatomy *59*, 127–8
Liverpool Museum of Anatomy *86*, 193–4
plastic models *see* anatomical models, plastic
Plasticine models 261, 311
plastination, *Body Worlds* exhibitions *see Body Worlds* exhibitions
Poe, Edgar Allan 270
poetics *see* anatomical poetics
A Polychrome Atlas of the Brain Stem (Krieg) *153*, 307–8
popular performance and entertainment links 255–9, 265
porter's house 206–7
portrait busts and plaster casts, dissecting room *29*, 67, 68–9, *89*, 161, 202
post-mortem
examinations and reactions to 35–6
photographs *15*, 34–5
preparations, anatomical 7, 24–6, *39*, *54*, 87, 115, 117–21, 123, *147*, 152–5
brain in thin slices (Hamilton) 311
preservation of (Hunter) *60*, 126, 128–30, 144
skull and neck *82*, 188–9
'wet' and 'dry' 130, 143–4, 188, 329
see also specimens
preservation 15, 60, 69, 81, 116–17, 164, 172–3, 179, 184–5, 187–8, 254, 318
and effects of time 81–2
formaldehyde 20, 58, 65–6, 204
head dissection *136*, 261, 274, 276
human foetus, Glasgow University 129
see also decay; embalming
private anatomical collections, memento mori 115–17
professor's private work room 206, 207
prosections, in dissecting room 74, 78–80

public viewing 24–5, 195–6
  see also anatomy theatres
Pugin, Augustus Charles, *Theatre of Anatomy*
  61, 131, 132

Quain, Richard, *Anatomy of the Arteries of the
  Human Body 68*, *139*, 147–8, 149, 285–7,
  296

racial differences, study of *109*, 183–4, 193,
  223–5, 227–37
Rackstrow, Benjamin, anatomical and
  curiosity collection 121–2, 130
rarities 37, 97, 104, 109–11, 113, 129, 131,
  154
  crocodile skeleton, defined as *71*, 153–4
RCSEd *see* Edinburgh, Royal Society of
  Surgeons of Edinburgh (RCSEd)
Read, Charles Hercules 228
reframing
  Anatomy Museum, reconfiguration
    327–34
  'wet' and 'dry' specimens *162*, *164*,
    329–30, 332
Reid, Robert William 11, 55, *94*, *96*, 136,
  208, 210
  Anatomy Museum *see* Aberdeen,
  Anatomy Museum development, Reid's
  professorship
  cataloguing and anatomical lists 319
  professional relationships and human and
    animal body acquisitions 222–4
  public lectures 235–6
Reimer's Anatomical Museum 194–5
relationships
  anatomical 12, 50, 51, 53, 71, 91–6,
    164, 231, 281–2, 303 *see also* dissecting
    room; intermediality; tactile engagement
  material 52–3, 85, 91, 307, 317 *see also*
    intermuseality
  social 19, 21, 31, 42–3, 37–8, 42, 51, 59,
    69, 99, 119, 134, 156, 158, 177–86, 200,
    204, 222–4, 228, 237, 339, 341, 350–51
  spatial 10, 19–20, 51–2, 77, 200, 205,
    317
  visual 52, 75, 221 *see also* intermediality;
    visual aids
relics 99–103
  authenticity 100
  convents producing 102–3
  display in reliquaries *46–7*, 100–103
  domestic settings 102–3
  and miracles 99–100
  saints' relics' materials 99–100
  spacial location 102–3
Rembrandt, *The Anatomy Lesson of Dr
  Nicolaes Tulp 23*, 54–5
remembrance *see* memorials
ritualized disposal 31–6, 99
Robb, John 184

Rome, Capuchin Crypt *11*, 31–2
Rose, Ian 231–2
Rouppert, N.
  exploded human skull *2*, 9, 10, 11, 12,
    191
  portal venous system 203
  wax anatomical model *146*, 296–8
  see also Maison Tramond
Rüff, Jakob, *De conceptu et generatione
  hominis 52*, 114, 115
Ruysch, Frederik
  anatomical collection 116–19, 120
  anatomical collection, preservation
    techniques 116–17
  *The Anatomy Lesson of Professor Frederik
    Ruysch* (Van Neck) *45*, 98–9
  Thesaurus animalium primus 54, 117–18
Ruysch, Rachel, *Still-life of Flowers on
  Woodland Ground 55*, 118, 119

Sarti, Signor, anatomical exhibitions 195
scale, large-scale exhibits *40*, 87–8, *121*, *147*,
  151, *164*, 189, 250, 299, 303, 304
Scratchley, James 285, 287
sculpture
  Bologna University, wooden sculptures
    (Lelli) 122
  Carey, Jodie *9*, 29
  classical 123–4
  funerary 113–14
  Trinity Cemetery memorial *166–70*,
    343–8, 349, 350–52
seeing *see* visual aids
self-dissection images, theatres of anatomy
  104, 108
self-knowledge, acquisition and mirrors,
  theatres of anatomy 112
Seligman, Charles 232
sensory histories of museums 48–53
  see also tactile engagement; visual aids
sewing, needlework 64, 269, 307,
Sheffield, Jo, organ waistcoat *1*, 6, 16
Sibson, Francis, *Medical Anatomy 72*, 164–5,
  166–7, 287
signage
  use of (1965) 319–20, 330–32, 333–4
  see also labelling
Sim, George (of Gourdas), insect collection
  81, 180, 181
Sim, George (taxidermist) *79–80*, 178–81
Simpson, Archibald 146
Simpson, William 184
Sinclair, David C. 55, 319–20, 347
  Anatomy Museum *see* Aberdeen,
  Anatomy Museum, reconfiguration,
  Sinclair's professorship
skeleton 63, 64–5, 200–203, 229
  articulation *31*, 72, 73, 95
  'giant' and 'dwarf' skeleton contrasts *123*,
    252, 259

skull *see under* head
spine *4*, 17, *31*, 72, *82*, 188, 189
see also bones
'Skeleton Jacket', Hunterian Museum of the
    Royal College of Surgeons, London 16
Skene, Charles 143
skin
    as cloth 306–7
    dermatomes *3*, 14, 15–16, *29*, 67, 68,
        154, 161, 203, 308, 309
    embalming 47, 57–8, 69–70, 99, 137
    removal 71, 123–4
    tactile engagement 46–50, 76–7, 207–8,
        211
skull *see* head
*Sleeping Beauty under Canopy in Slumber
    Room* (photograph) *15*, 34, 35
Slessor, Robert *91*, 205
slides *102–4*, 215, 216, 217–18, 232, 272–4
    circus performance *125*, 256, 257
    see also photography
Smith, Robert 155
social relationships 19, 21, 37–8, 42, 69, 99,
    119, 134, 177–86, 223–4
Somso models *26*, *28*, *32*, 61, *62*, 63, 73, 86,
    156, 312–13
South Africa, 'Bush-woman' and 'Bushman'
    plaster casts 20–21, *85*, *112*, 193–4, 203,
    232, 325
spatial relationships 10, 19–20, 51–2, 77
specimens 15, *162*, *164*, 188, 203–4, 329–30,
    332
    see also preparations
Spectacular Bodies exhibition (Hayward
    Gallery) *26*, *27*
spine *4*, 17, *31*, 72, *82*, 188, 189
    see also skeleton
Spittal, Robert Haig 224–5
Steger, Franz Josef, plaster model of head *38*,
    85, 191
Stephen, Donald J. 261
stereoscopic photographs *106–8*, 219–21,
    267–8, 298
    see also photography
Stonehaven, Viscountess 254–5, 322
store, museum 47, 56, 61–5, 85–6
Struthers, John 19, 55, 252
    anatomical lists 318–19
    Anatomical Museum *see* Aberdeen,
        Anatomical Museum growth, Struthers's
        professorship
    craniometer design 183
    infant skull specimen *103*, 173, 216,
        217
    international connections and reciprocity
        182–4
    Journal of Anatomy and Physiology articles
        190
    Osteological Memoirs 159
    praise in local newspapers 77, 171–2, 197

private collection *78*, 172, 173–4, 188,
    203, 255
public lectures 196–7
social relationships, and museum
    collecting 177–84
students
    bodies, measurement of 229, 233–4
    drawings, encouragement of 251
    former students' gifts 158, 183
    as 'living models' 47, 75–6, 265, 266
    note-taking 79, 149–52
    revision opportunities 86–91
Surrealist imagery 269–70
Suschitzky, Wolfgang, *Anatomy Class* 119,
    247
Susini, Clemente, wax anatomical model *57*,
    123–4, *125*
synoptic mazes, museums as 43–5

tactile engagement 46–50, 76–7, 207–8, 211
    see also sensory histories of museums
taxidermist 79–80, 177–82
teacher role 51, 144, 163, 204–5, 207–8, 219,
    241
technician role 43, 57–61, 64, 69, 79, *159*,
    163, 254, 319, 321, 323, 324, 328–32
Testut, Léo, *Traité d'anatomie humaine*
    100–101, 214, 215–16
textbooks
    authoritative books, use in theatres of
        anatomy 106
    divisible 288–9, 302–3
    illustrated textbooks, importance of
        260–65
    'paper anatomy' in *140*, *147*, 281, 287–9,
        298–9
    see also illustrations; individual
        publications
textile anatomy *1*, 6, 16, *155*, 308–10
theatres of anatomy *see* anatomy theatres
Thesaurus animalium primus (Ruysch) *54*,
    117–18
Thilesen, Patricia 312
Thompson, Arthur, *Anatomy of the Human
    Eye* 221
Thomson, Alexander, antiquities and
    curiosities collection 137–8, 147
Thomson, Allen 55, 147, 160, 187
Thomson, John Arthur 135–6, 283
threading and body fibres 123, 295, 306–10
three-dimensional models 91–6, 250, 261,
    282–3
    see also anatomical models
Topinard, Paul 227, 229
topographical studies of bodies 73, *105*, 147,
    164, 165, 166, 208, 218, 219, 320
touch *see* tactile engagement
Towne, Joseph 296
tracing 164–5, 218–19, 302, 306
    see also illustrations

transi tombs, memento mori 113–14, 115
transparent displays 10, 24, 60, 81, 95–6,
    311, 312, 331, 332
    body as transparent 250, 283
    layering sheets (Cheesman) 149, 301–2
    Perspex cases replacing glass 163, 329, 330
travel
    and colonial power 20–21, 37–8, 222,
        223–6, 232, 234–5, 254
    travelling menageries 175, 192–3, 322
tree metaphor see Aberdeen, Anatomical
    Museum growth Struthers's professorship
Turner, William 167–8, 187, 279
Tylor, Edward Burnett, *Anthropological Map*
    109, 223

University of Aberdeen Proceedings of the
    Anatomical and Anthropological Society
    (*PAAS*) 99, *102*, 212–13, 215, 216, 231
U.S. National Library of Medicine, 'Visible
    Human Project' 298
uterus
    dissection, theatres of anatomy *48*, 105,
        106–7
    study (Hunter) *59–60*, 126–30
    see also female body; foetus

Valverde de Hamusco, Juan 22, 108
Van Neck, Jan, *The Anatomy Lesson of*
    Professor Frederik Ruysch 45, 98–9
Van Rymsdyk, Jan 126
vanitas imagery, memento mori 115–16
variations 71, 75, *97*, 209–11
veins see under blood vessels
ventilators 206
Venus de' Medici 123
Verne, Jules 270
Vesalius, Andreas, *Fabrica see Fabrica*
    (*De humani corporis fabrica*)
Virchow, Rudolf 256
visual aids 242, 259–68
    colour use and three-dimensional
        appearance 261
    drawings see drawings
    illustrations see illustrations
    photography see photography
    slides see slides
    wallcharts *161*, 164–7, 328–9
    see also anatomy atlases; sensory histories
        of museums
visualization see anatomical visualization
vocabulary and anatomical terms 51–2
Von Bardeleben, Karl 256
Von Hagens, Gunther, *Body Worlds*
    exhibitions see *Body Worlds* exhibitions

wall 'book' *127*, 261, 263, 264
wallcharts *161*, 164–7, 328–9
war
    First World War effects on students 243

Second World War bombing of
    Hunterian Museum of the Royal College
    of Surgeons, London *117–18*, 243–5
war memorial 341
Waterston, David, *The Edinburgh Stereoscopic*
    Atlas of Anatomy 106–7, 221
wax models see anatomical models, wax
wax-injection techniques 121, 126
Weisker, Dr Rudolf, wax anatomical model
    84, 191
Wellcome Collection 26, 29
    labelling 330–31
Westminster Medical Society 289–91
'wet' and 'dry' specimens, reframing *162*, *164*,
    329–30, 332
whale study and dissection *87–9*, *159*, 175–8,
    182, 201, 202, 255, 270, 323, 324
    see also animals
Wilson, Cristina 234
Wilson, John, sternalis muscle drawing *97*,
    209, 210
Witkowski, Gustave Joseph, *Human Anatomy*
    and Physiology 147, 299
Woman's Own magazine clipping *134*, 274,
    275
Wombwell travelling menagerie 192–3, 322
women see female body
wooden models 60, 122, 178, 295
    see also anatomical models
workshop, anatomical parts, models and
    repairs *4*, 17, *25*, 59–61
Worm, Ole, *Museum Wormianum 51*, 111–12
writing (student note-taking) 79, 149–52

X-ray images *111*, 218, 226, 240, 242, 257–8,
    265–6

Yeates, Thomas 258
Youngson, William Coutts, memorial design
    347–8
Younie, Dr Dorothie 251

Ziegler studio 62, 203
Zoology Museum, Aberdeen 65, 85, *157*, 321,
    322–3, 326
    see also animals
Zumbo (Zummo), Gaetano Giulio, *Triumph*
    of Time 121